Analyzing Current Digital Healthcare Trends Using Social Networks

Sukanta Kumar Baral
Indira Gandhi National Tribal University, India

Richa Goel
Symbiosis International University, India

A volume in the Advances in Medical Technologies and Clinical Practice (AMTCP) Book Series

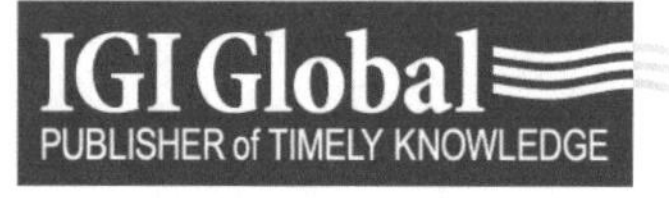

Published in the United States of America by
IGI Global
Medical Information Science Reference (an imprint of IGI Global)
701 E. Chocolate Avenue
Hershey PA, USA 17033
Tel: 717-533-8845
Fax: 717-533-8661
E-mail: cust@igi-global.com
Web site: http://www.igi-global.com

Library of Congress Cataloging-in-Publication Data

Names: Baral, Sukanta Kumar, 1966- editor. | Goel, Richa, 1980- editor.
Title: Analyzing current digital healthcare trends using social networks / edited by Sukanta Baral, Richa Goel.
Description: Hershey, PA : Medical Information Science Reference, [2024] | Includes bibliographical references and index. | Summary: "It is vital to define future policy orientations by understanding the link between stakeholders and industry-related concerns in order for digital health care solutions to be employed in practice. In order to analyze the network of the digital health care business, this book uses research articles, case studies, etc. that serve as the foundation for social discussions about such critical issues"-- Provided by publisher.
Identifiers: LCCN 2023054717 (print) | LCCN 2023054718 (ebook) | ISBN 9798369319345 (hardcover) | ISBN 9798369319352 (ebook)
Subjects: MESH: Digital Technology | Delivery of Health Care | Online Social Networking | Telemedicine | Electronic Health Records | Wearable Electronic Devices | Artificial Intelligence
Classification: LCC R859 (print) | LCC R859 (ebook) | NLM W 26.55.D4 | DDC 362.10285--dc23/eng/20240110
LC record available at https://lccn.loc.gov/2023054717
LC ebook record available at https://lccn.loc.gov/2023054718

This book is published in the IGI Global book series Advances in Medical Technologies and Clinical Practice (AMTCP) (ISSN: 2327-9354; eISSN: 2327-9370)

British Cataloguing in Publication Data
A Cataloguing in Publication record for this book is available from the British Library.

For electronic access to this publication, please contact: eresources@igi-global.com.

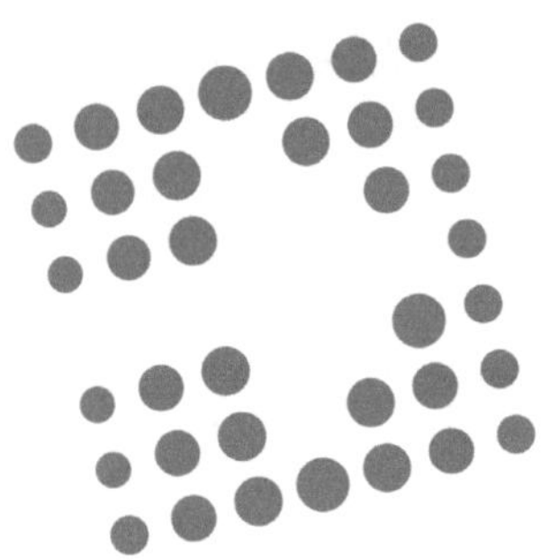

Advances in Medical Technologies and Clinical Practice (AMTCP) Book Series

Srikanta Patnaik
SOA University, India
Priti Das
S.C.B. Medical College, India

ISSN:2327-9354
EISSN:2327-9370

Mission

Medical technological innovation continues to provide avenues of research for faster and safer diagnosis and treatments for patients. Practitioners must stay up to date with these latest advancements to provide the best care for nursing and clinical practices.

The **Advances in Medical Technologies and Clinical Practice (AMTCP) Book Series** brings together the most recent research on the latest technology used in areas of nursing informatics, clinical technology, biomedicine, diagnostic technologies, and more. Researchers, students, and practitioners in this field will benefit from this fundamental coverage on the use of technology in clinical practices.

Coverage

- Telemedicine
- Biomechanics
- Patient-Centered Care
- Clinical Data Mining
- Biometrics
- Medical Informatics
- E-Health
- Neural Engineering
- Clinical Studies
- Nutrition

IGI Global is currently accepting manuscripts for publication within this series. To submit a proposal for a volume in this series, please contact our Acquisition Editors at Acquisitions@igi-global.com or visit: http://www.igi-global.com/publish/.

The Advances in Medical Technologies and Clinical Practice (AMTCP) Book Series (ISSN 2327-9354) is published by IGI Global, 701 E. Chocolate Avenue, Hershey, PA 17033-1240, USA, www.igi-global.com. This series is composed of titles available for purchase individually; each title is edited to be contextually exclusive from any other title within the series. For pricing and ordering information please visit http://www.igi-global.com/book-series/advances-medical-technologies-clinical-practice/73682. Postmaster: Send all address changes to above address.

Titles in this Series

For a list of additional titles in this series, please visit: http://www.igi-global.com/book-series/advances-medical-technologies-clinical-practice/73682

Multisector Insights in Healthcare, Social Sciences, Society, and Technology
Darrell Norman Burrell (Marymount University, USA)
Engineering Science Reference • © 2024 • 392pp • H/C (ISBN: 9798369332269) • US $545.00

Change Dynamics in Healthcare, Technological Innovations, and Complex Scenarios
Darrell Norman Burrell (Marymount University, USA)
Medical Information Science Reference • © 2024 • 331pp • H/C (ISBN: 9798369335550) • US $495.00

Intelligent Solutions for Cognitive Disorders
Dipti Jadhav (D. Y. Patil University (Deemed), Navi Mumbai, India & Ramrao Adik Institute of Technology, India) Pallavi Vijay Chavan (D. Y. Patil University (Deemed), Navi Mumbai, India & Ramrao Adik Institute of Technolgy, India) Sangita Chaudhari (D. Y. Patil University (Deemed), Navi Mumbai, India & Ramrao Adik Institute of Technology, India) and Idongesit Williams (CMI, Denmark & Aalborg University, Copenhagen, Denmark)
Medical Information Science Reference • © 2024 • 411pp • H/C (ISBN: 9798369310908) • US $355.00

Intelligent Technologies and Parkinson's Disease Prediction and Diagnosis
Abhishek Kumar (Chitkara University Institute of Engineering and Technology, Chitkara University, Punjab, India) Sachin Ahuja (Chandigarh University, India) Anupam Baliyan (Geeta University, India) Sreenatha Annawati (University of New South Wales, Australia) and Abhineet Anand (Chandigarh University, India)
Medical Information Science Reference • © 2024 • 390pp • H/C (ISBN: 9798369311158) • US $355.00

Innovations, Securities, and Case Studies Across Healthcare, Business, and Technology
Darrell Norman Burrell (Marymount University, USA)
Medical Information Science Reference • © 2024 • 555pp • H/C (ISBN: 9798369319062) • US $360.00

Handbook of Research on Advances in Digital Technologies to Promote Rehabilitation and Community Participation
Raquel Simões de Almeida (CIR, ESS, Polytechnic of Porto, Portugal) Vítor Simões-Silva (CIR, ESS, Polytechnic of Porto, Portugal) and Maria João Trigueiro (CIR, ESS, Polytechnic of Porto, Portugal)
Medical Information Science Reference • © 2024 • 513pp • H/C (ISBN: 9781668492512) • US $480.00

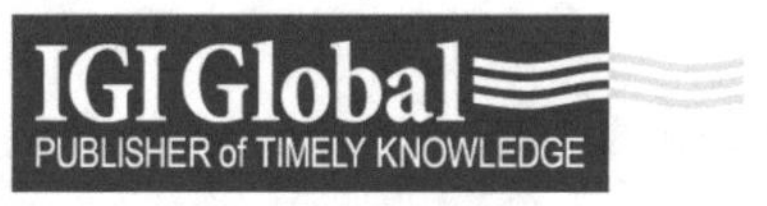

701 East Chocolate Avenue, Hershey, PA 17033, USA
Tel: 717-533-8845 x100 • Fax: 717-533-8661
E-Mail: cust@igi-global.com • www.igi-global.com

Dedication

This book is dedicated to the pioneers and visionaries in the field of digital healthcare, whose unwavering commitment to innovation has transformed the landscape of patient care to leveraging social networks for the betterment of healthcare has paved the way for a new era of collaboration, efficiency, and patient-centricity.

To the tireless authors and researchers who have contributed their expertise and insights to this volume to advancing our understanding of current digital healthcare trends is truly commendable. This book stands as a testament to showcase passion and dedication to improving healthcare through the lens of social networks.

We would also like to dedicate this book to the healthcare professionals, patients, and caregivers whose experiences and stories inspire us to continually explore new avenues for enhancing the delivery of healthcare services, resilience and determination are a driving force behind the transformative changes have been witnessed in the digital healthcare landscape.

Finally, a heartfelt dedication to our families and loved ones, whose unwavering support and understanding have been the foundation upon which this project was built a source of strength, and we are grateful for everyone's efforts, which have enabled us to contribute to the ever-changing field of digital health trends using social networks.

Table of Contents

Detailed Table of Contents

In overpopulated nations, the need for medical treatment is increasing along with the population; healthcare difficulties are becoming more common. The population's need for high-quality care is growing despite decreasing treatment costs. An internet of things (IoT) network is a group of hardware and software components, including sensors, gadgets, appliances, and software, that can share data and information among themselves without the assistance of a human. IoT benefits healthcare by enabling remote patient monitoring, telemedicine, medication management, resource optimization, infection control, and more. IoT is crucial in healthcare for remote monitoring, timely interventions, cost reduction, and data-driven care, ultimately improving patient outcomes and healthcare system efficiency. Nowadays, much advancement is taking place in the field of IoT especially in healthcare monitoring. Some of them are wearable IoT-enabled real-time health monitoring system, real-time remote health monitoring system driven by 5G MEC-IoT, which are further discussed in this chapter.

This chapter explores the synergy between digital health innovations and social networks, emphasizing their transformative impact on healthcare quality. Addressing challenges like access disparities, rising costs, and patient safety concerns, the author dissects telemedicine, EHRs, wearables, and AI, illustrating their contributions to healthcare improvement. Case studies highlight positive changes, from expanded access to informed decision-making. The role of social networks in facilitating adoption and ensuring patient engagement is crucial. The chapter introduces a framework with KPIs, underlining social networks as platforms for sharing best practices.

The world's top nations are working to find solutions to the complicated, multidimensional, and large-scale challenge of building smart cities. Control over critical aspects of the city's life cycle through computer technology and the ability to make wise operational decisions in an emergency are the two biggest benefits of a smart city. The digital transformation of healthcare, or the development of computerized clinics, communications, and intelligent systems for health monitoring and enhancing the quality of life of diverse population groups, is one of the main goals of creating a smart city. While IoT can improve human health, developing effective and safe data gathering methods for IoT healthcare monitoring systems still raises a number of restricting problems.

Foreword

In the rapidly evolving landscape of healthcare, the integration of digital technologies has become a transformative force, reshaping the way we approach patient care, research, and communication. Among the myriad tools that have emerged, social networks have proven to be particularly influential in driving change and fostering innovation within the healthcare sector.

This book, *Analyzing Current Digital Healthcare Trends Using Social Networks*, delves into the intersection of healthcare and social networking, exploring the dynamic relationship between these two realms. As the entire world navigates the complexities of the digital age, understanding and harnessing the power of social networks is essential for healthcare professionals, researchers, policymakers, and anyone involved in shaping the future of healthcare by examining the interconnected web of healthcare professionals, patients, researchers, and other stakeholders. This book is analyzing the impact of social networks on communication, collaboration, and knowledge sharing within the healthcare community by investigating how social networks empower patients to actively participate in their healthcare journey. Further, this book is discussing the utilization of social network data for health analytics and deriving meaningful insights and addressing challenges and opportunities in leveraging big data to enhance healthcare decision-making and policy formulation.

Further, this book aspires to be a comprehensive resource for readers seeking a deeper understanding of the dynamic interplay between digital technologies, social networks, and healthcare. Through insightful analyses, case studies, and thought-provoking discussions, and aiming to contribute to the ongoing dialogue surrounding the evolution of healthcare in the digital age with its rich contents of fifteen chapters.

As we all embark on this journey through the digital healthcare landscape, invite readers to critically engage with the content, challenge assumptions, and actively participate in shaping the future of healthcare through the lens of social networks.

Mohammad Saeed
Department of Business Administration, Minot State University, USA (Emeritus)

Preface

As editors of *Analyzing Current Digital Healthcare Trends Using Social Networks*, we are delighted to present this comprehensive reference book that delves into the intricate landscape of digital healthcare.

The year 2023 marked a pivotal moment for social media marketers who, despite the unpredictability of the digital landscape, found themselves in a position of relative security. With increasing portions of the marketing budget and greater control over their roles, the field of social media marketing has matured after more than a decade of growth. Successful social marketers have transitioned from broad strokes to precision, considering the long-term implications of their decisions. In this era, data-driven activities have become commonplace, shaping decisions across various organizational functions.

To propel the adoption of digital healthcare, a profound understanding of the industrial structure is imperative. The growing demand for mobile-based digital healthcare and the rapid evolution of digital technologies necessitate a closer look at telemedicine, data, and the business of healthcare. The establishment of a digital healthcare fee model, enhancing regulatory frameworks and cost-effectiveness, is essential for the sector's growth and institutionalization.

This book aims to bridge the gap in research concerning the industry structure, emphasizing the interconnectedness of digital healthcare goods with laws and policies. By unraveling the network of the digital healthcare business through research articles and case studies, we identify key players and pressing challenges, offering strategies to revitalize the sector.

Our target audience includes researchers, professors, executives, healthcare practitioners, entrepreneurs, and innovators. The book covers a spectrum of topics, ranging from emerging medical technologies to the integration of people, technology, and procedures in healthcare ecosystems. It explores social networks in assessing healthcare systems, the role of social media platforms in connecting medical professionals globally, and the impact of IoT networks on real-time healthcare monitoring.

We delve into the challenges of managing digital healthcare transformation, the management of technologies for social welfare, and the growth of emerging platforms in the global healthcare business transformation. This book serves as a beacon for those navigating the intricate landscape of digital healthcare, offering a comprehensive guide for individuals and entities contributing to the industry's continued evolution.

Chapter 1: Current Digital Healthcare and Wellness Tourism: Preliminary Study in the Cross-Border Context

Diana Marques, Teresa Pedreiro, Bruno Sousa

This chapter explores the inseparable relationship between advanced medical technologies, disruptive innovations, and digital communication in the context of "digital health." With a focus on the increasing significance of health and wellness tourism, the chapter investigates how relational marketing strategies can be applied to enhance health and wellness tourism. From an interdisciplinary perspective, the authors provide insights for marketing, tourism, and the economic development of territories, shedding light on the competitive landscape of thermalism as a sought-after product in cross-border contexts.

Chapter 2: Bridging the Gap: Theory of Change Guided Digital Health Implementation in Indonesian Primary Care

Rita Komalasari

Examining the potential of digital health deployment in Indonesian primary care, this chapter aligns digital health implementation with the Theory of Change (ToC) framework. By showcasing significant improvements in healthcare quality and evidence-based practice, the study emphasizes the transformative impact of ToC-guided digital health in low- and middle-income countries. The chapter serves as a guide for revolutionizing healthcare delivery and improving patient outcomes.

Chapter 3: Artificial Intelligence (AI) for Healthcare: Indian Retrospective

Vijay D. Joshi, Sukanta Baral, Manish Pitke, Rocky J. Dwyer

This chapter delves into the technological aspects of the healthcare services sector in India, focusing on the utilization of Artificial Intelligence (AI). Providing an overview of AI and its various subtypes, the authors explore the applications of AI in healthcare, including detection, diagnosis, data processing, and analysis. The chapter aims to offer readers a comprehensive understanding of AI's role in shaping the healthcare landscape in India.

Chapter 4: Digital Healthcare Current Trends: A Critical Review Through Cloud Computing

Bhubaneswari Bisoyi, Biswajit Nayak, Biswajit Das

Exploring the intersection of digital healthcare and cloud computing, this chapter addresses the emerging and fast-growing technology in healthcare industries. The authors highlight the role of cloud computing in providing a connected, accessible, and collaborative environment for healthcare stakeholders. Despite challenges, the chapter identifies the state of research, established frameworks, and addresses issues such as privacy, security, and accountability in the implementation of cloud computing in healthcare.

Chapter 5: Factors affecting Digital Healthcare Innovation in India: A Case Study of Delhi NCR

Pooja Mehra, Vanshika Verma

This chapter investigates the impact of psychological, socio-economic, and demographic factors on the awareness and adoption of digital healthcare schemes in India, with a focus on Delhi NCR. Utilizing Structural Equation Modelling, the study reveals insights into the lacking awareness in rural areas and the role of perception and income in urban areas. Recommendations include digital literacy programs and tailored awareness campaigns to bridge the gap in adoption.

Chapter 6: Implementation of the Internet of Things (IoT) in Remote Healthcare

Ajay N. Upadhyaya, Asma Saqib, J Vimala Devi, Sreekanth Rallapalli, S. Sudha, Sampath Boopathi

This chapter explores the emerging technology of remote patient monitoring using IoT devices and sensors. Highlighting the potential for IoT to transform the healthcare industry, the authors discuss different devices and sensors, hardware and software components, and future developments in IoT technology for remote patient monitoring. The use of IoT in healthcare is presented as a means to enhance efficiency, accuracy, and cost-effectiveness in healthcare delivery.

Chapter 7: Innovations in Robotic-Assisted Physiotherapy: Enhancing Rehabilitation and Recovery

Rabia Aziz, Anam Siddiqui, Habiba Sundus, Firdaus Jawed, Sohrab Khan

Examining the convergence of robotics and physiotherapy, this chapter navigates through avant-garde technologies and methodologies shaping a paradigmatic shift in patient care. From dexterous hand movements to robotic limbs, the authors explore how robotic-assisted physiotherapy is improving patient recovery outcomes and maximizing functional ability. The chapter highlights the transformative potential of this intersection in revolutionizing patient care and fostering holistic wellness.

Chapter 8: IoT Networks for Real-Time Healthcare Monitoring System

Venkat T, Lahari Mothukuri, Sangers Bhavana

Focusing on the application of Internet of Things (IoT) in healthcare, this chapter addresses the need for real-time healthcare monitoring systems. The authors discuss the benefits of IoT, including remote patient monitoring, telemedicine, medication management, and resource optimization. The chapter explores advancements in IoT for healthcare monitoring, such as Wearable IoT-enabled systems and Real-Time Remote Health Monitoring System Driven by 5G MEC-IoT.

Chapter 9: Digital Health Innovations to Significantly Improve the Quality of Services in Healthcare Systems

Tarun Kanade, Radhakrishna Batule

This chapter explores the synergy between digital health innovations and social networks, emphasizing their transformative impact on healthcare quality. The authors address challenges such as access disparities, rising costs, and patient safety concerns. Case studies illustrate positive changes resulting from telemedicine, Electronic Health Records (EHRs), wearables, and AI. The chapter introduces a framework with Key Performance Indicators (KPIs) and highlights social networks as platforms for sharing best practices.

Chapter 10: Disease Monitoring and Management: Healthcare Information Systems (HIS) in Smart Cities

Renugadevi R.

Focusing on the development of smart cities, this chapter explores the digital transformation of healthcare and the role of Healthcare Information Systems (HIS). The author discusses how IoT can improve human health and the challenges associated with data gathering methods for IoT healthcare monitoring systems. The chapter delves into considerations such as functionality, performance, data privacy, dependability, security, and stability in implementing IoT for healthcare in smart cities.

Chapter 11: Intelligent System for Predicting Healthcare Readmissions

Manu Banga

This chapter addresses the significant issue of healthcare readmissions and proposes a novel prediction model using machine learning. The model aims to predict readmissions for patients with disabilities and comorbidities, contributing to the reduction of healthcare costs. By analyzing data from the National Health Protection Mission in India, the chapter achieves a high level of correct prediction for readmissions, showcasing the potential of intelligent systems in healthcare.

Chapter 12: Impacts of 5G Machine Learning Techniques on Telemedicine and Social Media Professional Connection in Healthcare

P. Siva Satya Sreedhar, V. Sujay, Maderametla Roja Rani, L. Melita, Reshma S., Samp B.

Exploring the transformative impact of 5G connectivity, machine learning, and social media integration in healthcare, this chapter delves into the evolution of telemedicine and the role of social media in healthcare communication. The authors discuss the foundations of 5G technology, its implications for telemedicine, and ethical considerations of machine learning techniques in healthcare. The chapter envisions a future where these technologies integrate for efficient, ethical, and patient-centric healthcare.

Chapter 13: Understanding Digital Health Innovations to Improve the Quality of Services in Healthcare Systems: A Progressive Outlook

Dr. Vijit Chaturvedi

This chapter highlights developments in the healthcare industry, opportunities, challenges, and the role of various stakeholders in establishing a well-pronged healthcare infrastructure. The author discusses the role of technology in shaping digital healthcare systems and the shift from clinician-centric to patient-centric approaches. The chapter also addresses measures and strategies to avoid digital inequality and emphasizes the advancement in digital research.

Chapter 14: The Benefits of Social Media Platforms for Medical Practitioners: Building a Global Medical Network

Arpita Nayak, Atmika Patnaik, Ipseeta Satpathy, Sukanta Kumar Baral, B.C.M. Patnaik

This chapter provides an overview of the significant impact of social media platforms on medical practitioners, fostering global networking and collaboration. The authors explore how social media enhances healthcare and medical education, serving as a virtual center for professionals to search for global work opportunities. The chapter emphasizes the powerful promotional tools social media provides for medical meetings and conferences, attracting attendees worldwide and encouraging collaboration. It highlights the potential of social media to create a global network of subject matter experts in the medical field.

In the transformative year of 2023, social media marketers found themselves in a position of relative security, marking a mature phase in the field's growth. This book captures the essence of this maturation, highlighting the shift from broad strokes to precision and the incorporation of data-driven activities across various organizational functions. As we navigate the dynamic landscape of digital healthcare, a profound understanding of the industrial structure becomes imperative.

To propel the adoption of digital healthcare, a closer examination of telemedicine, data, and the business of healthcare is essential. This book serves as a bridge, addressing the gaps in research on the industry structure and emphasizing the interconnectedness of digital healthcare with laws and policies. By unraveling the network of the digital healthcare business through research articles and case studies, we identify key players and pressing challenges, offering strategies to revitalize the sector.

Our intended audience, ranging from researchers and professors to executives, healthcare practitioners, entrepreneurs, and innovators, will find a spectrum of topics covered. From emerging medical technologies to the integration of people, technology, and procedures in healthcare ecosystems, the book explores social networks in assessing healthcare systems, the role of social media platforms in connecting medical professionals globally, and the impact of IoT networks on real-time healthcare monitoring.

Each chapter in this book is a valuable contribution to the understanding of the intricate landscape of digital healthcare. From exploring the inseparable relationship between advanced medical technologies and digital communication to proposing novel prediction models for healthcare readmissions, the chapters collectively provide a comprehensive guide for individuals and entities contributing to the industry's continued evolution.

As editors, we are confident that this reference book will serve as a beacon for those navigating the intricate landscape of digital healthcare. It is our hope that readers find this collection a valuable resource in understanding innovative technologies, trends, and challenges in the field, ultimately contributing to the continued evolution of digital healthcare.

Sukanta Kumar Baral
Indira Gandhi National Tribal University, India

Richa Goel
Symbiosis International University, India

Acknowledgment

We would like to express my sincere appreciation to all the contributors who have played an instrumental role in the creation of this edited volume, *Analyzing Current Digital Healthcare Trends using Social Networks*. The collaborative effort and insightful contributions from each author have truly enriched the content and scope of this work.

We extend my heartfelt thanks to the authors for their dedication to exploring and dissecting the complexities of digital healthcare trends within the realm of social networks. Your expertise and commitment to advancing knowledge in this field have undoubtedly made a significant impact on the quality of this book.

We are also grateful to the reviewers whose constructive feedback and thoughtful suggestions have helped refine the chapters, ensuring the highest standards of academic rigor and relevance. Your valuable insights have been pivotal in shaping the overall coherence and depth of this volume.

Furthermore, we would like to express my gratitude to the editorial and production teams involved in bringing this book to fruition. Your professionalism, attention to detail, and commitment to excellence have been vital in transforming a wealth of diverse contributions into a cohesive and impactful publication.

Last but not least, we want to thank the readers and researchers who will engage with this book. It is our hope that the insights shared within these pages will stimulate further discourse and exploration in the dynamic field of digital healthcare trends and this collaborative effort has been a rewarding journey, and we are deeply thankful to everyone who has contributed to making this edited volume a reality.

Acknowledgment

Chapter 1
Current Digital Healthcare and Wellness Tourism:
Preliminary Study in the Cross-Border Context

Diana Marques
Polytechnic Institute of Cávado and Ave, Portugal

Teresa Pedreiro
https://orcid.org/0000-0001-8208-3660
University of Minho, Portugal

Bruno Sousa
https://orcid.org/0000-0002-8588-2422
Polytechnic Institute of Cávado and Ave (IPCA), Portugal

ABSTRACT

Under the term "digital health," advanced medical technologies, disruptive innovations, and digital communication have gradually become inseparable from providing best practice healthcare. With the increasing importance of health and wellness tourism, thermalism has become a very competitive product wanted by tourists who need treatments that are not available in their country due to lack of availability or because they are quite expensive. Since tourism is integrated in the services sector, a set of relational marketing strategies can be applied to establish and maintain relationships with tourists. Therefore, it is important to understand how relational marketing can improve health and wellness tourism. Based on a combination of theoretical and practical research, this chapter explores the dynamic system and mechanism of innovation and development of digital relational marketing strategies in specific contexts of tourism (i.e., health and wellness tourism) considering cross-border. From an interdisciplinary perspective, the chapter presents insights for digital relationship marketing and tourism (health and well-being) and for economic development.

DOI: 10.4018/979-8-3693-1934-5.ch001

1. INTRODUCTION

According to Mesko et al. (2017), a new phenomenon we call "digital health", and define as "the cultural transformation of how disruptive technologies that provide digital and objective data accessible to both caregivers and patients leads to an equal level doctor-patient relationship with shared decision-making and the democratization of care", initiated changes in providing care and practicing medicine. As technological innovations become inseparable from healthcare and as healthcare systems worldwide are becoming financially unsustainable, a paradigm shift is imminent. Therefore, the competitive market is intense, marked by the constant launch of everyday products, and companies navigate a dynamic environment characterized by continuous change. Consumers, accustomed to instant information and pressed for time, demand quick solutions, compelling organizations to make swift decisions. In consequence the relevance of marketing has increased, along with advances in technology and that changes the scenario of the market constantly, showing consumers increasingly stringent, sensitive not only to price but in search for products and services that offer differentials and aggregate values. Within a framework of strong renewals, we can say that the role of marketing is to make companies realize the importance of meeting customer needs (Bricci, Fragata, & Antunes, 2016). Relational marketing reflects a business philosophy and a strategic orientation that allows companies to focus on satisfying the needs of current customers to retain them instead of acquiring new ones (Rosario & Casaca, 2023). Relationship marketing focuses on forming and maintaining a relationship between the client and the company, based on the personalization of attention, data collection and fundamental support for the client, with the purpose of generating trust, satisfaction, a lasting relationship, important information for decision making, recommendation and expansion of the client portfolio, among others. It is concluded that the fundamental objective of relationship marketing is customer loyalty since it is the guarantor of a firm, satisfactory and lasting relationship with a view to increasing sales and the success, in general, of the company (Burbano-Perez, Velástegui-Carrasco, Villamarin-Padilla, & Novillo-Yaguarshungo, 2018).

Tourism is a dynamic, transversal relational phenomenon. It must therefore be analyzed and understood as a social phenomenon, understood from a systemic perspective. This requires tools to facilitate the analysis both of its different components and the relationships between them. However, this cannot be done from a single perspective, as tourism is such a complex phenomenon that such a procedure will depend on the objective of the analysis and study, always bearing in mind that the relationships between these components and dimensions should be considered key elements of analysis (Pulido-Fernández & Merinero-Rodríguez, 2018).

Mesko et al. (2017) argues that by the 2010s, the digitalization of healthcare became inevitable, the amount of medical knowledge continued to grow rapidly (3); and patients started to become empowered while stakeholders were not prepared (4). Physicians burn out easily under the burden of bearing with all the responsibility (5); patients become frustrated by looking for solutions in a mess of information and decision makers hesitate to change the system. Health and wellness tourism, more particularly, thermal tourism is currently a popular and growing option where tourists seek to access procedures that are either unavailable or because costs are high in their country of origin (Sousa & Barros, 2021). Like other emerging sectors of the modern economy, thermal tourism is a dynamic and constantly changing industry. Contemporary society has a broad and holistic perspective of what health and well-being are (Rodrigues, et al., 2022). The practice of health care and wellness management depends on successfully informing potential clients about procedural options, service excellence, treatment facilities, tourism opportunities, travel benefits and destination choice. As such, there is a growing need to understand consumer behavior in spa, wellness and health destinations (Sousa & Barros, 2021). Antunes (2012) states that spa institutions should seek to better identify their customers and develop individual and relevant relationships to understand their attitudes and changing needs to enhance their loyalty. Although tourist loyalty is crucial and timely in the emerging wellness tourism industry, little research has addressed this issue of destination loyalty in the wellness spa tourism sector (Han, Kiatkawsin, Jung, & Kim, 2018).

In terms of natural resources and thermalism, the Northwest Peninsular constitutes the territory with the most thermal resources in Europe, which has allowed the construction of a high number of thermal establishments, references in their sector. More precisely, in the tourist sector of the Euroregion North of Portugal and Galicia, thermal spa use constitutes a key activity for social, economic, and environmental development in these regions. The Euroregion is one of the areas of the Iberian Peninsula with the greatest wealth of mineral-medicinal waters (Amboage, Fernández, Boga, & Fernéndez, 2019). This research aims to contribute theoretically to the definition of a relational marketing strategy to enhance tourists' loyalty in specific tourism contexts . The proposed conceptual model suggests a relationship between the antecedents of relational marketing and tourist loyalty. The model will be empirically tested in the Euroregion North of Portugal and Galicia. This investigation will provide insights to strengthen business efficiency and economic growth in the two regions.

2. LITERATURE REVIEW

Digital Relationship Marketing

Digital technology has given rise to new economic models such as sharing economy and business structures such as omnichannel. Technological advancements also enable firms to build a one-on-one relationship with customers. Relationship marketers have access to an ever-increasing toolbox of technologies to manage their customer relationships, encompassing e-commerce and m-commerce channels, social networks, anthropomorphized agents, and big data.

According to Steinhoff and Palmatier (2021), the proliferation of the Internet and its dissemination into the commercial domain since the 1990s has revolutionized companies' way of doing business. As one major development, we have seen a multiplication of channels accessible to firms to distribute their products and services to customers. Marketeers were more concerned with selling and promoting products and less about building ongoing relationships with consumers. With the emergence of technological advances, producers began to interact directly with many consumers and due to a variety of organizational development processes the direct relationship between producers and consumers returned to consumer and industrial markets, leading to a greater relational orientation among marketers (Sheth, Parvatiyar, & Sinha, 2012). The hegemony of marketing management of mass-produced and distributed consumer goods was challenged and a relational approach to marketing in general was spread. Service companies and government organizations began to understand the need for marketing and service management and professionals developed new strategies (Gummesson & Gronroos, 2012). This is how relational marketing emerges, dubbed as the new paradigm (Antunes & Rita, 2007; Christopher, Payne, & Ballantyne, 2013; Gbadamosi, 2019) representing the milestone of the transition from a traditional marketing approach oriented towards masses, shifting their central focus to building stable and lasting relationships with their customers (Antunes & Rita, 2007).

Lupton (2013) argues that regarding hardware, internet access, mobile phone and smartphone penetration has been increasing. Medical technologies such as artificial narrow intelligence, robotics, genomics, telemedicine, virtual and augmented reality are becoming disruptive. Regarding the software/information component, an enormous amount of medical information, peer support and open access clinical studies and guidelines are becoming widely available. It does not only lead to potentially better quality and a larger quantity of information being obtained in healthcare but also to the opportunity for self-care.

Relationship marketing is an umbrella term for a loose collection of ideas and concepts that emerged in different empirical contexts from the late 1970s. Informed by diverse research traditions, it represented at the same time an extension of existing ideas within marketing management and a very different way of thinking about marketing (O'Malley, 2014). This type of marketing requires that a firm offers more resources and activities than a core product (goods or services) in order to satisfy the long-term value needs of its customers (Grönroos, 1997).

Kotler (2000, p.35) considers that relationship marketing establishes solid economic, technical and social links between the parties. Furthermore, it reduces the money and time invested in transactions. In successful cases, transactions stop being negotiated from time to time and become routine. In this way, the concept of relational marketing emphasizes post-sales relationships. Its essence represents the establishment of balance between marketing efforts to achieve new customers and maintain relationships with existing customers even after sales. The main theories of relationship marketing are not just about customer acquisition and sales transactions, but also about customer continuity and the importance of increasing the number of customers (Yegin, 2021).

Commercial relationships based on the relationship marketing paradigm promote knowledge exchange and, therefore, innovation (Arosa-Carrera & Chica-Mesa, 2020).In recent years, several factors have contributed to the rapid development and evolution of relationship marketing. This includes the increasing process of disintermediation in many industries due to the advent of sophisticated new computer and telecommunications technologies that allow producers to interact directly with end customers and the direct marketing databases and tools that provided producers with the means to individualize their marketing efforts. As a result, producers do not need the functions previously performed by intermediaries. Even consumers are willing to assume some of the responsibilities of direct ordering, personal merchandising, and services related to product use with little help from producers. The process of disintermediation and consequent prevalence of relationship marketing is also due to the growth of the service economy. As services are normally produced and provided by the same institution, consequently the role of intermediaries is minimized (Sheth, Parvatiyar, & Sinha, 2015; Sheth, Parvatiyar, & Sinha, 2012).

The concept of relationship marketing has been discussed among marketing academics and managers since the early 1980s. Instead of reaching its maturity stage, relationship marketing is nowadays encountering its next upsurge. Due to a confluence of trends driving the global business world—including the transition to service-based economies, faster product commoditization, intensified competition worldwide, growth among emerging markets, aging populations, advertising saturation, and (above all) the digital age—strong customer relationships are more than ever vital to company strategy and performance (Palmatier & Steinoff, 2019). Online interactions have emerged as a dominant exchange mode for companies and customers. Cultivating online relationships—defined as relational exchanges that are mediated by Internet-based channels—presents firms with challenges and opportunities. In turn, online relationships feature five unique aspects, relative to offline relationships: they are more seamless, networked, omnichannel, personalized, and anthropomorphized. The toolkits for engaging customers in continuous relational exchanges also have become increasingly elaborate and sophisticated, moving well beyond mere e-commerce strategies (Steinhoff, Arli, Weaven, & Kozlenkova, 2019). In this era, social media platform is integrated into the marketing strategy. This new technology sets out new mechanisms and communication tools that companies can rely on to interact and engage with actual and potential customers. Social media marketing is an integral part of online marketing strategies that enhances the brand performance. It is associated with customer-relationship marketing and its positive influences on customer loyalty and therefore generating more sales and profit (Ebrahim, 2020).

Cross-Border Regions and Health Tourism

Tourism has assumed a decisive strategic role in the development of the Euroregion Galicia-North of Portugal (Liberato, Alén, & Liberato, 2018). This should be discussed as an important strategic sector for the Euroregion economy and, in particular, for the dry borders economy, providing benefits in a sustainable way. Border regions have been the target of some investment interventions at EU level, to allocate infrastructure and equipment considered essential to boost the territory, attracting investments to settle residents. The symbolic capital of this region lies precisely in its natural and architectural landscapes, as well as in various products from the region that are globally classified as endogenous resources (Liberato, Alén, & Liberato, 2020). However, in terms of tourism, the regions of Galicia and the North of Portugal do not promote themselves together (Pereira D., 2020).

In the tourist sector of Galicia and the North of Portugal, thermal spa use is a fundamental activity for the social, economic, and environmental development of the place. The Euro-region is one of the areas of the Iberian Peninsula with the greatest wealth of mineral-medicinal waters, in terms of quality and number of springs. For this reason, thermal tourism presents itself as an attractive tourist model, capable of generating employment and attracting tourists from different parts of Spain, Portugal and the rest of Europe (Amboage, Fernández, Boga, & Fernández, 2019). Furthermore, it contributes to regional wealth and represents a growth opportunity that has not yet been maximized. Thermalism in this Euro-region is guided by several entities and is subject to different technical and administrative procedures. However, it is crucial that there is a strategic alignment of existing thermal laws throughout the Euro-Region to promote its sustainable growth. In this way, legislators could help promote a more favorable environment for the development and reinforcement of thermalism in the Euroregion (Ladeiras, Mota, & Pardo, 2015).

The Euro-region makes up the territory with the most thermal resources in Europe. This fact is corroborated by the number of mineral water springs that appear in the geography, in addition to the quality and variety of their waters. This quantity of mineral water allows the construction of many spas, which are a reference in this sector (Sánchez-Amboage, Martínez-Fernández, Juanatey-Boga, & Rodríguez-Fernández, 2017).

Tourist destinations in the context of healthcare and medical tourism can be managed together with the study of the tourist consumer behavior and should focus on aspects that reinforce relationship marketing to the site, as planning services excellence, communication strategies, promotion services, integrated experiences and combating seasonality (Sousa & Alves, 2019).

3. METHODOLOGY

The present (preliminary) research was conducted using mixed method research using quantitative data (i.e., surveys) and qualitative data (i.e., interviews) to understand not only the perspective of consumers but also of professionals on the research problem.

The proposed conceptual model presents a relationship between the variables satisfaction, commitment, trust and loyalty. Through this model it can be observed that satisfaction is an antecedent of commitment and trust, and loyalty is presented as a consequence of these two variables. Based on the theme of this research, this conceptual model aims to study the influence of satisfaction of tourists from the Euro-Region on trust and commitment they feel towards the thermal spas they visit and understand whether these variables are determinants of the level of loyalty the tourist feels towards the thermal spas.

The sampling process used to distribute questionnaire surveys was a non-probabilistic process. The surveys were made available online through the Google Forms platform, and were subsequently distributed on social networks (Facebook, LinkedIn and Instagram) in private and non-private groups, email addresses, with free access to anyone. Considering the research topic being directed exclusively to the Northern Euro-Region of Portugal and Galicia, two research questionnaires were prepared, one in Portuguese and the other in Spanish, considering the target audience, which is mostly from Portuguese or Spanish nationality. In addition to the questionnaire survey, a set of exploratory semi-structured interviews were carried out with entities in the Euro-region, with the intention of obtaining opinions from the different interviewees on the potential of creating a commun product (i.e, thermal cluster) in the Euro-region North of Portugal and Galicia and that what has to be done to make tourists loyal to the product in this same destination. The constitution of the sample considered the knowledge of the research topic on the part of the interviewees who, for professional reasons, the positions they hold or the research they have been developing, have knowledge about the problems and potential of the Euro-region, in economic, social, tourist, cultural, territorial terms. Individual interviews were carried out with three entities, one in the North of Portugal and two in Galicia. These interviews were carried out online since it was a flexible method taking considering the availability of the interviewees, and also due to the greater ease in terms of logistics of time and space.

Considering the data obtained by the surveys, it was possible to observe using Pearson's correlation coefficient, that there is a confirmation of the positive correlation among the variables put to test in the conceptual model. A direct relationship was found, although in different degrees from that hypothesis. All variable measurement scales, except for 'satisfaction' inherent to the Portuguese survey, present values greater than 0.9, which means that the reliability of the variable scales is very good. Regarding the reliability value of the scale measuring the variable 'satisfaction' in the first survey, it corresponds to 0.857, that is, the coefficient is greater than 0.8 and therefore the reliability of the scale is good. In general, all values are positive, which means that all scales are reliable and suitable for measuring the variables.

4. PRELIMINARY ANALYSIS OF RESULTS

Through the analysis of the interviews, it was possible to understand that tourists who visit the spas in the North of Portugal and Galicia represent a heterogeneous and quite diverse public, representing a demanding and concerned niche that seeks peace and the best way to take care of themselves and their body. Furthermore, it is possible to notice a demand for this type of tourism among younger people who want a healthier lifestyle. As for the older public, they seek this type of treatments to treat chronic illnesses. To promote the creation of a common product across the Euro-region, the interviewees proposed the creation of a thermal cluster so that there can be an exchange of knowledge and to value endogenous resources and de-seasonalize summer tourism, reinforcing the continuous training of professionals and promote job creation in the regions. It is essential to create a relational marketing strategy within the management of spa resorts to create relationships with tourists and increase their loyalty. Digital tools become important to promote resort information and create a close connection with tourists.

Considering the growing importance of health and wellness tourism, this research aimed to promote the study of the profile of the tourist who looks for an experience in this type of tourism and their motivations. The results reveal that most tourists who visit thermal areas in the Euro-region are female, aged between 25 and 34 and have secondary education. Tourists take the initiative to visit spas in the Euroregion mostly on their own initiative, for their own well-being being, being the main motivation. Furthermore, most tourists have already visited the thermal areas in these regions more than once.

Through a quantitative approach, the developed empirical research permitted the verification of the authenticity of the formulated hypotheses in the proposed conceptual model. Thus, based on the results obtained by Pearson's demonstration analysis we were able to test and confirm the study hypotheses of the conceptual model. Furthermore, it is then possible to answer the starting question of the research. It is notable that there is a relationship between the study variables, with satisfaction being directly related to tourists' commitment and trust and these two variables being directly related to loyalty of tourists towards thermal spas. More specifically, satisfaction ends up influencing tourists' loyalty through trust and commitment.

From these results it is possible to affirm that tourists who show loyalty towards the spa they frequent are those who are more satisfied and consequently more committed and more confident with the spa. There is a great influence on tourists' commitment to loyalty, as can be seen in the values presented in the two surveys.

5. CONCLUSIONS, LIMITATIONS, AND FUTURE RESEARCH

Healthcare is a robust industry, which is tightly related to other sectors such as travel and tourism, wellness and information, communication and technology. The merging of health care and travel sectors has seen it become a prominent movement in the past decade or so. It has created a phenomenal enhancement in human mobility worldwide. In fact, the concept of healthcare travel has its history dating back to the ancient times when people travelled places, searching far and wide, for the best healthcare services (Wong & Hazley, 2021). For instance, healthcare know-how and technologies are available in many parts of the world. The availability of IR 4.0 technologies also enhances expert mobility (e.g. doctors, nurses, professors and care takers) virtually and further enhances the readiness of developing nations to receive its health tourists with an open hand (Wong & Hazley, 2021). In this chapter, digital relational marketing is explored in the context of thermalism in the Northern Euroregion of Portugal and Galicia, where thermal waters are not only sources of well-being, but also unique and rigorous experiences. Throughout this research, it became clear that relationship marketing plays a crucial role in the sustainability and growth of the thermal industry. A deep understanding of customers' needs and expectations proves to be fundamental to establishing solid and lasting bonds between thermal establishments and their visitors. The Euroregion, with its rich thermal heritage, offers a useful solid base for the application of relationship marketing strategies. The personalization of services, adaptation to cultural preferences and the promotion of different experiences are the pillars of this approach, where thermal waters are not only linked to their physical benefits, but also to the history and identity of the region.

It is notable that the increase in satisfaction is entirely interconnected with the increase in other relational constructs such as commitment and trust, which, in turn, are related to the intensification of loyalty to the spa. This reflects the importance of spa centers working on a relational marketing strategy. The implementation of this strategy will increase the likelihood of making tourists more satisfied with the service provided, more committed and confident with the spa they visit and, consequently, more loyal, that is, more likely to revisit and recommend it.

The results of the survey data analyze revealed that all correlations carried out for the analysis of the conceptual model are statistically significant, highlighting the correlation between trust and commitment between tourists and thermal centers, which suggests that marketeers should be concerned about develop strategies that promote tourist satisfaction and trigger a feeling of pride and priority on tourists in choosing the thermal spa they visit compared to other possible choices. By applying this strategy, as the results demonstrate, the likelihood of revisiting and recommending of the spa is greater.

Although the defined methodology allowed the proposed objectives of this research to be achieved, some limitations were felt throughout the research. The first limitation is since the sample of respondents is non-probabilistic in nature, which does not allow the generalization of the results across the population related to the study context. The second limitation corresponds to the exploratory interview method, which led to the interviewee presenting their own elements and opinions that do not meet the topic in question. We sought to overcome this situation, relating the results of the interviews with aspects that were considered interesting in this chapter. Another limitation is the fact that data collection was carried out through a survey made available online and had public access, which makes effective control of responses difficult, and the questionnaire may have been answered by people who do not meet the criteria defined for the representative sample of the study. This chapter presents some limitations of sampling nature and analysis and discussion of results. As for future research, it may lead to other interesting relationships by including different variables in the study, in addition to those that are already covered in this work, making the study more complete.

REFERENCES

Amboage, E. S., Fernández, V. A., Boga, O. J., & Fernández, M. M. (2019). Redes sociales y promoción de destinos turísticos termales de la Eurorregión Galicia-Norte de Portugal. *Observatorio (OBS*), 13*(1), 137-152. doi:10.15847/obsOBS13120191108

Anaya-Aguilar, R., Gemar, G., & Anaya-Aguilar, C. (2021). Usability Analysis of Andalusian Spas' Websites. *Sustainability (Basel), 13*(4), 1–14. doi:10.3390/su13042307

Antunes, J., & Rita, P. (2007). O marketing relacional e a fidelização de clientes - Estudo aplicado ao termalismo português. *Global Economics and Management Review, 12*(2), 109–132.

Arosa-Carrera, C., & Chica-Mesa, J. C. (2020). La innovación en el paradigma del marketing relacional. *Journal of Management and Economics for Iberoamerica, 36*(154), 114–122. doi:10.18046/j.estger.2020.154.3494

Bricci, L., Fragata, A., & Antunes, J. (2016). The Effects of Trust, Commitment and Satisfaction on Customer Loyalty in the Distribution Sector. Journal of Economics. *Business and Management*, *4*(2), 174–177. doi:10.7763/JOEBM.2016.V4.386

Burbano-Perez, Á. B., Velástegui-Carrasco, E. B., Villamarin-Padilla, J. M., & Novillo-Yaguarshungo, C. E. (2018). El marketing relacional y la fidelización del cliente. *Polo del conocimiento, 3*(8), 579-590. doi:10.23857/pc.v3i8.683

Christopher, M., Payne, A., & Ballantyne, D. (2013). *Relationship Marketing*. Elsevier. doi:10.4324/9780080516042

Cristobal-Fransi, E., Daries, N., del Rio-Rama, M., & Fuentes-Tierno, M. G. (2023). The challenge of digital marketing in health tourism: The case of Spanish health resorts. *Quality & Quantity*. Advance online publication. doi:10.1007/s11135-023-01744-2

Dillete, A. K., Douglas, A. C., & Andrzejewski, C. (2020). Dimensions of holistic wellness as a result of international wellness tourism experiences. *Current Issues in Tourism*, *24*(6), 794–810. doi:10.1080/13683500.2020.1746247

Ebrahim, R. S. (2020). Articles The Role of Trust in Understanding the Impact of Social Media Marketing on Brand Equity and Brand Loyalty. *Journal of Relationship Marketing*, *19*(4), 287–308. doi:10.1080/15332667.2019.1705742

Gbadamosi, A. (2019). Marketing: The Paradigm Shift. In A. Gbadamosi (Ed.), *Contemporary Issues in Marketing* (pp. 1–480). SAGE.

Global Welness Institute. (2018). *The global wellness tourism economy report.* Obtido de https://globalwellnessinstitute.org/industry-research/global-wellness-tourism-economy/

Grönroos, C. (1997). Value-driven relational marketing: From products to resources and competencies. *Journal of Marketing Management*, *13*(5), 407–419. doi:10.1080/0267257X.1997.9964482

Gül, M., & Gül, K. (2016). Innovative Planning in Thermal Tourism Destinations: Balikesir-Güre Thermal Tourism Destination Case Study. In *Global Issues and Tourism* (pp. 149-162). Academic Press.

Han, H., Kiatkawsin, K., Jung, H., & Kim, W. (2018). The role of wellness spa tourism performance in building destination loyalty: The case of Thailand. *Journal of Travel & Tourism Marketing*, *35*(5), 595–610. doi:10.1080/10548408.2017.1376031

Heung, V. C., & Kucukusta, D. (2013). Wellness Tourism in China: Resources,Development and Marketing. *International Journal of Tourism Research*, *15*(4), 346–359. doi:10.1002/jtr.1880

Kotler, P. (2000). *Marketing Management, Millenium Edition*. Prentice-Hall.

Ladeiras, A., Mota, A., & Pardo, M. C. (2015). A Comparative Study of Thermal Legislation in the Galicia–North Portugal Euroregion. In Health and Wellness: Emergence of a New Market Segment (pp. 1-20). Springer. doi:10.1007/978-3-319-11490-3_1

Leandro, M., Nogueira, F., & Carvalho, A. (2015). Diversity and Interconnection: Spas, Health and Wellness Tourism. In Health and Wellness Tourism (pp. 153-164). doi:10.1007/978-3-319-11490-3_10

Liberato, D., Alén, E., Liberato, P., & Domínguez, T. (2018). Governance and cooperation in Euroregions: Border tourism between Spain and Portugal. *European Planning Studies*, *26*(7), 1347–1365. doi:10.1080/09654313.2018.1464129

Lupton, D. (2013). The digitally engaged patient: Self-monitoring and self-care in the digital health era. *Social Theory & Health*, *11*(3), 256–270. doi:10.1057/sth.2013.10

Meskó, B., Drobni, Z., Bényei, É., Gergely, B., & Győrffy, Z. (2017). Digital health is a cultural transformation of traditional healthcare. *mHealth*, *3*, 3. doi:10.21037/mhealth.2017.08.07 PMID:29184890

Moreira, A. C., & Silva, P. M. (2015). The trust-commitment challenge in service quality-loyalty relationships. *International Journal of Health Care Quality Assurance*, *28*(3), 253–266. doi:10.1108/IJHCQA-02-2014-0017 PMID:25860922

Nilashi, M., Samad, S., Manaf, A. A., Ahmadi, H., Rashid, T. A., Munshi, A., ... Ahmed, O. H. (2019). Factors influencing medical tourism adoption in Malaysia: A DEMATEL-Fuzzy TOPSIS approach. *Computers & Industrial Engineering*, *106005*. Advance online publication. doi:10.1016/j.cie.2019.106005

O'Malley, L. (2014). Relational marketing: Development, debates and directions. *Journal of Marketing Management*, *30*(11-12), 1220–1238. doi:10.1080/0267257X.2014.939592

Palmatier, R., & Steinoff, L. (2019). *Relationship Marketing in the Digital Age*. Routledge. doi:10.4324/9781315143583

Pereira, D. (2020). *Estratégias e ações de marketing para o destino Galiza e Norte de Portugal: um contributo para a sua valorização turística*. Instituto Politécnico de Viana do Castelo.

Philip, K. (2000). *Marketing Management*. Academic Press.

Pulido-Fernández, J. I., & Merinero-Rodríguez, R. (2018). Destinations' relational dynamic and tourism development. *Journal of Destination Marketing & Management*, *7*, 140–152. doi:10.1016/j.jdmm.2016.09.008

Rodrigues, C., Ferreira, F., Costa, V., Alves, M. J., Vaz, M., Fernandes, P. O., & Nunes, A. (2022). User's profile of thermal establishments: A literature Review. *Proceedings of the 5th International Conference on Tourism Research,* 15, 344-350. 10.34190/ictr.15.1.129

Romanova, G., Vetitnev, A., & Dimanche, F. (2015). Health and Wellness Tourism. In Tourism in Russia: A Management Handbook. Emerald.

Rosario, A. T., & Casaca, J. A. (2023). Marketing relacional y satisfacción del cliente: Una revisión sistemática de la literatura. *Estudios Gerenciale*, *39*(169), 516–532. doi:10.18046/j.estger.2023.169.6218

Sánchez-Amboage, E., Martínez-Fernández, V.-A., Juanatey-Boga, O., & Rodríguez-Fernández, M.-M. (2017). Modelos de Gestión de los Balnearios de la Eurorregión Galicia-Norte de Portugal. *Revista Portuguesa de Estudos Regionais*, (44), 5–21. doi:10.59072/rper.vi44.455

Sheth, J. N., & Parvatiyar, A. (1995). The Evolution of Relationship Marketing. *International Business Review*, *4*(4), 397–413. doi:10.1016/0969-5931(95)00018-6

Sheth, J. N., Parvatiyar, A., & Sinha, M. (2012). The Conceptual Foundations of Relationship Marketing: Review and Synthesis. *The European Electronic Newsletter*, *13*(3), 4–26.

Sousa, B. B., & Barros, C. (2021). Encouraging Relational Marketing in the Wellness and Thermalism Segments. *Економічний вісник Національного технічного університету України «Київський політехнічний институт»,* (28), 98-102. doi:10.20535/2307-5651.18.2021.240453

Sousa, B. M., & Alves, G. M. (2019). he role of relationship marketing in behavioural intentions of medical tourism services and guest experiences. *Journal of Hospitality and Tourism Insights*, *2*(3), 224–240. doi:10.1108/JHTI-05-2018-0032

Steinhoff, L., Arli, D., Weaven, S., & Kozlenkova, I. V. (2019). Online Relationship Marketing. *Journal of the Academy of Marketing Science*, *47*(3), 369–393. doi:10.1007/s11747-018-0621-6

Steinhoff, L., & Palmatier, R. W. (2021). Commentary: Opportunities and challenges of technology in relationship marketing. *Australasian Marketing Journal*, *29*(2), 111–117. doi:10.1016/j.ausmj.2020.07.003

Wong, B. K. M., & Hazley, S. A. S. A. (2020). The future of health tourism in the industrial revolution 4.0 era. *Journal of Tourism Futures*, *7*(2), 267–272. doi:10.1108/JTF-01-2020-0006

World Health Organization. (2020). *Constitution of the World Health Organization*. Obtido de https://www.who.int/about/who-we-are/constitution

Yegin, T. (2021). Brand Loyalty in Creating Relationship Marketing Practices: A Study on GMS Operators. *Electronic Journal of Social Sciences*, *20*(77), 201–216. doi:10.17755/esosder.661291

Zhang, J. Z., Watson, G. F., Dant, R. P., & Palmatier, R. W. (2016). Dynamic Relationship Marketing. *Journal of Marketing*, *80*(5), 53–75. doi:10.1509/jm.15.0066

KEY TERMS AND DEFINITIONS

Cross-Border Regions: A cross-border region is a territorial entity that is made of several local or regional authorities that are co-located yet belong to different nation states. Cross-border regions exist to take advantage of geographical conditions to strengthen their competitiveness.

Digital Healthcare: The broad scope of digital health includes categories such as mobile health (mHealth), health information technology (IT), wearable devices, telehealth and telemedicine, and personalized medicine. From mobile medical apps and software that support the clinical decisions doctors make every day to artificial intelligence and machine learning, digital technology has been driving a revolution in health care. Digital health tools have the vast potential to improve our ability to accurately diagnose and treat disease and to enhance the delivery of health care for the individual.

Relationship Marketing: Is a strategy of Customer Relationship Management (CRM) that emphasizes customer retention, satisfaction, and lifetime customer value. Its purpose is to market to current customers versus new customer acquisition through sales and advertising.

Chapter 2
Bridging the Gap:
Theory of Change-Guided Digital Health Implementation in Indonesian Primary Care

Rita Komalasari
https://orcid.org/0000-0001-9963-2363
Yarsi University, Indonesia

ABSTRACT

This chapter explores the potential for digital health deployment to improve primary care in Indonesia using the theory of change (ToC) framework. By aligning digital health implementation with the ToC framework, the study demonstrates significant improvements in healthcare quality and evidence-based practice within the Indonesian primary care context. The research emphasizes the potential of ToC-guided digital health to revolutionize healthcare delivery and improve outcomes for patients in low- and middle-income countries.

INTRODUCTION

As with many other countries in a similar economic bracket, Indonesia faces the "60-30-10 challenge," highlighting the critical need for creative solutions to transform healthcare (Keikhosrokiani, 2022). One potential strategy for improving healthcare quality and safety in the face of these problems is digital health and, more specifically, electronic health record (EHR) systems (Gatiti et al., 2021). This chapter's goal is to examine how primary care in Indonesia might be significantly enhanced via the use of digital health. We want to show how a contextually sensitive approach to digital health might bridge the gaps in evidence-based practice and healthcare quality in middle-income countries, guided by the Theory of Change (ToC) paradigm. The methodology employed in this chapter relies on a comprehensive literature study, providing a foundation for our exploration. We examine the global landscape of digital health implementation and delve into the nuances of the Theory of Change methodology within healthcare. By doing so, we aim to uncover insights that can inform a strategic and contextually sensi-

DOI: 10.4018/979-8-3693-1934-5.ch002

tive approach to digital health implementation in Indonesian primary care. The subsequent sections of this chapter will unfold in a structured manner. First, the author will lay the groundwork theoretically by surveying the literature on healthcare IT transformation and the Theory of Change approach (Rhodes et al., 2019). Building on this foundation, we will present the methodology employed in our exploration, emphasizing the rigor and depth of our system. Following this, the results and conclusions of our pilot study will be outlined, highlighting the significant improvements observed in healthcare quality and evidence-based practice within the Indonesian primary care context. As we delve into the details of our study, it will become clear that a powerful solution to the problems caused by the "60-30-10 challenge" may be achieved by strategically aligning the deployment of digital health with the Theory of Change framework (Hamdani et al., 2021). The chapter will conclude by synthesizing the most salient findings from our pilot study, accompanied by proposals to increase access to digital health services in middle-income countries. This research underscores the transformative potential of the Theory of Change-guided digital health, offering a pathway to revolutionize healthcare delivery and improve outcomes for patients in low- and middle-income countries.

BACKGROUND

As of 2023, Indonesia faces substantial challenges in its healthcare system, characterized by limited access to quality healthcare services, uneven distribution of healthcare resources, and a growing burden of both communicable and non-communicable diseases (World Bank, 2023). The "60-30-10 challenge" emphasizes that 60% of health outcomes are determined by social and environmental factors, 30% by individual behavior, and only 10% by healthcare services (Braithwaite et al., 2020). This underscores the need for innovative solutions beyond traditional healthcare delivery models (da Rosa, 2021). More and more people throughout the world are turning to digital health technology. From 2019 to 2025, the worldwide digital health industry is expected to expand from an initial valuation of $86.4B in 2018 at a CAGR (Rolfe & Hooper, 2020) of 25.9 percent. Digital health relies heavily on the widespread use of EHRs, or electronic health records. Electronic health records (EHRs) enhance healthcare quality, patient safety, and evidence-based practice, according to research by Tubaishat, (2019). New research, like that of Neves et al. (2020), shows that digital health interventions positively affect primary care, leading to better patient outcomes, better communication between healthcare practitioners, and more efficient healthcare delivery overall. Healthcare treatments that use the Theory of Change (ToC) paradigm are becoming more popular. The value of ToC in healthcare settings for designing, executing, and assessing complicated treatments is shown by McGill et al. (2021) research. The Indonesian government is serious about using technology to improve healthcare. According to the Indonesian Ministry of Health (2021), there is a deliberate effort to enhance healthcare using technology. Examples of such initiatives are the National Health Information System (NHIS) and the Indonesia Health Card (KIS). There is a chance for digital health solutions to be widely adopted in Indonesia due to the country's rising mobile phone usage. Indonesia has more than 175 million smartphone users as of 2021, which opens up possibilities for mobile health interventions (Mariana & Yusuf, 2021).This study can potentially enhance Indonesia's healthcare environment by generating new information that may benefit many stakeholders. The study's findings may be used by the following persons and organizations: Medical practitioners, nurses, and other primary care providers may use the results to improve their practices. greater patient care, more efficient workflows, and more effective communication across healthcare teams may result from a greater understanding of how digital health can be effectively implemented, driven by the Theory of Change. Indonesian policymakers and government officials may benefit from the study's findings. Policymakers may benefit from understanding how digital health strategies correspond with the Theory of Change framework to push for the broad implementation of electronic health record (EHR) systems and other digital health solutions, which will improve healthcare nationally. The study's findings may help healthcare facility administrators understand how to implement digital health technology. With this information, primary care settings may better integrate EHR systems, which in turn help optimize the allocation of resources and the delivery of healthcare services. With these studies' results, digital health solution providers and developers in Indonesia can better meet the demands of the country's primary care system. This may involve developing user-friendly interfaces, ensuring interoperability, and addressing the unique considerations highlighted by the Theory of Change approach. Researchers and academics in healthcare, digital health, and implementation science can build upon the study's methodology and findings. The research contributes to the academic discourse by showcasing the effectiveness of applying the Theory of Change framework in guiding digital health interventions, providing a basis for further exploration and refinement of implementation strategies. Patients and the general public stand to benefit from improved healthcare quality and evidence-based practices resulting from the successful implementation of digital health solutions. People may be more involved in their healthcare management if they have greater access to accurate health information, can communicate with their healthcare professionals better, and have better healthcare experiences. The study's findings may help foreign assistance and development organizations better understand how to help other middle-income nations with healthcare reform efforts dealing with comparable issues. The findings add to the existing information on digital health's potential in contexts with limited resources. This study adds to the existing body of knowledge on improving healthcare delivery in middle-income nations via digital health technology and the Theory of Change framework while simultaneously tackling the unique problems encountered by Indonesia's healthcare system. Through its practical implications and theoretical contributions, the study has the potential to catalyze positive changes, influencing policies, practices, and innovations in the healthcare field.

In more than one manner, this study's findings could shake up the practical realm and add to what is already known about applied research: Informed choices on using digital health solutions in healthcare practices may be made by healthcare practitioners using the findings. Insights into the effective alignment of these technologies with the Theory of Change can guide practitioners in optimizing workflows, improving patient care, and enhancing overall healthcare delivery. Policymakers can leverage the research findings to formulate and implement policies that support the strategic adoption of digital health in primary care. The study provides evidence of the positive impact of such implementations, offering a foundation for developing policies that promote integrating digital health solutions into broader healthcare strategies. Healthcare administrators can utilize the results to enhance the management and administration of healthcare institutions. This includes optimizing resource allocation, improving interoperability of digital health systems, and addressing specific challenges identified in the Theory of Change framework, ultimately leading to more efficient and effective healthcare delivery. Developers of digital health solutions can refine their products based on the study's findings. Developers may better serve healthcare providers and institutions in Indonesia by learning about the unique primary care environment, the difficulties practitioners face, and the results achieved using the Theory of Change methodology. This study adds to the literature on implementation science by shedding light on real-world examples of using the Theory of Change paradigm in healthcare. In the field of digital health, this has the potential to spark further scholarly investigation, debate, and progress on the role of theoretical frameworks in facilitating the effective execution of complicated treatments. Examining the difficulties and triumphs of implementing digital health in a middle-income nation like Indonesia offers valuable cross-cultural insights. This information may be used to understand better how digital health methods and the Theory of Change framework can be used globally in comparable circumstances. The study's findings guide the tactics of international assistance and development organizations that aim to enhance healthcare in middle-income nations. To create interventions and programs that are more focused and effective, the lessons learned from the Indonesian context might be applied to other places that are dealing with comparable problems. Based on the findings, patient-centered reforms may be implemented, including better two-way communication between patients and healthcare professionals, more accessible access to health records, and patient empowerment in health management. This aligns with global efforts to shift towards more patient-centric healthcare models. The results of this research have immediate practical implications for Indonesia's healthcare landscape and contribute valuable knowledge to the broader field of applied research. The study's insights can guide practitioners, policymakers, and researchers in making evidence-based decisions, fostering positive changes in healthcare practices, and contributing to advancing implementation science in healthcare contexts worldwide.

Method

A literature study forms the methodological backbone of our exploration, offering a comprehensive examination of the global landscape of digital health implementation. This method involves scrutinizing various scholarly articles, reports, and studies published from 2018 onwards. By synthesizing existing knowledge, we gain insights into the trends, challenges, and successes in digital health, providing a foundation for our investigation into its potential in Indonesian primary care. Our methodology includes meticulously analyzing the literature and extracting key themes, trends, and empirical evidence. This qualitative synthesis enables us to distill relevant information, identify gaps in current understanding, and establish a robust foundation for our subsequent exploration into the Theory of Change-guided digital health deployment in Indonesia.

THEORY OF CHANGE GUIDED DIGITAL HEALTH IMPLEMENTATION

This section discusses the Theory of Change (ToC) and other health informatics paradigms that form the basis of this research (Hanley et al., 2021). A project's "how" and "why" may be defined using the ToC method, which originates in theory-driven and theory-based assessment. It is both a procedure and an end result, generating iterative maps and components with logical relationships. The Theory of Constraints (ToC) is described by the UK's Department for International Development (DFID) as a critical thinking approach to program and initiative design, execution, and assessment that aims to enable change in specific situations (Amlung et al., 2020). This research introduces electronic health record (EHR) installation in a primary healthcare setting to effect change. As a process and a product, ToC starts when stakeholders establish a long-term objective and work backward to discover prerequisites and describe assumptions that will lead to the intended results. Specific elements, including beliefs, interventions, long-term goals, inputs, and outputs, should be included in high-quality ToCs. For this kind of program or research to have a ToC that is considered successful, It has to be reasonable, achievable, and tested to be implemented for electronic health records. The credibility of a TOC is supported by a mix of practitioners' experiences, literature evidence, results from past implementations, and the program designer's implicit reasoning (Brenas & Shaban, 2020). There is no universally applicable set of assumptions; instead, they serve as theories that direct the many components of the ToC and the interactions between them. They change depending on the intervention and the circumstance. Actions taken in the vicinity of the intervention will produce outcomes, which may be quantified as indicators, assuming the assumptions are correct. This will help win over the appropriate stakeholders. The Theory of Constraints (ToC) is more of a technique than a theory since it is based on various research methodologies, including interviews, RCTs, and workshops. It lays the framework for integrating multiple methods and helps direct the project towards its objectives. According to Sapci (2020), because it is based on assumptions and ideas about preconditions, inputs, outputs, and outcomes—which impact people's behavior—ToC is both a strategy and a theory. It is possible to gauge the efficacy or influence of other components of the ToC, however, including outputs and intermediate outcomes. A method that has developed over the years to account for the ever-changing complexity of international development initiatives, the Theory of Change (ToC) is a product and a process with origins in theory-driven and theory-based assessment.

Positivist, interpretivist, and pragmatic research are the three primary schools of thought in philosophical thought. The positivist paradigm—which holds that reality is objective and not subjective—is widely used in health informatics and information systems (Kim et al., 2023). But the social world—people, groups, and organizations—is best studied differently. An issue with IS research is that the development and implementation of IT in businesses are deeply influenced by social settings defined by factors such as time, place, politics, and culture. If these factors are disregarded, the events occurring in information systems may not be fully understood. The interpretative paradigm mitigates some of positivism's negative aspects by positing that human interactions shape and reinforce social constructions rather than objective facts (Burns et al., 2020). Subjective meanings or realities are emphasized by this viewpoint. To comprehend the efficacy and use of digital health in providing healthcare services to mothers and children, this research considered this viewpoint. Research may include many paradigms from a pragmatic standpoint. Research may use positivist ontologies as a starting point but then use interpretivist ontologies to examine its assumptions (Ugwu et al., 2021). Because of this, the approaches and procedures employed in this research will be unique. The research may take a scientific tack by creating a digital app without human participants and testing its effects in the real world using quantitative or qualitative techniques. Due to its focus on the social processes involved in creating and interpreting digital health systems, this study is considered part of the interpretive tradition. This insight reveals the reciprocal influence of IS and its societal setting.

The social processes involved in creating electronic health record systems and implementing them in Indonesia's primary care settings were thought to be best studied using this paradigm (Harahap et al., 2022). Qualitative approaches predominated because research issues need in-depth analyses relevant to the study's setting. In this chapter, we look at the survey to discover how EHRs helped in Indonesia. The study's methodology is enhanced with success criteria to guarantee the assessment rigor of the research results and the philosophical foundations of the research are offered. Electronic health record (EHR) system deployment at Festac Primary Health Centre (PHC), Indonesia, is the subject of this research. The pilot study used the Theory of Change (ToC) methodology to determine what circumstances were necessary to achieve the long-term objective. Starting with the end in mind, the ToC method decided the inputs and mediating components needed to reach the long-term goals.

The research repeatedly created and updated ToC maps with pertinent parts because of the intricate nature of an EHR deployment. To what extent does using electronic health records (EHRs) improve the provision of mother and child health services in Indonesia? This was the primary objective of the research question. As part of the literature study, we drafted the ToC map, analyzed the process and risks, and conducted a readiness assessment. To strengthen the SR evidence and the EHR system's influence on maternity and child healthcare (MCH) at Festac PHC, the author's ToC was used in programming design and assessment. Funders, lawmakers, and implementers might find this approach's thorough, evidence-based conclusions helpful when making decisions about digital health deployment. Drawing on lessons learned from developing and wealthy countries, the research also investigated what makes digital health implementation last for maternity and child healthcare. Lessons learned from the implementation were further influenced by existing EHR literature and performance reports, and the EHR deployment at Festac PHC was assessed using known success criteria. Definitions of the ToC components are as follows. Change with an eye on the future: This is the end that all parties involved aim for. Stakeholders have identified several problems with the present paper-based health records system. Those who have a vested interest in the outcome of the EHR deployment, whether they are directly or indirectly engaged, are called stakeholders. These are the assumptions that explain why the ToC pieces are connected logically. Inputs are the things that are done in the context of the intervention. Interventions are the steps taken to affect the intended results; in this case, the EHR sustainability and implementation plans. Seventh, the concrete results of the inputs and the intervention are called outputs. More broadly applicable advantages: the generally applicable guidelines showing the stakeholders how feasible the change is in the long run.

Literature reviews, discussions with the regional HIM, and lessons learned from other EHR rollouts created the initial ToC map. Everyone at Festac PHC, from doctors to administrators, had a hand in creating, launching, and assessing the electronic health record system. A new ToC map was designed to incorporate post- and during EHR implementation adjustments. Relevant stakeholders interested in implementing this kind of intervention in comparable situations outside of Surabaya, Indonesia, may use a generic version of the ToC map that reflects a comprehensive framework as a toolbox (Adian & Budiarto, 2020). Considering the specifics of such contexts, stakeholders may modify it for use in primary care EHR installations. One way to measure how well an EHR rollout went is with the help of the ToC method. Problems with theory, measurement, testing, and interpretation are obstacles it must overcome. The research modified the success criteria used by Sari et al. (2020) and Macabasag et al. (2023) to evaluate the implementation's maturity. Organizational management, ethics, regulations, cultural factors, political health policies, available funds, software architecture, user interfaces, data standards, privacy/security, training abilities, and long-term viability are all factors that go into determining whether an EHR implementation is successful.

Ensuring evidence-based practice and delivering high-quality treatment poses a tremendous challenge to the healthcare environment in middle-income nations like Indonesia. The urgency of this challenge becomes evident in the context of the "60-30-10 challenge," a paradigm that delineates the intricate web of determinants influencing health outcomes. According to this model, 60% of health outcomes are shaped by social and environmental factors, 30% by individual behavior, and 10% by direct healthcare services (Crear et al., 2021). This stark distribution accentuates the critical need for innovative solutions to transform healthcare services effectively. In response to this imperative, digital health emerges as a beacon of promise, with Electronic Health Record (EHR) systems standing out as a pivotal component. These technological advancements will likely improve healthcare delivery while decreasing costs and increasing patient safety. A comprehensive literature study forms the bedrock of our exploration, revealing a global imperative for digital health transformation. Wright and Zascerinska, (2023), forecasts a substantial growth trajectory in the digital health market worldwide, signifying a collective recognition of its potential benefits. Electronic health records (EHRs) steadily improve healthcare quality, patient safety, and evidence-based practice, according to research like Classen et al. (2020). This robust body of evidence underscores the centrality of digital health, specifically EHR systems, in addressing the challenges faced by middle-income countries in delivering high-quality healthcare. The "60-30-10 challenge" encapsulates the multifaceted nature of health determinants, emphasizing the influence of social and environmental factors that extend beyond the traditional healthcare setting. This contextual challenge necessitates a nuanced and adaptive approach, prompting the exploration of digital health strategies tailored to the specific needs of middle-income countries. Digital health, with its cornerstone in EHR systems, emerges as a transformative force capable of reshaping the healthcare landscape. These technologies offer improved efficiency in data management and a comprehensive view of patient information, empowering healthcare practitioners to make evidence-based decisions. To tackle the complicated "60-30-10 challenge" using digital health, this chapter lays the groundwork for thoroughly examining the Theory of Change (ToC) paradigm as a guiding principle. The chapter's body delves into the confluence of challenges and solutions. As we delve into the nuances of ToC methodology and its application in healthcare, the subsequent sections will unveil how this approach can bridge existing gaps in evidence-based practice and healthcare quality in middle-income countries, specifically focusing on Indonesia.

A pivotal aspect of our investigation lies in comprehending the global landscape of digital health implementation. Extensive literature scrutiny serves as the bedrock of this exploration, revealing compelling trends and projections that underscore the transformative potential of digital health technologies. Notable research from Mathews et al., (2019) gives a comprehensive picture of the international digital health industry. Between 2019 and 2025, the results show a significant upward trend, with a predicted CAGR of 25.9 percent (Jakovljevic et al., 2022). The widespread recognition of the potential advantages of digital health solutions in many healthcare settings is shown in their rapid proliferation, indicating their rising acceptance. The study identifies critical drivers propelling this growth, including the escalating demand for improved healthcare access, the ubiquity of smartphones, and the imperative to enhance healthcare efficiency. These factors collectively contribute to the momentum behind digital health implementation on a global scale.

Furthermore, the research emphasizes the diverse spectrum of digital health technologies contributing to this growth, encompassing electronic health records (EHRs), mobile health (mHealth), telehealth, and health information systems (Istepanian, 2022). This diversity underscores the multifaceted nature of digital health solutions, each playing a distinctive role in reshaping the global healthcare landscape. The recognition of such trends on a worldwide scale reinforces the relevance and timeliness of our exploration into the potential of digital health deployment in the specific context of Indonesian primary care. It establishes a broader context for understanding the shared challenges and opportunities across various healthcare systems and economies, laying the groundwork for a nuanced examination of the Indonesian scenario within this global framework. The evidence gleaned from the global landscape of digital health implementation sets the stage for a focused study of how these overarching trends align with and contribute to the specific challenges faced by middle-income countries like Indonesia. It forms a critical foundation for our subsequent discussions on the Theory of Change (ToC)-guided digital health deployment, aiming to bridge gaps in evidence-based practice and healthcare quality within the Indonesian primary care context. The profound impact of Electronic Health Records (EHRs) on healthcare quality, patient safety, and evidence-based practice constitutes a key pillar in our exploration of the potential of digital health, especially in the context of middle-income countries like Indonesia. A series of studies, including the notable work by Hansen and Baroody, (2023), consistently underscore the transformative role of EHRs in shaping contemporary healthcare delivery.

Research conducted by Sriram and Subrahmanian, (2020) has demonstrated a compelling association between the adoption of Electronic Health Records (EHRs) and marked improvements across critical dimensions of healthcare. The study reveals a positive correlation with enhanced healthcare quality, underlining the pivotal role of digital health technologies, particularly EHR systems, in elevating the standards of care provision. The findings elucidate improvements in patient safety attributable to EHR adoption. Enhanced documentation, streamlined communication among healthcare providers, and reduced medication errors emerge as tangible outcomes. This speaks to the potential of EHRs in mitigating risks and resonates with the broader goal of ensuring safe and reliable healthcare practices.

Furthermore, the research by Marx and Padmanabhan, (2020) consistently showcases the positive impact of EHRs on evidence-based practice. The digitization of health records facilitates seamless access to comprehensive patient information, fostering informed decision-making among healthcare practitioners. This alignment with evidence-based practices contributes significantly to healthcare delivery's overall efficacy and efficiency. These findings are significant in middle-income countries struggling to deliver high-quality healthcare. The transformative potential of EHRs in addressing these challenges becomes apparent, signaling a shift toward more advanced and technologically supported healthcare systems. Notably, the consistency of these findings across studies and contexts establishes a robust evidence base, reinforcing the relevance of our exploration. It not only substantiates the theoretical underpinnings of the potential benefits of digital health, specifically EHRs, but also provides a practical foundation for understanding the tangible improvements that can be realized through their adoption. The body of evidence surrounding the role of Electronic Health Records (EHRs) is a compelling testament to the transformative impact of digital health technologies (Nashwan & Hani, 2023). As we delve deeper into the context-specific application of EHRs, guided by the Theory of Change framework, the foundation laid by these studies becomes instrumental in elucidating how this transformative potential can be harnessed to address the unique challenges faced by Indonesian primary care.

Our exploration's core lies in a strategic approach to digital health implementation, guided by the Theory of Change (ToC) framework. This section delves into the rationale behind employing ToC as a guiding framework, emphasizing its systematic and participatory nature and highlighting its potential to offer a nuanced, contextually sensitive solution to the challenges faced by Indonesian primary care. The "60-30-10 challenge" encapsulates the multifaceted nature of health determinants, emphasizing the influence of social and environmental factors that extend beyond the traditional healthcare setting (Zurynski et al., 2020). This contextual challenge necessitates a nuanced and adaptive approach, prompting the exploration of digital health strategies tailored to the specific needs of middle-income countries. The Theory of Change (ToC) framework, emphasizing understanding the underlying assumptions and causal pathways of interventions is well-suited to address the complexity of contextual challenges (Rice et al., 2020). By engaging stakeholders in a participatory process, ToC ensures that the digital health strategy is informed by evidence and attuned to the socio-cultural and economic nuances of the Indonesian primary care context. Digital health, with its cornerstone in EHR systems, emerges as a transformative force capable of reshaping the healthcare landscape. These technologies offer improved efficiency in data management and a comprehensive view of patient information, empowering healthcare practitioners to make evidence-based decisions. However, realizing the transformative potential of digital health requires a deliberate and well-informed strategy. The Theory of Change (ToC) framework serves as a guiding light, ensuring that each step of the digital health deployment aligns with the desired outcomes. It helps map out the logical sequence of events, clarify assumptions, and foster a shared understanding among stakeholders regarding the pathway to improved healthcare delivery. The "60-30-10 challenge" underscores the multifactorial nature of health outcomes. By strategically aligning digital health implementation with the ToC framework, the study aims to address the various determinants of health, particularly the social and environmental factors that contribute significantly to the overall health of individuals (Piras et al., 2022). This alignment is crucial in overcoming the challenges posed by the "60-30-10 challenge" and creating a comprehensive healthcare solution. The Theory of Change framework provides a structured approach to identifying and addressing each challenge component, ensuring that the digital health strategy goes beyond the traditional healthcare paradigm and incorporates a holistic understanding of health determinants. The deployment of digital health, guided by the Theory of Change framework, is not merely a technical solution but a strategic endeavor to address the complex challenges inherent in the Indonesian primary care context. The arguments presented here establish the rationale for this approach, emphasizing its suitability for navigating the intricate landscape of healthcare transformation in middle-income countries.

Strategic Alignment for Overcoming the "60-30-10 Challenge"

The "60-30-10 challenge" delineates a paradigm where 60% of health outcomes are shaped by social and environmental factors, 30% by individual behavior, and only 10% by direct healthcare services (Bennett & James, 2022). This intricate web of determinants underscores the multifactorial nature of health outcomes and necessitates a strategic approach to digital health implementation. By aligning this implementation with the Theory of Change (ToC) framework, our study seeks to navigate and overcome the challenges posed by the "60-30-10 challenge," specifically focusing on addressing the various determinants of health (Wynne et al., 2021). The "60-30-10 challenge" prompts a reevaluation of the conventional understanding of healthcare, highlighting the influence of factors beyond the purview of traditional medical interventions. Social determinants, such as economic status, education, cultural context, and environmental factors, collectively contribute to most health outcomes. Recognizing this complexity is the first step in developing a comprehensive healthcare solution. The Theory of Change (ToC) framework becomes instrumental in strategically aligning digital health implementation with the multifactorial nature of health outcomes. ToC is not merely a theoretical construct but a practical guide that maps out the logical sequence of events leading to desired results. It involves a participatory process, engaging stakeholders to identify and articulate the digital health strategy's assumptions and causal pathways underpinning it. The strategic alignment with ToC allows for a targeted approach to addressing health's social and environmental determinants. The digital health strategy becomes contextually sensitive by involving key stakeholders, including communities, policymakers, and healthcare providers. This approach acknowledges and integrates the unique challenges posed by social and environmental factors in the Indonesian context, ensuring that the healthcare solution goes beyond the confines of clinical care. Overcoming the challenges posed by the "60-30-10 challenge" requires a comprehensive healthcare solution that extends beyond traditional medical interventions (Castral et al., 2023). The strategic alignment with ToC facilitates the identification of critical leverage points within the healthcare system and broader societal context. This ensures that the digital health implementation is technically sound and addresses the root causes contributing to the multifactorial nature of health outcomes. The strategic alignment of digital health implementation with the Theory of Change framework is a deliberate effort to create a holistic and contextually sensitive healthcare solution. It acknowledges the multifactorial nature of health outcomes, addresses social and environmental determinants, and fosters a collaborative approach beyond the traditional healthcare delivery boundaries. Through this alignment, our study aims to contribute to the evolution of healthcare practices in middle-income countries, such as Indonesia, by creating a transformative and comprehensive approach to primary care.

SOLUTIONS AND RECOMMENDATIONS

In light of our findings, we recommend formulating and adopting policies that encourage and support the strategic alignment of digital health initiatives with the Theory of Change framework. Policymakers should recognize the multifaceted nature of health determinants and prioritize integrating ToC principles in the planning, implementing, and evaluating digital health strategies. This approach ensures that policies are informed by evidence and responsive to the unique challenges faced by middle-income countries striving to enhance healthcare quality and delivery.

FUTURE RESEARCH DIRECTIONS

While this study provides a foundation for understanding the potential of the Theory of Change-guided digital health in middle-income countries, future research endeavors should delve deeper into this approach's practical implications and scalability. Investigating the long-term impact of ToC-aligned digital health initiatives on patient outcomes, healthcare practitioner satisfaction, and overall healthcare system efficiency would contribute significantly to the evolving discourse on healthcare transformation. Additionally, exploring variations in applying ToC in diverse cultural and socioeconomic contexts will enhance the generalizability of findings, informing more tailored strategies for regions facing similar challenges. The strategic alignment of digital health with the Theory of Change framework is not merely a theoretical construct but a pragmatic and actionable approach. It sets the stage for transformative changes in healthcare delivery, offering a nuanced solution to the intricate challenges posed by the multifactorial nature of health outcomes in middle-income countries. Through thoughtful policy considerations and continued research efforts, the journey toward comprehensive and contextually sensitive healthcare solutions continues, aiming to improve primary care and patient outcomes in diverse global settings.

CONCLUSION

In conclusion, the strategic alignment of digital health implementation with the Theory of Change (ToC) framework emerges as a pivotal approach in addressing the complexities posed by the "60-30-10 challenge" within the healthcare landscape of middle-income countries like Indonesia. The multifactorial nature of health outcomes, influenced by social and environmental determinants, necessitates a nuanced strategy beyond conventional healthcare paradigms. Through the integration of ToC, our study aims to navigate and overcome these challenges, recognizing the significance of aligning digital health initiatives with the diverse and context-specific factors shaping health. This section underscores the imperative of strategic alignment in digital health deployment, emphasizing the need for a targeted approach that acknowledges and addresses the various determinants of health. By weaving the Theory of Change framework into the fabric of our exploration, we aim to comprehend the multifactorial nature of health outcomes and pave the way for a comprehensive and contextually sensitive healthcare solution in Indonesian primary care.

REFERENCES

Adian, Y. A. P., & Budiarto, W. (2020). Literature Review: The Implementation of E-Health At Primary Healthcare Centers in Surabaya City. *Jurnal Administrasi Kesehatan Indonesia*, *8*(1), 40. Advance online publication. doi:10.20473/jaki.v8i1.2020.40-55

Amlung, J., Huth, H., Cullen, T., & Sequist, T. (2020). Modernizing health information technology: Lessons from healthcare delivery systems. *JAMIA Open*, *3*(3), 369–377. doi:10.1093/jamiaopen/ooaa027 PMID:33215072

Bennett, C. L., & James, A. H. (2022). quality improvement. *Clinical Leadership in Nursing and Healthcare*, 337-353. doi:10.1002/9781119869375.ch16

Braithwaite, J., Glasziou, P., & Westbrook, J. (2020). The three numbers you need to know about healthcare: The 60-30-10 challenge. *BMC Medicine*, *18*(1), 1–8. doi:10.1186/s12916-020-01563-4 PMID:32362273

Brenas, J. H., & Shaban-Nejad, A. (2020). Health intervention evaluation using semantic explainability and causal reasoning. *IEEE Access : Practical Innovations, Open Solutions*, *8*, 9942–9952. doi:10.1109/ACCESS.2020.2964802

Burns, M., Bally, J., Burles, M., Holtslander, L., & Peacock, S. (2022). Constructivist grounded theory or interpretive phenomenology? Methodological choices within specific study contexts. *International Journal of Qualitative Methods*, *21*, 16094069221077758. doi:10.1177/16094069221077758

Castral, T. C., Bueno, M., Carvalho, J. C., Warnock, F., Sousa, J. C. G. D., Ribeiro, L. M., & Mendonça, A. K. M. S. (2023). Implementation of a knowledge translation and exchange intervention for pain management in neonates. *Acta Paulista de Enfermagem*, *36*. Advance online publication. doi:10.37689/acta-ape/2023ARSPE024073

Classen, D. C., Holmgren, A. J., Newmark, L. P., Seger, D., Danforth, M., & Bates, D. W. (2020). National trends in the safety performance of electronic health record systems from 2009 to 2018. *JAMA Network Open*, *3*(5), e205547–e205547. doi:10.1001/jamanetworkopen.2020.5547 PMID:32469412

Crear-Perry, J., Correa-de-Araujo, R., Lewis Johnson, T., McLemore, M. R., Neilson, E., & Wallace, M. (2021). Social and structural determinants of health inequities in maternal health. *Journal of Women's Health*, *30*(2), 230–235. doi:10.1089/jwh.2020.8882 PMID:33181043

da Rosa, V. M., Saurin, T. A., Tortorella, G. L., Fogliatto, F. S., Tonetto, L. M., & Samson, D. (2021). Digital technologies: An exploratory study of their role in the resilience of healthcare services. *Applied Ergonomics*, *97*, 103517. doi:10.1016/j.apergo.2021.103517 PMID:34261003

Gatiti, P., Ndirangu, E., Mwangi, J., Mwanzu, A., & Ramadhani, T. (2021). Enhancing healthcare quality in hospitals through electronic health records: A systematic review. *Journal of Health Informatics in Developing Countries*, *15*(2), 1.

Hamdani, S. U., Huma, Z. E., Suleman, N., Warraitch, A., Muzzafar, N., Farzeen, M., Minhas, F. A., Rahman, A., & Wissow, L. S. (2021). Scaling-up school mental health services in low resource public schools of rural Pakistan: The Theory of Change (ToC) approach. *International Journal of Mental Health Systems*, *15*(1), 1–10. doi:10.1186/s13033-021-00435-5 PMID:33436049

Hanley, T., Sefi, A., Grauberg, J., Prescott, J., & Etchebarne, A. (2021). A theory of change for web-based therapy and support services for children and young people: Collaborative qualitative exploration. *JMIR Pediatrics and Parenting*, *4*(1), e23193. doi:10.2196/23193 PMID:33749615

Hansen, S., & Baroody, A. J. (2023). Beyond the boundaries of care: Electronic health records and the changing practices of healthcare. *Information and Organization*, *33*(3), 100477. doi:10.1016/j.infoandorg.2023.100477

Harahap, N. C., Handayani, P. W., & Hidayanto, A. N. (2022). Barriers and facilitators of personal health record adoption in Indonesia: Health facilities' perspectives. *International Journal of Medical Informatics*, *162*, 104750. doi:10.1016/j.ijmedinf.2022.104750 PMID:35339888

Istepanian, R. S. (2022). Mobile health (m-Health) in retrospect: The known unknowns. *International Journal of Environmental Research and Public Health*, *19*(7), 3747. doi:10.3390/ijerph19073747 PMID:35409431

Jakovljevic, M., Lamnisos, D., Westerman, R., Chattu, V. K., & Cerda, A. (2022). Future health spending forecast in leading emerging BRICS markets in 2030: Health policy implications. *Health Research Policy and Systems*, *20*(1), 23. doi:10.1186/s12961-022-00822-5 PMID:35183217

Keikhosrokiani, P. (Ed.). (2022). *Big data analytics for healthcare: datasets, techniques, life cycles, management, and applications*. Academic Press.

Kim, E. D., Kuan, K. K., Vaghasiya, M. R., Penm, J., Gunja, N., El Amrani, R., & Poon, S. K. (2023). Passive resistance to health information technology implementation: The case of electronic medication management system. *Behaviour & Information Technology*, *42*(13), 2308–2329. doi:10.1080/0144929X.2022.2117081

Macabasag, R. L. A., Mallari, E. U., Pascual, P. J. C., & Fernandez-Marcelo, P. G. H. (2023). Catching up with rapid technology implementation: Mobilities, electronic medical records, and primary care work in the Philippines. *Applied Mobilities*, *8*(2), 97–112. doi:10.1080/23800127.2022.2087014

Mariana, C. D., & Yusuf, D. (2021). Building Timeless. co Brand Awareness Through Influencer and Internet Marketing. *Management and Sustainable Development Journal*, *3*(1), 75–92. doi:10.46229/msdj.v3i1.247

Marx, E. W., & Padmanabhan, P. (2020). *Healthcare digital transformation: How consumerism, technology and pandemic are accelerating the future*. CRC Press. doi:10.4324/9781003035695

Mathews, S. C., McShea, M. J., Hanley, C. L., Ravitz, A., Labrique, A. B., & Cohen, A. B. (2019). Digital health: A path to validation. *NPJ Digital Medicine*, *2*(1), 38. doi:10.1038/s41746-019-0111-3 PMID:31304384

McGill, E., Er, V., Penney, T., Egan, M., White, M., Meier, P., Whitehead, M., Lock, K., Anderson de Cuevas, R., Smith, R., Savona, N., Rutter, H., Marks, D., de Vocht, F., Cummins, S., Popay, J., & Petticrew, M. (2021). Evaluation of public health interventions from a complex systems perspective: A research methods review. *Social Science & Medicine*, *272*, 113697. doi:10.1016/j.socscimed.2021.113697 PMID:33508655

Nashwan, A. J., & Hani, S. B. (2023). Transforming cancer clinical trials: The integral role of artificial intelligence in electronic health records for efficient patient recruitment. *Contemporary Clinical Trials Communications*, *101223*. Advance online publication. doi:10.1016/j.conctc.2023.101223 PMID:38034843

Neves, A. L., Freise, L., Laranjo, L., Carter, A. W., Darzi, A., & Mayer, E. (2020). Impact of providing patients access to electronic health records on quality and safety of care: A systematic review and meta-analysis. *BMJ Quality & Safety*, *29*(12), 1019–1032. doi:10.1136/bmjqs-2019-010581 PMID:32532814

Piras, S., Tobiasz-Lis, P., Currie, M., Dmochowska-Dudek, K., Duckett, D., & Copus, A. (2022). Spatial justice on the horizon? A combined Theory of Change scenario tool to assess place-based interventions. *European Planning Studies*, *30*(5), 952–973. doi:10.1080/09654313.2021.1928057

Rhodes, R. E., McEwan, D., & Rebar, A. L. (2019). Theories of physical activity behaviour change: A history and synthesis of approaches. *Psychology of Sport and Exercise*, *42*, 100–109. doi:10.1016/j.psychsport.2018.11.010

Rice, W. S., Sowman, M. R., & Bavinck, M. (2020). Using Theory of Change to improve post-2020 conservation: A proposed framework and recommendations for use. *Conservation Science and Practice*, *2*(12), e301. doi:10.1111/csp2.301

Rolfe, D., & Hooper, N. (2020). Startup don't stop. *Company Director*, *36*(4), 65–68.

Sapci, A. H., & Sapci, H. A. (2020). Artificial intelligence education and tools for medical and health informatics students: Systematic review. *JMIR Medical Education*, *6*(1), e19285. doi:10.2196/19285 PMID:32602844

Sari, P. K., Handayani, P. W., & Hidayanto, A. N. (2020, July). Security value issues on eHealth implementation in Indonesia. In IOP Conference Series: Materials Science and Engineering (Vol. 879, No. 1, p. 012040). IOP Publishing. doi:10.1088/1757-899X/879/1/012040

Sriram, R. D., & Subrahmanian, E. (2020). Transforming health care through digital revolutions. *Journal of the Indian Institute of Science*, *100*(4), 753–772. doi:10.1007/s41745-020-00195-0 PMID:33132546

Tubaishat, A. (2019). The effect of electronic health records on patient safety: A qualitative exploratory study. *Informatics for Health & Social Care*, *44*(1), 79–91. doi:10.1080/17538157.2017.1398753 PMID:29239662

Ugwu, C. I., Ekere, J. N., & Onoh, C. (2021). Research paradigms and methodological choices in the research process. *Journal of Applied Information Science and Technology*, *14*(2), 116–124.

Wright, D. W. M., & Zascerinska, S. (2023). Becoming immortal: Future wellness and medical tourism markets. *Journal of Tourism Futures*, *9*(2), 168–195. doi:10.1108/JTF-05-2021-0119

Wynne, R., Davidson, P. M., Duffield, C., Jackson, D., & Ferguson, C. (2021). Workforce management and patient outcomes in the intensive care unit during the COVID-19 pandemic and beyond: A discursive paper. *Journal of Clinical Nursing*, jocn.15916. Advance online publication. doi:10.1111/jocn.15916 PMID:34184349

Zurynski, Y., Smith, C. L., Vedovi, A., Ellis, L. A., Knaggs, G., Meulenbroeks, I., & Braithwaite, J. (2020). *Mapping the learning health system: a scoping review of current evidence*. Australian Institute of Health Innovation and the NHMRC Partnership Centre for Health System Sustainability.

KEY TERMS AND DEFINITIONS

Digital Health: Digital health uses digital technologies, information, and communication tools to improve health and healthcare delivery. It encompasses many applications, including electronic health records, mobile health (mHealth), telehealth, health information systems, and wearable devices, to enhance healthcare access, efficiency, and patient outcomes.

Electronic Health Records: (EHR): Electronic Health Records (EHR) are digital versions of patients' paper charts. EHRs contain a patient's medical history, diagnoses, medications, treatment plans, immunization dates, allergies, radiology images, and laboratory test results. They provide a comprehensive and real-time view of a patient's health information and facilitate secure data sharing among healthcare providers.

Indonesia: Indonesia is a Southeast Asian country with thousands of volcanic islands. It is known for its diverse cultures, rich biodiversity, and significant economic growth. The country faces healthcare challenges related to access, infrastructure, and the burden of diseases, and it is actively exploring digital health solutions to address these issues.

Primary Care: Primary care is the first point of contact for individuals seeking healthcare services. It involves the provision of comprehensive, continuous, and coordinated care for a range of health needs. Primary care providers, such as general practitioners and family physicians, play a central role in preventive care, diagnosis, treatment, and management of common health conditions.

Theory of Change: (ToC): The Theory of Change (ToC) is a systematic and participatory approach to planning, implementing, and evaluating social interventions. In the context of this research, ToC provides a framework for understanding the underlying assumptions, causal pathways, and expected outcomes of digital health implementation, guiding a contextually sensitive approach to healthcare transformation.

Chapter 3
Artificial Intelligence (AI) for Healthcare:
India Retrospective

Vijay D. Joshi
Dr. Ambedkar Institute of Management Studies and Research, India

Sukanta Kumar Baral
https://orcid.org/0000-0003-2061-714X
Indira Gandhi National Tribal University, India

Manish Pitke
S.P. Mandali's Prin L.N Welingkar Institute of Management, India

Rocky J. Dwyer
College of Management and Human Potential, Walden University, Canada

ABSTRACT

The present world and economy are driven by technological changes and innovation-keen individuals across all areas. Given the speed at which machine learning, AI, and deep learning have developed as of late, these new advances are without a doubt expected to influence how we live and work. One region where this worldview may stand apart today as well as in what is in store is the 'medical care and related management' that empowers the utilization of these technology-based tools and techniques to detect (identify), diagnose (conclude), handle information (processing of data), and examine (analysis of data) rapidly. The objective of this chapter is to provide the reader with an idea about the technological aspects (and their related components) involved in the healthcare services sector in India. This is specifically in the context of the use of artificial intelligence (AI) in the healthcare sector. This chapter outlines the fundamental ideas behind artificial intelligence (AI), as well as its various subtypes and medical-related applications.

DOI: 10.4018/979-8-3693-1934-5.ch003

1. INTRODUCTION

Here you can see what this chapter is about and its scope. The scope of this chapter includes an understanding of the origin and key aspects of the term Industry 4.0, knowledge of its relationship with Healthcare 4.0, various technologies used in Healthcare 4.0, and the use of artificial intelligence (AI) in healthcare. It also provides some insights about Industry 4.0, and the Indian and global scenario of AI in healthcare, etc.

2. WHAT IS INDUSTRY 4.0? (CARVALHO & CAZARINI, 2020)

Industry 4.0 is a framework for faster, smarter, and more advanced manufacturing. This framework has three elements viz. smart plant, smart, production, and smart logistics to achieve the desired goals.

2.1 Industry 4.0: Origin

The term "Industry 4.0" comes in the context of a new industrial revolution that has an emphasis on automation and integration. It includes state-of-the-art technological innovations and helps in both customized and faster production (of goods) (Kagermann, et al., 2016). This term originated in Germany in 2011, referring to changes directly linked to automation fields integrated with information technology (Carvalho and Cazarini, 2020).

Furthermore, this Fourth Industrial Revolution aims to manufacture products through automation. The aim is to improve productivity through "intelligent devices." A hallmark of this Fourth Industrial Revolution is the (systematic and planned) integration of the Internet and production processes using smart devices (such as small sensors), and artificial intelligence on machines (Schwad, 2016).

2.2 Industry 4.0: Key Aspects

Industry 4.0 is a junction of three general aspects to consider: smart plant, smart production, and smart logistics (Carvalho and Cazarini, 2020), (Zhou et al., 2016).

Figure 1 shows the interconnection between these three aspects.

Figure 1. Key Aspects of Industry 4.0.
Source: Adapted from Carvalho and Cazarini (2020)

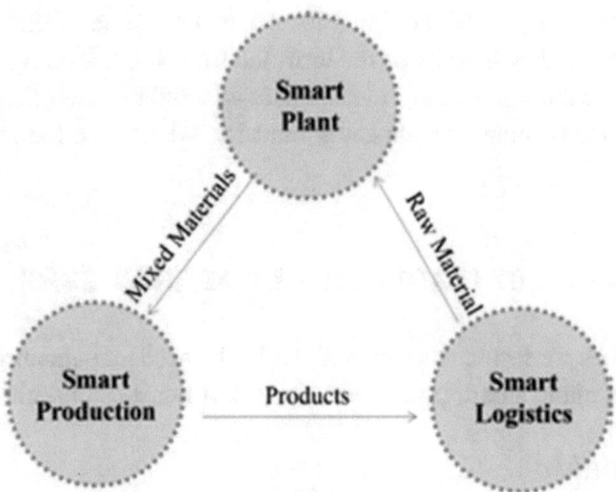

"Smart Plants" can be seen as an extension of digital factories. This is a key component of future smart infrastructure. We focus on strong and efficient production setups and processes, and the performance of network distribution in production facilities that make up the factory layout (Kagerman, 2015).

Further, (Kagermann, 2015) stated that logistics management and industry-wide production are related to "intelligent production." Human-to-machine (H2M) interaction as well as the application of 3D/4D technology in industrial processes are supported by this. These processes are part of a high-capacity industrial chain with aspects like personalization, flexibility, and active participation (in a network).

The Internet supports "Intelligent Logistics." The network can get a service match for logistical support if it interacts with the high performance of logistics resource efficiency on both the supply and demand side. (Anderl, 2014) believes that there are three parameters comprising Industry 4.0 – the plant, production, and logistics, and are independent of each other. The purpose of smart manufacturing is to create customized products for customers.

3. INDUSTRY 4.0 AND MEDICAL/HEALTHCARE SERVICES

Artificial intelligence, human psychology, the Internet of Things, machine learning, big data mining, and augmented reality are just a few of the modern technologies used in the healthcare sector. Some factors need more consideration, but Industry 4.0 is ready to take the next step. Indeed, it is causing a paradigm change in the healthcare sector (Popov et al., 2022).

The healthcare sector can be made simpler by Industry 4.0. This could be done by improving and enabling remote monitoring systems. Fast communication, instant measurement of any type of quantity, deployment, and assistance from cloud-based record systems, are some indicators of the most noticeable advancement. Another advantage of Industry 4.0 (technologies) is the ability to transfer data from one place to another (Aceto et al., 2020).

The fourth industrial revolution is the most notable one that introduced cyber-physical systems consisting of useful technology-based resources and techniques. These may include the Internet of Things (IoT), Big Data Analytics (BDA), Cloud Computing, blockchain, and Artificial Intelligence (AI). Indeed, this fourth revolution was triggered by the development of information technology (IT) (Aceto et al., 2020), (Javaid and Haleem, 2019).

According to (Haleem et al., 2022), at the forefront are emerging technologies such as the Internet of Things (IoT), blockchain, Cloud Computing, and Artificial Intelligence (AI). These have resulted in the upgradation of the healthcare systems. Industry 4.0, because it has reduced time, and costs, resulted in the development (and availability) of better solutions in healthcare.

Many industries and sectors are benefitting from Industry 4.0, according to (Haleem et al., 2022), but healthcare is seen as the biggest winner. By giving patients faster access to medicines, constant technological advances mean medical breakthroughs become more effective and better. The fourth medical revolution, known as Medical 4.0, uses cutting-edge technologies to vastly improve healthcare. As life expectancy increases, the need for better healthcare for older adults increases. Medical 4.0 addresses the idea of a highly networked health system (Haleem et al., 2022). The Internet of Things (IoT) makes it possible to use patient data from connected hospital beds.

In addition to being innovative, (Haleem et al., 2022), claimed that Medical 4.0 will not only benefit emerging markets (by providing comprehensive, high-quality healthcare) but also help reduce the healthcare burden in developed countries. Technological advances in the medical field that support patient-centered care procedures are referred to as "Medical 4.0." This digital transformation replaces physician-centered procedures with patient-centered care steps. In this case, patient data is collected electronically and used by technology to provide better understanding and diagnosis.

3.1 Artificial Intelligence (AI) in Healthcare 4.0.

3.1.1 Where Does Artificial Intelligence (AI) Come In (Healthcare/Medical Services)?

SigTuple CEO Tathagato Dastidar says "*We are dealing with the problem of shortage of pathologists, especially in the Tier-II/III cities. When it comes to microscopy, it is difficult for a pathologist to work around the clock to identify and report with accuracy. Across the world, digital pathology is still in its nascent stage. This is where AI comes in.*" (Mabiyan, 2022)

Geetha Manjunath, CEO, and Founder of Niramai says "*Radiologist to general population ratio is 1:1,00,000 in India. There is a huge backlog of imaging that needs to be assessed by doctors. This results in delays in diagnosis and the interpretation of the results. In turn, this may result in the spreading of the disease and increased complications. Therefore, AI in radiology is very important.*" (Niramai, 2022)

Some of the challenges in the Indian Healthcare system are:

- Low doctor-to-patient ratio: A major issue facing India's healthcare system is the lack of doctors in rural areas. One doctor is thought to be present for every 1511 Indians on average. The doctor-to-patient ratio in India's villages is significantly lower than the WHO standard of 1:1000 because the majority of doctors work in urban areas (Jha, 2022).
- No uniform distribution of the available expertise across the geography (of the country): Given the differences in the degree of regional development, India shows that medical professionals are

primarily concentrated in urban areas. This is an illustration of a lopsided distribution in the provision of services and healthcare to individuals (Selvaraj et al., 2022).

- Healthcare is becoming expensive now, not affordable: Only the private sector provides high-quality healthcare facilities in the Indian environment. Because of their poor income and lack of access to basic health insurance, the rural population cannot afford these amenities. However, India's public healthcare system lacks digitally-led services and solutions as well as basic infrastructure (Adani, 2022).
- Lack of trained manpower (to handle this technology): The pricing, accessibility, and quality of India's healthcare systems are severely flawed. It is evident that the majority of the personnel and manpower employed in the healthcare industry lack proper training or are out of date concerning their specific areas of expertise. There are notable differences in medical care delivery between rural and urban areas as a result of this shortage of qualified labor and qualified health professionals (Kumar, 2022).
- Old procedures and practices prone to errors (diagnostics-related) resulting in delayed detection: The use of old procedures and methods will make the detection of a disease a time-consuming process. This will even delay the initial diagnosis and the start of preliminary treatment (STPI, 2022).

Some of the Challenges of Using AI in Healthcare

Some of the challenges in using AI in healthcare are (Emeritus, 2023), (Rosen, 2023), (Pongtriang et al., 2023):

Data Privacy (and Security) Concerns: A vast amount of patient data (or medical data) is what motivates the usage of AI in healthcare. Concerns around the security and privacy of data are growing as a result of this. In this particular situation, it is imperative to guarantee that patient data is safeguarded against unauthorized access and disclosure of any type.

Ethical Considerations: Accompanying the aforementioned is the consideration of data ethics. Since different data may be used by many AI systems, it is necessary to use this data "ethically", and to protect it. The lack of a common ethical framework for rules about the usage of AI in healthcare makes it challenging to determine or define accountability.

The Need for Regulatory Framework: Clear laws and policies governing the application of AI in healthcare are currently lacking. This may create a problem for healthcare service providers in understanding how to use the technology responsibly. Stakeholders in the healthcare sector, including practitioners, patients, and industry leaders, lack knowledge; many do not know how AI can be integrated into current procedures and practices. To address this, an appropriate structure must be in place to allow all parties involved (in the healthcare sector) to successfully integrate AI.

3.1.2 The Framework of Artificial Intelligence (AI) in Healthcare 4.0?

AI in healthcare has an active role at every step of the healthcare value chain; different types of AI include vision, conversational, sense, and decision AI. (See Table 1)

Table 1. Different Types of AI

Sr. No.	Type of AI	Features/Description	Representative Image
1	Vision AI	Generates information from images, videos, or documents. It uses sensors, cameras, neural networks, and machine learning (ML) algorithms. Applications are facial recognition, object recognition, etc.	
2	Conversational AI	As the name suggests, it is based on dialogue. It is capable of voice-based and text-based conversations. It generates information in an instant. It automates conversations and provides information instantly. Applications are chatbots, virtual assistants, etc.	
3	Sense-based AI	It makes use of various human emotions that may take different forms of communication. It extracts information from human emotions such as expressions, and speech. It collects and analyses data using sensors and hardware. Applications are wearables, smart home devices, etc.	
4	Decision-based AI	It can make any decision. It automates the processes with relevant (and accurate) decision-making capabilities by analyzing retrieved data. For accurate decision-making, it uses ML and optimization algorithms. It has a reasoning and prediction ability like humans. Applications are supply chain management, healthcare, etc.	

Source: Compiled by the authors from various literature related to Artificial Intelligence in the Healthcare Sector.

The definitions of relevant terms in AI and virtual components of AI will be described subsequently. Typically, the healthcare value chain has the following areas/elements (See Table 2):

Table 2. Elements of the Healthcare Value Chain

Sr. No.	Area of the Value Chain	Aimed At
1	Keeping Well: Self-care, prevention, and wellness.	Improvement in Public Health Management
2	Triaging: Triaging for efficient emergency response.	Improvement in Public Health Management
3	Detection and Diagnostics: Early detection, and identification of any unwanted things in the human body.	Training and capacity building of the healthcare workforce
4	Decisioning: Deciding about the treatment, Clinical Decision Support	Sharpening research and innovation
5	Care Delivery: Assisted surgery and post-operative care.	
6	Chronic Care: Condition management e.g., diabetes, cardiac care.	Improving operations in terms of their functionality (better, faster, and cheaper)
7	Remote Care: Long-term care.	

Source: Compiled by the authors from various literature related to Artificial Intelligence in the Healthcare Sector.

Gradually, AI has started to address some of the problems in the healthcare sector. AI has the potential to help people keep well, make care accessible, improve quality, and make care cheaper. This is shown in Table 3.

Table 3. AI is Addressing Problems in the Healthcare Value Chain

Sr. No.	Area of the Value Chain	Challenge or Problem Area	How It Is Addressed (by AI)?
1	Keeping Well	Increased longevity and chronic ailments requiring personal care at home.	Providing tracking and monitoring solutions. This may be in the form of sensors, smart wearable devices, or providing an option for smart exercising.
2	Triaging	Non-availability of staff or trained manpower increases the patient load on the healthcare establishments.	Enabling enterprises to prioritize on a real-time basis (e.g., COVID-19). Implementing practices of risk-based identification for reducing complications such as the possibility of heart attacks
3	Detection and Diagnostics	Not possible to reach healthcare expertise outside any urban area. This increases the turnaround time.	Use of mechanical image analysis (such as pathology and radiology). It may use critical illness diagnostics and personal medication based on genome analysis.
4	Decisioning	Non-uniform availability (uneven spread) of doctors in urban areas and quality of doctors (in terms of services provided by them).	Development and establishment of clinical decision support systems for primary care. It is also set up for advanced care such as oncology.
5	Care Delivery	Limited availability of skilled and trained manpower due to specific requirements such as varying levels of skillsets and standards of care.	Use of VR (virtual reality) techniques in teaching/educating surgeons. This is used to teach new procedures and determine their competency levels. Use of systems to support post-surgery recuperation or recovery. Systems help in providing decision support for treatment planning.
6	Chronic Care (Administrative and Automation)	Providing personalized health management with an emphasis on refraining from hospitalization by systematic management of chronic care.	Use of monitoring devices such as continuous glucose level monitoring and insulin dosage adjustment. Measurement of stress levels and using the same for effective management.
7	Remote Care	High cost of medical services when admitted to hospital. Offering convenience by providing home-based care.	Use of smart devices such as smart wearables, and deploying tracking and monitoring mechanisms (as required).

Source: Compiled by the authors from various literature related to Artificial Intelligence in the Healthcare Sector.

3.1.3 Understanding Different Categories Wherein Artificial Intelligence (AI) Goes Into Healthcare 4.0

Different categories wherein AI goes into healthcare are shown in Table 4.

Table 4. Different categories of healthcare wherein AI may be used

Sr. No.	Category	What Is It About?
1	Clinical Trials	Emphasis on clinical trial management by building more robust datasets.
2	Compliances	Development of AI-driven privacy solutions or frameworks (such as secure transfer of patient data), for healthcare authorities/administrators.
3	Drug Discovery	Leveraging AI to find the most effective combinations of drug compounds, reduces the time and capital required in drug discovery. In this context, there are two ways of doing business. The first is – biotechnology-based organization have their internal R&D to discover new drugs. Another one is the pureplay SaaS (software-as-a-service) organizations selling analytics software to pharmaceutical companies (as per their needs).
4	Fitness	AI-driven wellness applications that let consumers track their health and fitness metrics.
5	Genomics	Deployment of AI for personalized healthcare, genome sequencing, and CRISPR research.
6	Hospital Decision Support	This is about leveraging AI to improve decision-making for hospitals. This may be achieved by assessing healthcare quality with quantifiable, data-driven metrics. This also includes the use of robotic process automation to streamline hospital operations.
7	Imaging and Diagnostics	Use of AI software to detect and diagnose diseases at an early stage.
8	Mental Health	Developing algorithms to track and diagnose mental health challenges.
9	Nutrition	As the name suggests, it is about using artificial intelligence to develop nutritional foods and supplements. This also includes the delivery of personalized health plans (including diets, and vitamins) to consumers.
10	Predictive Analysis and Risk Scoring	This is about analyzing and combining health data from many sources (such as health records, medical pictures, and genetic data) using machine learning and natural language processing (NLP) to identify at-risk patients. It also gives insurers a clearer view of prospective medical expenses and gives professionals better data with which to make the diagnosis.
11	Remote Monitoring	As the name suggests, it is about deploying AI-driven software to collect and analyze data from wearables, sensors, or FDA-approved home devices. This may include the use of a proprietary software analytics layer and smart sensors.
12	Virtual Assistant	Building voice and text-based AI assistants that interact with patients and analyze their responses.

Source: Compiled by the authors from various literature related to Artificial Intelligence in the Healthcare Sector.

3.1.3.1 Applications AI in Healthcare 4.0

World Economic Forum (WEF) says "*NITI Aayog, a public policy think tank in India is currently validating the use of AI as a screening tool in eye care, by comparing its diagnostic accuracy with that of retina specialists. Here, AI integration with portable screening devices (such as 3Nethra) is explored.*" (Nair and Sethumadhavan, 2022)

For most of the hospitals and organizations that are developing AI tools specifically for the healthcare sector, the journey started four years ago, mostly with radiology (Ghosh, 2022). COVID-19 firmed up AI's role in healthcare, with hospitals using it to detect lung damage in the second wave. From radiology, it is now expanding to preventive healthcare too.

"The initial use of AI was in radiology. We started using AI for image identification and have made arrangements with the companies to validate the findings. During the COVID-19 pandemic, especially during the second wave, we used AI to analyze CT scans to find out the degree of lung infection." said Dr. Bharat Aggarwal, Chief Technology Officer, Max Healthcare, New Delhi (Ghosh, 2022).

3.1.3.2 Uses of AI in the Fight Against COVID-19

Artificial Intelligence (AI) can be used to identify any issues the patient is having right away in an emergency. In China, AI-based video surveillance using Healthcare 4.0 technology was deployed during the COVID-19 period. This is used to monitor the actions of patients who are infected with COVID-19 and to stop the transmission of the virus (Petropoulos, 2020).

Drug and vaccine clinical trials can be improved with the use of AI (Javaid et al., 2020). The said study reviewed healthcare applications in Industry 4.0.

This sub-section made an effort to integrate the advantages of Healthcare 4.0 and its many technologies during the COVID-19 pandemic. Virtual reality can be used to provide robotics-based treatment to patients as this will minimize the risks posed to clinicians (Javaid and Haleem, 2019), (Riffat et al., 2021), (Ren et al., 2020), (Ahsan et al., 2021).

In the medical industry during the pandemic, AI has also aided in supply chain management (Ruan et al., 2020).

Artificial intelligence can be used to find viral pneumonia. A robot has been used as a police officer. This was used to make sure that people were following the (lockdown) procedures. Artificial intelligence was used to control the amount of human interaction during the pandemic (Ienca and Vayena, 2020).

Even though there is a pandemic, health data security must be maintained. It was possible to have remote execution and this was possible mainly due to AI (Hathaliya and Tanwar, 2020).

Figure 2 highlights some of the uses of AI in the fight against COVID-19.

Figure 2. Uses of AI in the Fight Against COVID-19
Source: Javaid and Haleem (2019)

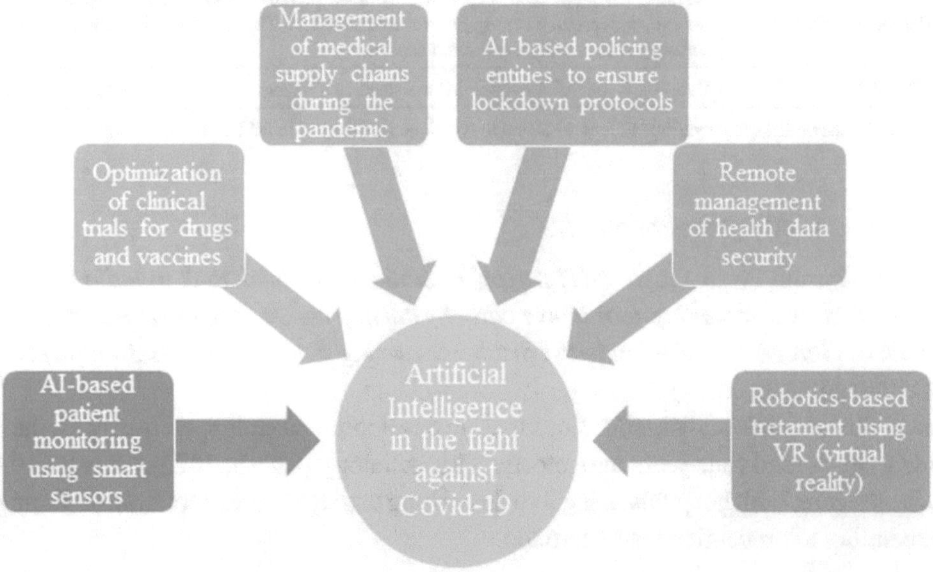

3.1.3.3 State-of-the-Art AI in Healthcare 4.0/Upcoming Technologies

Dr. Prateek Sharma is a renowned gastroenterologist and is the first chair of the ASGE – American Society for Gastrointestinal Endoscopy. In an interview with Durgesh Nandan Jha, he says "*AI has shown benefits in a whole range of specialties. In the field of gastroenterology, AI has helped in the detection of polyps during colonoscopy and the detection of cancer in the GI tract. Other medical fields like cardiology and radiology are experiencing growth as AI is helping to detect and diagnose diseases."* (Jha, 2022)

Due to the availability of large databases and recent improvements in deep learning, the performance of artificial intelligence systems reaches or even exceeds human levels for an increasing number of complex tasks (Goliner, 2022). According to Sabrina Golnier, this is a new field of research called XAI – eXplainable Artificial Intelligence. She says "X*AI can be described as a bridge between human-computer interaction (HCI) and artificial intelligence. The focus of XAI is to explain the interaction to the end-user to create a trustworthy environment. From early detection to diagnosis, the role of AI is now expanding to provide decision support."* (Goliner, 2022)

Artificial Intelligence can reconstruct MRI (magnetic resonance imaging) scans into high-quality images with the same diagnostic value as traditional scans. This was stated in a study undertaken by the NYU Grossman School of Medicine and Meta AI Research (NewsMedical, 2023). Michael P. Recht, Chair of the Department of Radiology at NYU Grossman School of Medicine, in an interview with NewsMedical, says "*Our new study conveys the use of AI in radiology. FastMRI has the potential to dramatically change how we do MRI and increase the accessibility of MRI to more patients."*

Patricia M. Johnson, Ph.D., Assistant Professor in the Department of Radiology at NYU Grossman School of Medicine, says "*The said study truly paves the way for more innovation and advancements in the future. This research represents exciting progress towards translating AI accelerated imaging into clinical practice."* The FastMRI method, used in this study, can be completed in less than five minutes, making the examination time for MRI comparable to X-rays or CT scans (Johnson et al., 2023). It is stated that as compared to the conventional methods of reconstruction, deep learning reconstruction (of prospectively accelerated knee MRI) has enabled a considerable reduction in scan time, enhanced image quality, and equivalent diagnostic utility.

3.1.3.4 Emerging Trends and Potential Benefits of Using AI in Healthcare

In this context, let us look at some of the emerging trends of using AI in healthcare and the potential benefits of using AI in healthcare.

Emerging Trends of Using AI in Healthcare

Some of the emerging trends in AI in healthcare research and development are (Emeritus, 2023), (UNF, n.d.), (Infante, 2024), (Nathan, 2023):

Predictive Analytics: AI can also be used to forecast possible illnesses based on a patient's lifestyle, genetic makeup, and medical history. Artificial Intelligence (AI) evaluates patient-related electronic medical records (EMR) data in real-time, and forecasts treatment outcomes as a result. Put differently, predictive analytics can be defined as nothing more than the application of artificial intelligence to analyze, and forecast data from the past and present.

AI-driven Genomics: Genomic analysis is an area in which artificial intelligence is essential. A lot of generic data is processed and interpreted by AI techniques such as machine learning (ML), and deep learning (DL). Based on training from the vast datasets, these algorithms can recognize patterns, forecast outcomes, and categorize genetic variants. AI is becoming a powerful tool for finding genetic alterations. This cutting-edge technology makes it easier to identify mutations, which opens the door to customized medicine and focused therapy.

Robotics in Surgeries: AI-powered tools can facilitate more efficient processes and steer surgical procedures. In addition to gathering a wealth of data from which to draw conclusions and create fresh approaches, robotic surgery reduces surgeon stress.

Potential Benefits of Integrating AI into Healthcare

Some of the key benefits of integrating AI into healthcare are (Emeritus, 2023), (Rosen, 2023):

Improved Accuracy in Diagnosis: Large volumes of medical data can be used and analyzed by AI systems. This is leading to an early and precise diagnosis. Healthcare professionals can handle enormous volumes of data with ease because of the use of technologies like artificial intelligence (AI) and cloud computing platforms. Since AI enables physicians to diagnose patients more quickly and accurately, accuracy is improved.

Efficiency in treatment: With faster turnaround time, AI provides quick diagnosis of test results. Further, AI is also able to analyze genomic, metabolomic, and bioinformatic data of individuals in less time. This will not only save costs but also ensure timely (and efficient) treatment.

Personalized care: AI has the potential to be helpful in the development of customized drugs for certain medical issues. Human disease conditions, symptoms, and treatment outcomes differ according to their physiology, behaviour, and genetic makeup. Therefore, it is imperative to offer tailored care to each individual. The application of AI in healthcare institutions personalized treatments and pharmaceutical programs for patients.

3.1.4 Artificial Intelligence: Definition of Relevant Terms and Virtual Components

Globally, multiple applications are emerging that use AI/ML/DL to make the healthcare sector better in terms of product development and delivery of services.

Figure 3 shows the interconnection between AI/MI/DL.

Figure 3. Interconnection AI/ML/DL
Source: STPI (2022)

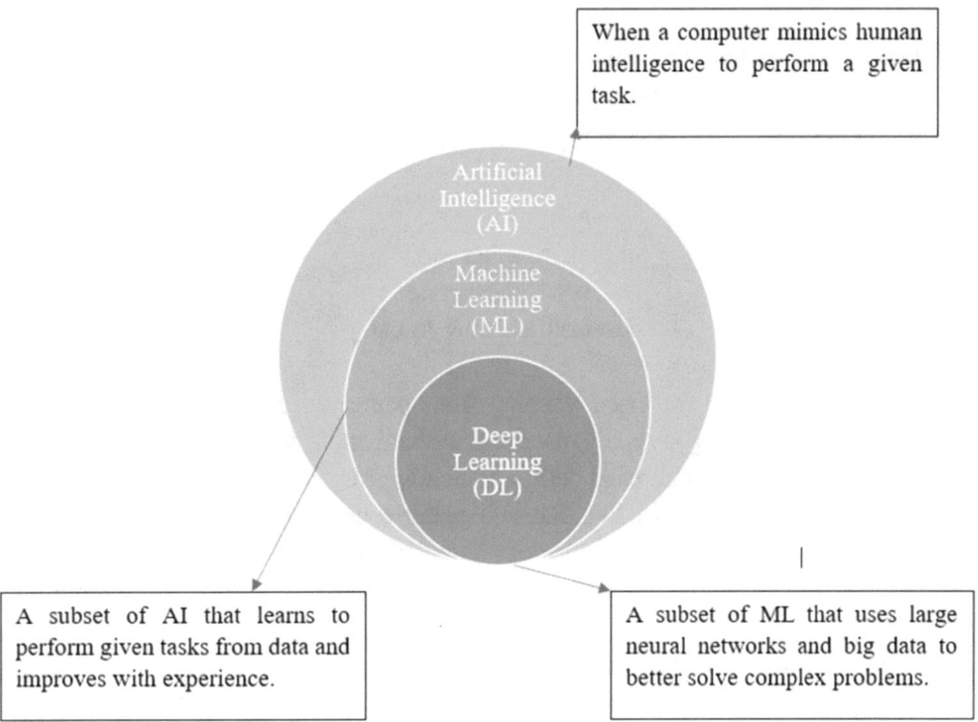

In this context, let us look at some of the definitions of relevant terms and virtual components of AI.

Definitions of Relevant Terms

Some of the definitions of relevant elements in the context of AI in healthcare, as presented by (UNF, n.d.), (Keserer, 2023), are reproduced herewith.

Machine Learning (ML): This is a subfield of AI where computer systems are given the ability to learn and improve from the experience without being explicitly programmed. This is usually accomplished by training the system with large amounts of data. For example, Amazon uses recommendation systems, which suggest products based on a user's browsing and purchasing history.

Deep Learning (DL): It is a subset of machine learning where artificial neural networks and algorithms are inspired by the human brain, and learn from large amounts of data. Deep learning networks are composed of many layers. The depth of the network is important because it allows the network to learn complex patterns in the data.

Artificial Neural Networks (ANN): ANN is a computing system designed to simulate the way the human brain works, analyses, and processes information. It is the foundation of artificial intelligence and solves complex problems. For example, OCR (Optical Character Recognition) uses ANN to recognize handwritten or printed text in digital images.

Natural Language Processing (NLP): This is a subset of AI that deals with the understanding and manipulation of human language. NLP is used in a variety of applications, such as text classification, sentiment analysis, and machine translation. Google Translate, Siri, Alex, and all the other examples of personal assistants are examples of applications that use NLP.

Virtual Components of Artificial Intelligence

Virtual components of artificial intelligence are supervised learning, unsupervised learning, and reinforcement learning (Saba and Faheem, 2023), (UNF, n.d.), (Keserer, 2023)

Supervised Learning: In supervised learning, pre-existing labeled data is utilized. This is done to get the appropriate conclusions from the incoming data or samples. The machines' ability to draw conclusions increases with the quantity of samples. In other terms, we may state that it is a type of machine learning where the model is trained on a labeled dataset i.e., where the "correct" answers are provided. Spam filters, for example, employ supervised learning to categorize emails as spam or not based on previous instances.

Unsupervised Learning: Unsupervised learning finds patterns that are either nonexistent or were previously missed. They are categorized by machines without any external direction. Following a comparison and classification of the unlabeled data, it logically groups the information. Stated differently, it is a form of machine learning in which a dataset's patterns and correlations are found by the model without the need for labels or preconceived ideas about what to search for. For example, clustering algorithms automatically group the buyers based on their purchase patterns without providing explicit grouping information.

Reinforcement learning: Positive and negative reinforcement is essential for rewarding machine learning in this deep learning technique. The science of making decisions is known as reinforcement learning, in which the computer learns from its own experiences without the need for pre-labeled data to provide a favorable result. Put differently, it can be described as a form of machine learning in which an agent gains decision-making skills through action and the possibility of rewards or punishments. For example, DeepMind's AlphaGo defeated world champions in the game of Go after learning how to play it through reinforcement learning.

3.1.5 Understanding of the Global and Indian Scenario: Artificial Intelligence (AI) in Healthcare

As stated by Precedence Research, the global artificial intelligence in healthcare market size was estimated at US$ 11 billion in 2021 and US$ 15 billion in 2022. It is expected to grow at a CAGR (compounded annual growth rate) of ~37% from 2022 to 2030, to reach ~US$ 188 Billion in 2030 (Precedence, n.d.).

As stated in the STPI report, the HealthTech market in India is at a nascent stage. It is expected to grow at a healthy CAGR in the years to come to grow in the future. Some of the major sub-segments in the Indian HealthTech market are E-pharmacy, B2B HealthTech, B2B Medical Supplies, Tele-medicine/Tele-consultation, E-diagnostics, etc.

3.1.6 Healthcare Artificial Intelligence (AI) Companies/Start-Ups to Watch...

Regarding various categories of the healthcare value chain (listed in sub-section 3.1.2), different companies and start-ups are working. Just have a look at them. (See Table 5a for some of the global companies and Table 5b for some of the Indian companies in this domain.)

Table 5. A Few Global Companies in the AI Domain

Sr. No.	Area of the Value Chain	Company	Country	What Is It Doing?
1	Keeping Well	Spring Health	USA	AI-based mental assistance program for mental well-being.
		workrise	USA	Employee wellness and tracking platform.
		TONAL	USA	AI-based digital full-body motion analysis and training.
		verily	USA	AI-based suite solutions for health management.
2	Triaging	iodine	USA	AI-based documentation solution for efficient and quick response time.
		LinkDoc	China	Providing oncology-focused medical records and data solutions for quick and effective response.
3	Detection and Diagnostics	Dental Monitoring	France	Dental monitoring technology to detect tooth movements.
		XtalPi	China	Developer of tool to predict the crystal structure of a drug.
		Benevolent AI	UK	Enhancing research and innovation: AI-based computational drug discovery platform.
		ICarbonX	China	Health management and drug development bioinformatic platforms for better research and innovation practices.
4	Decisioning	Olive	USA	Clinical decision support with intelligent automation.
		Modernizing Medicine	USA	Clinical, financial, and, operational software products.
		YITU	China	Provider of AI-based intelligent platform for multiple sectors.
		Komodo Health	USA	Cloud-based business analytics platform for life sciences companies.
5	Care Delivery	mindmaze	Switzerland	VR-based solution provider for neuro-rehabilitation.
		ORCAM	Israel	Provider of AI-based devices for the visually impaired.
6	Chronic Care (Administrative and Automation)	----	-----	-----
7	Remote Care	innovaccer	USA	Cloud and AI-based telehealth solutions.
		k-health	USA	Online healthcare services platform.

Source: Compiled by the authors from various literature related to Artificial Intelligence in the Healthcare Sector.

Table 6. A few Indian Companies in the AI Domain

Sr. No.	Area of the Value Chain	Company	City	What Is It Doing?
1	Keeping Well	----	-----	-----
2	Triaging	qure.ai	Mumbai	Deep learning technology for automated interpretation of radiology exams.
		Tricog	Bengaluru	Cloud-connected device for the interpretation and analysis of ECG results.
3	Detection and Diagnostics	Niramai	Bengaluru	Developer of AI-based early-stage breast cancer screening devices.
		SigTuple	Bengaluru	AI-based healthcare diagnostic solutions.
		CELLIX	Hyderabad	Innovative ways for drug design and development of therapeutics.
4	Decisioning	HealthPlix	Bengaluru	Clinical decision support via artificial intelligence and cloud-based electronic medical record (EMR) management solutions.
		Synapsica	New Delhi	Decision support is provided by the development of AI-assisted radiology tools for workflow and practice management.
5	Care Delivery	BLUSEMI	Hyderabad	Provider of IoT-based solutions to manage healthcare.
		dozee	Bengaluru	A_-based contactless remote patient monitoring and early-warning system.
6	Chronic Care (Administrative and Automation)	----	-----	-----
7	Remote Care	wysa	Bengaluru	AI-based chatbot and evidence-based cognitive behavioural techniques for managing mental health.

Source: Compiled by the authors from various literature related to Artificial Intelligence in the Healthcare Sector.

3.1.7 Potential in India: Artificial Intelligence (AI) in Healthcare

Depth of Focus: AI in India

It is observed that across the healthcare value chain, two areas are important for three countries. These are Triaging, detection, and diagnostics. These areas have been receiving the high focus and high impact areas for AI in healthcare across three countries, covered in the STPI Report. This is shown in Table 6a.

Table 7. A Qualitative Overview of Depth of Focus in AI

Sr. No.	Area of the Healthcare Value Chain	Depth of Focus		
		India	China	USA
1	Keeping Well	Medium	Low	High
2	Triaging	High	High	High
3	Detection and Diagnostics	High	High	High
4	Decisioning	Medium	High	High
5	Care Delivery	Medium	Medium	High
6	Chronic Care (Administrative and Automation)	Low	Medium	High
7	Remote Care	Medium	Medium	High

Source: Compiled by the authors from various literature related to Artificial Intelligence in the Healthcare Sector. These include the STPI Report on Artificial Intelligence in the Healthcare Sector, October 2022, the Centre for Security and Emerging Technologies, the NASSCOM Adoption Index Report, Primary conversations with the industry representatives, Secondary Research, and PGA Labs Analysis.

STPI report suggests that India has high potential in all the areas of AI application. The AI maturity level reveals that the latent value from the use of AI is waiting to be unlocked. All sectors are looking to scale up their ongoing AI initiatives. The focus is on cost efficiencies and business growth opportunities with the use of AI.

Maturity and Adoption of AI as a Solution: AI in India

A qualitative overview of the Maturity and Adoption of AI is shown in Table 6b.

Table 8. A Qualitative Overview of the Maturity and Adoption of AI

Sr. No.	Area of the Healthcare Value Chain	Maturity and Adoption of AI as a Solution		
		India	China	USA
1	Keeping Well	Low	Medium	Low
2	Triaging	Medium	High	Medium
3	Detection and Diagnostics	Low	Very High	Very High
4	Decisioning	Medium	High	Medium
5	Care Delivery	Low	High	Medium
6	Chronic Care (Administrative and Automation)	Low	Medium	Medium
7	Remote Care	Medium	High	Medium

Source: Compiled by the authors from various literature related to Artificial Intelligence in the Healthcare Sector. These include the STPI Report on Artificial Intelligence in the Healthcare Sector, October 2022, the Centre for Security and Emerging Technologies, the NASSCOM Adoption Index Report, Primary conversations with the industry representatives, Secondary Research, and PGA Labs Analysis.

According to NASSCOM's Adoption Index report, among healthcare companies:

- About one out of two companies have a well-defined AI strategy.
- About seven out of ten companies have active Proof of Concept (PoC) or defined use cases.

- About two out of three companies have a focus on cost optimization with AI.
- About six out of ten companies are leveraging AI in product/service development.
- About seven out of ten companies have allocated less than 10% of their IT budget to AI projects.

AI in Education: In India

In this context, the NEP - National Education Policy of 2020 is playing a pivotal role in spreading AI culture. It has a special emphasis on the inclusion of AI in education.

Table 9. The Extent of AI in Education

India	China	USA
Medium	Very High	High

- India
    - Most of the leading institutions such as IITs, IIMs, NIT, etc. – have started including AI in their curricula.
    - Under the National Education Policy 2020, AI has been made a part of the Class IX curriculum – the policy places special emphasis on AI.
    - The NPTEL platform offers ~10 certificate courses on AI. In 2021, there were ~15,000 AI/ML graduates in the country.
- China
    - The Chinese Government has mandated AI education in high school curricula. In this context, AI companies are partnering with schools and universities to train students.
    - Since 2018, the Chinese government has approved 340+ universities to offer an AI major, and at least 34 universities have launched their own AI institutes.
- USA
    - Around 200+ AI/ML courses are available across universities, including the top Ivy League universities.
    - The US places a heavier emphasis on computer science education. It has been experimenting with AI education curricula and industry partnership initiatives, although in a fragmented or disconnected way that varies as per the laws of each state.

Research and Development: In India

In this context, the NEP - National Education Policy of 2020 is playing a pivotal role in spreading AI culture. It has a special emphasis on the inclusion of AI in education.

Table 10. The Extent of Research and Development

India	China	USA
Low	Very High	High

Source: Compiled by the authors from various literature related to Artificial Intelligence in the Healthcare Sector. These include the STPI Report on Artificial Intelligence in the Healthcare Sector, October 2022, NASSCOM, RNAip, World Intellectual Property Organization, Secondary Research, and PGA Labs Analysis.

- India
    - Organizations have a limited focus on AI patents and research with many AI patents being filed by research or academic institutes.
    - In India, patents have grown at ~40% compounded annual growth rate (CAGR). However, the total AI patents in India is 75x lower than in China.
    - Long lead time for patent processing - an average Indian patent examiner sees 3x more applications.
    - Patent processing in India is ~30% longer than in the US/ China.
- China
    - In the past decade, China has filed ~350K patents in the field of AI, accounting for ~75% of the global total, and the US has filed ~280K. On the other hand, ~5K AI patents have been filed in India in the same period.

3.1.8 Initiatives to Support Artificial Intelligence (AI) in Healthcare in India

STPI report suggests that in the Indian context, apart from funding, most founders cite data availability for training and validation and market access as the top areas where start-ups need support. Some of the areas mentioned by the companies and start-ups and the support required are presented in Table 7.

Table 11. Focus Areas and Support required as mentioned by companies/start-ups

Sr. No.	Area in Which Support Is Needed (by a Start-Up)	Extent of Requirement	The extent of Support Available	Task Ahead	Description
1	Data for training, and validation of the models	Very High	Low	Getting access to data as well as its procurement. Addressing data security and privacy concerns. On-the-field trials and validation.	Reliable and good-quality datasets are required to train and test AI-based systems. Access and support for field validation (of AI-based models).
2	Funding or Financial Assistance	Very High	Low	No availability of liquid assets/cash. Start-ups may be overvalued or undervalued.	Just a POC – proof of concept will not bring funds. Early-stage funding is not enough for the long run. Needs credit line to meet working capital requirements.
3	Market Reach or Access	Very High	Low	A tough task to go through the regulatory framework and have initial deployment.	Start-ups are locked in the 'ethical clearance' required to obtain data. Support is needed for testing and deployment. There is a need for pilot programs and certifications to demonstrate market validity.
4	Infrastructure	High	High	Limited access to labs and advanced equipment.	Difficulty in finding a proper infrastructure to establish a team, and start day-to-day work.
5	Marketing	Medium	Medium	Marketing expertise available on time. Need for stringent IP rights.	Marketing channels have insufficient knowledge and thus offer limited help. The high cost required to file patents.
6	Mentorship	Medium	Medium	Suitable and systematic guidance. Academic partnerships. Need for professional networking.	Getting the right person to guide you at the right time is not an easy task. Establishing academic partnerships is a challenge for nascent start-ups. There is difficulty in reaching the faculty members.

Source: Compiled by the authors from various literature related to Artificial Intelligence in the Healthcare Sector. These include the STPI Report on Artificial Intelligence in the Healthcare Sector, October 2022, Primary Conversations, Secondary Research, and PGA Labs Analysis.

3.1.9 Key Insights From the Government Initiatives to Support Artificial Intelligence (AI) in Healthcare in India

An overview of the opinions of government officials is presented herewith. (See Table 8)

Table 12. An Overview of Some of the Opinions of Government Officials

Sr. No.	Name of the Person	Designation	Organization	Views and Opinions About the Use of AI in India
1	Shri Alkesh Kumar Sharma	Secretary	Ministry of Electronics and Information Technology	The government has been proactively introducing AI initiatives, policies, and schemes in the healthcare sector. AI-based solutions are booming in the Indian health-tech sector making healthcare services more accessible, affordable, and effective.
2	Shri Bhuvnesh Kumar	Additional Secretary	Ministry of Electronics and Information Technology	India is a country with demographic diversity. Hence, the effective use of AI in the medical and healthcare sector (in India), can be a game-changer in many ways. It can make services accessible in remote areas, easy availability of the same for underprivileged people, and more effective for the entire community.
3	Shri Arvind Kumar	Director General	Software Technology Parks of India	AI is one of the emerging technologies of today, and it holds an immense future in the Indian context. AI will help in resolving some of the major problems in the Indian healthcare system such as delayed and incorrect diagnosis, low doctor-to-patient ratio, affordability, inadequately trained staff, etc. It will bring down the cost of medical services soon.
4	Dr. Harpreet Singh	Scientist and Head, Division of Biomedical Informatics	Indian Council of Medical Research (ICMR)	In India, the AI ecosystem for health can bring a paradigm shift in the delivery of healthcare services (to people). ICMR will facilitate the development of highly curated datasets for the researchers. This will help them to develop better AI algorithms/applications.
5	Dr. Pravin Gedam	Additional Chief Executive Officer	National Health Authority	ABDM – Ayushman Bharat Digital Mission is to support integrated digital health infrastructure in the country.
6	Mansukh Mandaviya	Union Health Minister	Government of India	India's G-20 presidency is creating a fairer global health architecture (GHA). It envisages equipping countries to face the next health emergency with robust healthcare systems.

Source: Compiled by the authors from various literature related to Artificial Intelligence in the Healthcare Sector.

3.1.10 Select Case Studies: Artificial Intelligence (AI) in Healthcare in India

In this context, it is proposed to enlist some companies in India working in the AI domain. The names of the organizations provided in this sub-section are examples. These are used for representation purposes only.

Indian start-ups: Niramai & SigTuple are working on software-based imaging and democratizing microscopy respectively, by leveraging AI (STPI, 2022).

Table 13. Indian Start-Ups: Nirami and SigTuple

Company Name	Established In	Geographical Presence
Niramai	2016	India, USA, Europe
Founder/s	Investors	Patents
Geetha Manjunath Founder & CEO • 25+ years in IT & innovation • Ex - Xerox Research India, Hewlett Packard India	Axilor, Dream Incubator, Ankur Capital, Pi Ventures, BEENEXT, etc.	Niramai has 27 granted patents across different countries, with 11 of them granted in the US and 11 of them in India.
Company Overview	NIRAMAI has developed a novel software-based medical device to detect breast cancer at a much earlier stage than traditional methods of self-examination. • Radiation-free imaging method, non-touch, not painful, and works for women of all ages. • Low-cost, accurate, automated, portable cancer screening tool that can be operated in any clinic or from home.	
Product/Service Offerings	•Thermalytix: A computer-aided breast cancer detection system powered by AI. • XraySetu: An AI-driven X-ray analysis for Covid interpretation via WhatsApp. • Niramai FeverTest: Simple screening for Covid symptoms.	
SIG{(·)}TUPLE	2015	India, USA
Founder/s	Investors	Patents
Tathagato Dastidar, Founder & CEO • 21+ years in tech & software • Ex- Tribune Digital, American Express Ashes Ganguly, Chief Technology Officer • 20+ years in healthcare • Ex – GE Healthcare, Abbott Labs, Samsung Healthcare	Accel, Microsoft Accelerator, Trifecta Capital, Chiratae Ventures, etc.	SigTuple has 19 patents granted in the US & India.
Company Overview	•SigTuple democratizes microscopy by automating it through advanced AI and robotics. •AI-assisted digital microscopy, enabled through the cloud, provides a smart alternative to the current process. •Use of robotics and AI to digitize any biological sample on a glass slide to enable AI-empowered remote review.	
Product/Service Offerings	• AI100: An in-vitro diagnostic device that is designed to automate manual microscopy using robotics and AI. • Shonit: An AI application to analyze blood cell morphology. • Shrava: An AI application to analyze and pre-classify multiple elements in urine sediment.	

Source: Information has been taken directly from the company website.

Indian start-ups: Qure.ai & Tricog are working on automated radiology interpretation, and virtual cardiology services respectively, by leveraging AI (STPI, 2022).

Table 14. Indian Start-Ups: Qure.ai & Tricog

Company Name	Established In	Geographical Presence
qure.ai	2016	India, USA, UK
Founder/s	Investors	Patents
Prashant Warrier, Co-Founder & CEO • 19+ years in AI & deep learning, data science • Ex- Imagna, Fractal Analytics Chranjiv Singh, Chief Commercial Officer • 21+ years in healthcare & marketing • Ex – GE Healthcare, Adidas	Sequoia, MSD, fractal, HEALTH QUAD, novo holdings, etc.	Qure.ai has filed 12 patents. The three most popular patent topics are Artificial Neural Networks, Machine Learning, and Medical Imaging.
Company Overview	•Qure.ai leverages deep learning technology to provide automated interpretation of radiology examinations like X-rays, CT, and •Ultrasound scans for time and resource-strapped healthcare professionals. Enabling them to do faster analysis and provide speedy treatment.	
Product/Service Offerings	•qXR: Chest X-ray interpretation powered by AI. •qER: AI for neuro-critical care – detects abnormalities in the brain. •qCT-Lung: AI for lung nodule detection and analysis. •qVH: AI for ultrasound imaging (cardiovascular diseases). •qMSK: AI for musculoskeletal X-rays. •qTrack: Lung Health Management Platform. •qRemote: AI-enabled telehealth solution.	
tricog	2014	India, Singapore, China, Malaysia
Founder/s	Investors	Patents
Charit Bhograj, Founder & CEO • 23+ years as a Cardiologist • Ex- Vikram Hospital, Fortis Hospitals Zainul Charbiwala, Founder & CTO • 17+ years in healthcare, ML, and energy efficiency. • Ex – IBM India, Qualcomm	UTEC, Dream Incubator, SG, BLUME, Inventus Capital, Partners, etc.	Tricog Health has filed for 5 patents.
Company Overview	•With robust AI technologies, backed by human expertise, Tricog is a leader in the MedTech space solving critical Cardiovascular conditions by identifying them using AI. •The company leverages its deep medical and technology expertise to provide 'Virtual Cardiology Services' to remote clinics. •AI data store exhibits 200+ cardiac conditions, which significantly enhances the detection of cardiac disorders. •Predictive Healthcare Analytics backed by a highly experienced team.	
Product/Service Offerings	• Insta ECG: It is the flagship product of the company. It is a cloud-connected device that makes the interpretation and analysis of an ECG report quick and easy. • Insta Echo: it helps in quick and accurate echocardiogram diagnosis, and helps in reducing the treatment time and saving critical lives.	

Source: Information has been taken directly from the company website.

Apart from the above, there are some Indian companies appeared in the headlines in the recent past.

This is an attempt to make a passing reference to a few of them.

Example 1

"Over the last six years, the event has generated over 1,400 ideas and has resulted in many path-breaking solutions and automation initiatives". Sunil Singh, Senior Director, IQVIA (IQVIA, 2023).

IQVIA is a healthcare IT and clinical research company with 23,000 employees in India. The sixth edition of the company's hackathon held recently saw 150 ideas and solutions being submitted by its employees (as teams). Teams used technologies like AI, ML, natural language processing (NLP), and IoT to solve complex healthcare challenges. One of the members of the winning team says that they have developed an AI-powered virtual avatar that can do live interactions with patients and providers. This will enable healthcare to reach remote and underdeveloped areas, where trained healthcare professionals are scarce (IQVIA, 2023.

Example 2

"I have learned a lot in Silicon Valley. Empowering employees to deliver is the culture there. At KareExpert, my team feels that they are contributing to society as they are addressing a major societal need." Nidhi Jain, Founder & CEO, KareExpert (KareExpert, 2023).

KareExpert is a Reliance Jio-funded venture. The company is helping hospitals to become digital. The company's platform-centric approach has been recognized by NASSCOM, Google, and AWS. Google selected it for its accelerator program. Nidhii says the program helped a lot in understanding how to use AI, ML, UI, and UX. It has been just 18 months since KareExpert started its commercial operations and it already has over 200 hospitals as customers. These include Apollo Group, Reliance Group, and Mahindra Group's CFS (Care for Sight) (KareExpert, 2023).

Example 3

"Artificial intelligence, machine learning, virtual reality, augmented reality, and wearable technology are gradually becoming critical for healthcare (service) providers and organizations to perform (themselves) more efficiently." Dr. Rajneesh Wadhwa, Dean, SGT University (Tiwari, 2023).

According to Dr. Wadhwa, a competency-based medical curriculum must emphasize practical learning as suggested and prioritized by the National Medical Commission (NMC). Emerging technologies are now transforming medical education in the form of simulation-based medical training. In this case, AI-controlled mannequins remove the constraints that practicing on real patients has. This shift to a competency-based approach has demanded the integration of simulation-based techniques in the curriculum (Tiwari, 2023).

"Artificial intelligence is used in medical training and is transforming medical education now. This simulation-based medical training has become essential because hands-on training in the medical world has many challenges. Going ahead, we expect every college will adopt this new-age technology." Dr. Sumer Sethi, Managing Director, Delhi Academy of Medical Sciences (DAMS) (Tiwari, 2023).

4. WAY FORWARD

As stated by the Union Health Minister, Mansukh Mandaviya, India's G-20 presidency is creating a fairer global health architecture (GHA). It has three priorities (GHA, 2023). The first one is strengthening national capacities (in the healthcare sector). This is mainly to prevent, prepare for, and respond to any outbreaks. The second priority (of GHA) is reinforcing cooperation with the pharmaceutical sector. This is required to improve equitable access to quality vaccines, therapeutics, and diagnostics. The third priority is digital health innovations and solutions to provide universal health coverage. COVID experience has demonstrated how digital technologies can help in remote data capture, medical diagnostics, and virtual care. Now, India plans to draw a framework for the 'Global Initiative on Digital Health,' and harness the potential of artificial intelligence (AI) in building more resilient infrastructure.

In their study, (Sikandar et al., 2022) stated that digital technologies have great potential and can change healthcare (services delivery) and drug development. This will be accomplished by changing the way we collect, process, and visualize health data. (Sikandar et al., 2022) believe that there is a growing trend of using social media, big data analytics, and AI in the healthcare industry to improve healthcare and medical awareness. Now, AI and ML have revolutionized the way health organizations use social media. The management of an enormous volume of data generated through social media can be a daunting task for organizations. In this context, AI, and ML can help organizations in effective management of the information to improve telehealth, remote patient monitoring, and the well-being of individuals and communities.

In the healthcare industry, social media analytics pertains to the systematic approach of gathering, evaluating, and interpreting information from various social media platforms. According to Hootsuite (n. d.), these factors can assist healthcare companies in gathering important information and making defensible judgments. According to a blog post by (Hootsuite, n.d.), social media analytics can assist managers in combating disinformation, identifying patient patterns, saving time, and preserving the reputation of their company when utilized properly.

(Ohme et al., 2023) share similar opinions regarding the collection of digital trail data and its application in three areas of communication study. They are well-being, algorithmic bias, and false information. All of this has to do with answering the question of how to gather unprocessed data on social media content and use the most recent techniques for data gathering to get relevant findings and decisions.

Over the past 20 years, the integration of cutting-edge technologies has progressed Healthcare 4.0, according to a study by (Krishnamoorthy et al., 2023). As a result, the medical sector is producing services that are superior in terms of quality and delivery. The authors contend that technology such as remote health monitoring, disease prediction, and surgical help represent a substantial advancement in healthcare service delivery over in-person patient-doctor interactions. Several state-of-the-art technologies have made a substantial contribution to this integration. How can new technologies be used by healthcare systems to facilitate the creation of next-generation apps? are issues that will be taken into consideration while creating new health systems.

This may involve the use of emerging technologies such as Telehealthcare, Software-Assisted Networking, Machine Learning, Cloud Computing, the Internet of Things, Big Data Analytics, and many more. The healthcare industry will have a tonne of chances thanks to these cutting-edge technologies. (Krishnamoorthy et al., 2023) added a warning, saying that security and privacy must be established in future healthcare systems.

Artificial Intelligence (AI) is transforming the healthcare industry in India, (Jayapriyanka, 2023). According to a World Economic Forum Report, India's economy is expected to add US$ 1 trillion to its GDP by 2035. The market for artificial intelligence in healthcare is expected to grow to US$ 102 billion by the end of the decade. Experts say that artificial intelligence will improve the quality of healthcare facilities (in India), but security questions remain unanswered.

REFERENCES

Abantika, G. (2022, April 2). *How AI is changing India's healthcare — it is reading scans, predicting risks & a lot more.* The Print. https://theprint.in/health/how-ai-is-changing-indias-healthcare-its-reading-scans-predicting-risks-a-lot-more/896495/

Abid, H., Mohd, J., Pratap, S. R., & Rajiv, S. (2022). Medical 4.0 technologies for healthcare: Features, capabilities, and applications. *Internet of Things and Cyber-Physical Systems, 2*, 12-30. doi:10.1016/j.iotcps.2022.04.001

Aceto, G., Persico, V., & Pescapé, A. (2020). Industry 4.0 and health: Internet of things, big data, and cloud computing for healthcare 4.0. *Journal of Industrial Information Integration, 18*, 100129. doi:10.1016/j.jii.2020.100129

Ahsan, M. M., Ahad, M. T., Soma, F. A., Paul, S., Chowdhury, A., Luna, S. A., Yazdan, M. M. S., Rahman, A., Siddique, Z., & Huebner, P. (2021). Detecting SARS-CoV-2 From Chest X-Ray Using Artificial Intelligence. *IEEE Access : Practical Innovations, Open Solutions, 9*, 35501–35513. doi:10.1109/ACCESS.2021.3061621 PMID:34976572

Anderl, I. (2014, October 9). Industrie 4.0 – advanced engineering of smart products and smart production, technological innovations in product development. *19th International Seminar on High Technology*, 1-14.

Carvalho and Cazarini. (2020). *Industry 4.0 - What Is It?* Núbia Gabriela Pereira Carvalho and Edson Walmir Cazarini. IntechOpen., doi:10.5772/intechopen.90068

Deliana, I. (2024, Jan. 12). *AI-Powered Genomic Analysis: Revolutioning the Detection of Genetic Mutations.* News Medical. https://www.news-medical.net/health/AI-Powered-Genomic-Analysis-Revolutioning-the-Detection-of-Genetic-Mutations.aspx

Ekin, K. (2023, Nov. 24). *The Six main subsets of AI: (Machine Learning, NLP, and more).* https://www.akkio.com/post/the-five-main-subsets-of-ai-machine-learning--nlp-and-more

Emeritus. (2023, July 21). *(Some of the) Benefits of AI in Healthcare and How It Improves Patient Care.* https://emeritus.org/blog/ai-andml-benefits-of-ai-in-healthcare/

GHA. (2023, January 17). Because both rich and poor countries deserve good health…. *Times of India*, p. 12.

Hathaliya, J. J., & Tanwar, S. (2020). An exhaustive survey on security and privacy issues in Healthcare 4.0. *Computer Communications, 153*, 311–335. doi:10.1016/j.comcom.2020.02.018

Hootsuite. (n.d.). *Social Media Analytics in Healthcare: A Complete Guide*. https://blog.hootsuite.com/social-media-analytics-healthcare/amp/

Howard, R. (2023, Feb. 7). *(Some of the) Opportunities and Challenges of AI in Healthcare*. Forbes Business Council. https://www.forbes.com/sites/forbesbusinesscouncil/2023/02/07/top-five-opportunities-and-challenges-of-ai-in-healthcare/amp/

Ienca, M., & Vayena, E. (2020). On the responsible use of digital data to tackle the Covid-19 pandemic. *Nature Medicine*, *26*(4), 463–464. doi:10.1038/s41591-020-0832-5 PMID:32284619

IQVIA. (2023, January 11). IQVIA techies build AI avatar for remote healthcare. Times Techies supplement. *Times of India,* p. 15.

Jacob, O., Theo, A., Deen, F., Ram, N., & Bryan, R. (2023, February 27). Digital Trace Data (DTD) Collection for Social Media Effects Research: APIs, Data Donation, and (Screen) Tracking. *Communication Methods and Measures*, 1–18. Advance online publication. doi:10.1080/19312458.2023.2181319

Javaid, M., & Haleem, A. (2019). Industry 4.0 applications in the medical field: A brief review. *Current Medicine Research and Practice*, *9*(3), 102–109. doi:10.1016/j.cmrp.2019.04.001

Javaid, M., Haleem, A., Vaishya, R., Bahl, S., Suman, R., & Vaish, A. (2020). Industry 4.0 technologies and their applications in fighting the Covid-19 pandemic. *Diabetes & Metabolic Syndrome*, *14*(4), 419–422. doi:10.1016/j.dsx.2020.04.032 PMID:32344370

Jayaprinkya, J. (2023, June 30). Artificial Intelligence in Indian Healthcare: A promising future with challenges. *Hindu Business Line*. https://www.thehindubusinessline.com/news/science/artificial-intelligence-in-indian-healthcare-a-promising-future-with-challenges/article67015361.ece/amp/

Jha Durgesh Nandan. (2022, December 29). AI is a force multiplier in medicine, but it is not about to replace doctors. *Times of India*, p. 10.

Johnson, P. M., Lin, D. J., Zbontar, J., Zitnick, C. L., Sriram, A., Muckley, M., Babb, J. S., Kline, M., Ciavarra, G., Alaia, E., Samim, M., Walter, W. R., Calderon, L., Pock, T., Sodickson, D. K., Recht, M. P., & Knoll, F. (2023, January 17). Deep learning reconstruction enables prospectively accelerated clinical knee MRI. *Radiology*, *307*(2), e220425. Advance online publication. doi:10.1148/radiol.220425 PMID:36648347

Joseph, N. (2023, Feb. 15). *Four Ways Artificial Intelligence Can Benefit Robotic Surgery*. Forbes Technology Council. https://www.forbes.com/sites/forbestechcouncil/2023/02/15/four-ways-artificial-intelligence-can-benefit-robotic-surgery/amp/

Kagermann, H. (2015). *Change through digitization - value creation in the age of Industry 4.0. Management of Permanent Change*. Springer. doi:10.1007/978-3-658-05014-6_2

Kagermann, H., Anderl, R., Gausemeier, J., Schuh, G., & Wahlster, W. (2016). *Industrie 4.0 in a Global Context: Strategies for Cooperating with International Partners (Acatech Study).* https://www.acatech.de/wp-content/uploads/2018/03/acatech_STU_engl_KF_Industry40_Global_01.pdf

KareExpert. (2023, January 13). How Nidhi Jain is helping hospitals become digital. Times Techies supplement. *Times of India*, p. 11.

Krishnamoorthy, S., Dua, A., & Gupta, S. (2023, January). The Role of Emerging Technologies in the Future of IoT-driven Healthcare 4.0: A Survey, Current Challenges, and Future Directions. *Journal of Ambient Intelligence and Humanized Computing*, *14*(1), 361–407. doi:10.1007/s12652-021-03302-w

Nair Mohit and Sethumadhavan Arathi. (2022, October 18). *AI in healthcare: India's trillion-dollar opportunity*. World Economic Forum. https://www.weforum.org/agenda/2022/10/ai-in-healthcare-india-trillion-dollar/

News Medical. (2023, January 17). *Reconstructing MRI scans with AI promises to expand MRI access to more patients*. https://www.news-medical.net/news/20230117/Reconstructing-MRI-scans-with-AI-promises-to-expand-MRI-access-to-more-patients.aspx#:~:text=Reconstructing%20MRI%20scans%20with%20AI%2C%20which%20is%20four%20times%20faster,for%20appointments%2C%20the%20study%20says

Niramai. (2022). *Niramai announces 'Easy launch kits' for NGOs to enable Community Screening*. A blog article on their website. September 28, 2022. https://www.niramai.com/blog/

Nitesh. (2022, September 10). AI to transform the Indian Healthcare Sector. *Business World*.

Petropoulos, G. (2020). Artificial Intelligence in the Fight against. https://www.bruegel.org/2020/03/artificial-intelligence-in-the-fight-against-covid-19/

Popov, V. V., Kudryavtseva, E. V., Katiyar, N. K., Shishkin, A., Stepanov, S. I., & Goel, S. (2022). Industry 4.0 and Digitalisation in Healthcare. *Materials (Basel)*, *15*(6), 2140. Advance online publication. doi:10.3390/ma15062140 PMID:35329592

Praditporn, Aranya, Jiang, & Yi. (2023, July 31). Challenges in Adopting Artificial Intelligence to Improve Healthcare Systems and Outcomes in Thailand. *Central. Healthc Inform Res.*, 280–282. . doi:10.4258/hir.2023.29.3.280

Precedence Research. (n.d.). *Global artificial intelligence in the healthcare market is growing at ~37% CAGR from 2022 to 2030*. https://www.precedenceresearch.com

Rashmi, M. (2022, May 31). Worldwide, less than 4% of the labs have adopted digital pathology: SigTuple CEO. *The Economic Times, Health World.*

Ren, J., Zhang, A. H., & Wang, X. J. (2020). Traditional Chinese medicine for COVID-19 treatment. *Pharmacol. Res., 155*, 104743. https://www.ncbi.nlm.nih.gov/pubmed/32145402 doi:10.1016/j.phrs.2020.104743

Riffat, M., Yasir, A., Naheen, I. T., Paul, S., & Ahad, M. T. (2021). Augmented Reality for Smarter Bangladesh. *Proceedings of the 2020 IEEE Green Technologies Conference (GreenTech),* 217–222. 10.1109/GreenTech46478.2020.9289699

Ruan, Q., Yang, K., Wang, W., Jiang, L., & Song, J. (2020). Clinical predictors of mortality due to COVID-19 based on an analysis of data from 150 patients from Wuhan, China. *Intensive Care Medicine*, *2020*(46), 846–848. doi:10.1007/s00134-020-05991-x PMID:32125452

Saba and Faheem. (2023). *Types of Artificial Intelligence and Future of Artificial Intelligence in Medical Sciences. Saba Noor Us and Faheem Mohd. June 2023.* IntechOpen. doi:10.5772/intechopen.112056

Sabrina, G. (2022, July 26). *State of the art of Explainable AI in healthcare in 2022*. https://medium.com/@thinkdata/state-of-the-art-of-explainable-ai-in-healthcare-in-2022-c02225deba1

Schwab, K. (2016). *The Fourth Industrial Revolution*. Currency.

Selvaraj, S., Karan, K. A., Srivastava, S., Bhan, N., & Mukhopadhyay, I. (2022). India Health System Review. New Delhi: World Health Organization, Regional Office for South-East Asia. 2022. *Health Systems in Transition*, *11*(1).

Siddarth, T. (2023, January 6). How simulation technology will transform medical education. Times Techies supplement. *Times of India*, p. 13.

Sikandar, H., Abbas, A. F., Khan, N., & Qureshi, M. I. (2022). Digital Technologies in Healthcare: A Systematic Review and Bibliometric Analysis. *International Journal of Online and Biomedical Engineering*, *18*(8), 34–38. doi:10.3991/ijoe.v18i08.31961

Srushti, A. (2022, June 14). Creating quality and affordable healthcare for every Indian. *Times of India*, p. 14.

STPI. (2022). *Artificial Intelligence in the healthcare sector*. STPI KnowledgeUp Series.

UNF. (n.d.). *Artificial Intelligence Definitions*. Office of Faculty Excellence, University of North Florida. https://www.unf.edu/ofe/ai/definitions.html

Zhou, K., Liu, T., & Liang, L. (2016). From cyber-physical systems to industry 4.0: Make future manufacturing become possible. *International Journal of Manufacturing Research*, *11*(2), 167–188. doi:10.1504/IJMR.2016.078251

Chapter 4
Digital Healthcare Current Trends: A Critical Review Through Cloud Computing

Bhubaneswari Bisoyi
KIIT University, India

Biswajit Nayak
Sri Sri University, India

Biswajit Das
KIIT University, India

ABSTRACT

Cloud computing is an emerging and fast-growing technology in the field of healthcare industries. It provides a connected, accessible, and collaborative environment for all the stakeholders of the healthcare system. In the present time, health organizations are focusing towards increasing the quality of patient care or health information systems through digitalization. Despite several risks in implementation, compliance, availability, security, etc., cloud computing plays a major role in healthcare due to high storage capability, scalability, collaboration, and most importantly, provisioning of information when required without any delay. The performance of the healthcare system always depends on accessibility, sharing, storage, processing, and analysis of data. This chapter identifies the state of the research and identifies the established framework. This chapter addresses the different challenges and opportunities of adopting a cloud environment as well as related issues like privacy, security, and accountability.

DOI: 10.4018/979-8-3693-1934-5.ch004

1. INTRODUCTION

The cloud computing environment in the healthcare industries makes easier and safer sharing of medical records, automates the backend operations, and provides the health care data to increase the efficiency health care system. Cloud computing majorly accelerates the health care analysis, automates the data processing and scalability, reduces risk of data loss, and increases the patent data accessibility.

Cloud Computing Application mostly active in different divisions of health care system listed in the Figure 1.

Figure 1. Cloud Computing Applications in Health Care

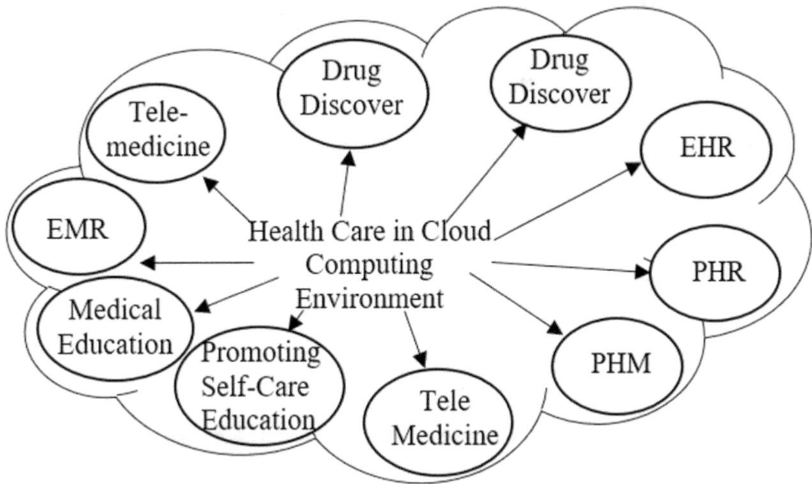

2. HEALTHCARE SYSTEM

Health care industry has always been underutilized, digitization of health care information system to access the information between department and application have always depended on notes and records. But this wastes a huge amount (in millions) in each year.

Not only the academic researchers but also the software companies heavily invested in the cloud computing environment with some new health care services and information online. The reason is to provide easy access to the information irrespective of the place where it is but there should be the availability of internet facility (Nayak et al., 2019, Nayak et al., 2018).

According to the Precedence Research organization shown in Figure 2., the global cloud market size was calculated as USD 30.5 billion in the year 2021and predicted year wise report till 2030 and estimated around 127 billion.

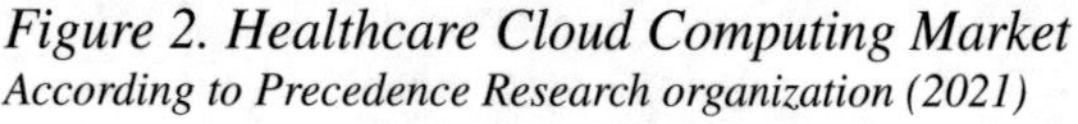

Figure 2. Healthcare Cloud Computing Market
According to Precedence Research organization (2021)

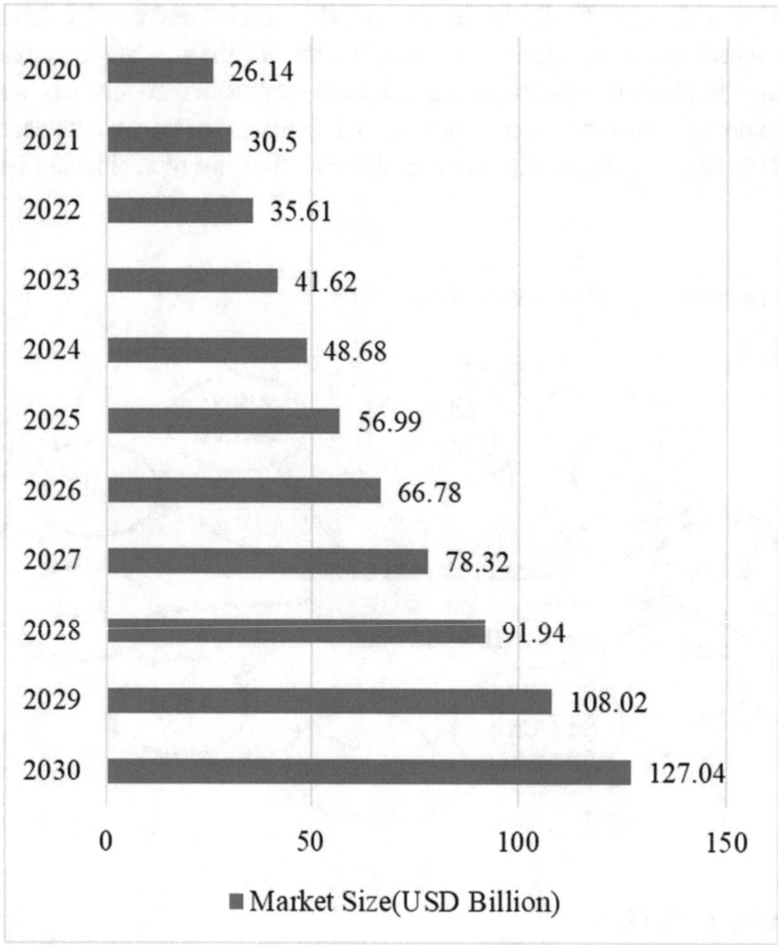

As the industry is related to health and wellbeing of the patient, the accountability for all the stakeholders is the primary objective. It is vital that the health care professionals of the organization are held accountable to their work and profession. Otherwise, the health and wellbeing of patient as well the stakeholder shall suffer drastically from life-threatening consequences. Improved performance always ensures quality management of all the resources like human, physical and technical resources. The optimum benefit to the stakeholders is always necessary and how to fit into the health care system and its requirement. Cloud computing identifies the connections or relationship between actors of the health care system and estimates the capability of supply and demand information. Improving performance is through compliance with standard and procedure. Health care system focuses on demonstrating and accounting for performance based on services and its result. These can be assessed in terms of several purposes like, controlling misuse of resources, ensuring that resources are implemented under proper standard and procedure, and supporting improved delivery of services through resource management. It is possible to reduce the misuse and overuse or underuse of resources while providing greater optimality in service.

3. CLOUD-BASED REMOTE HEALTHCARE SYSTEM

Traditional System: The traditional system introduced to overcome the problem arising due to the limited number of resources available to people. The problem mainly arises in remote places and it cannot be ignored. It is always important to reduce the information gap between people and the lack of resource. Building infrastructure with the concept of the traditional system requires a huge investment not only for the technical resources but also for the infrastructure required for those technical resources.

Figure 3. Traditional Model Used in the Healthcare System
Source: Padhy et al. (2012)

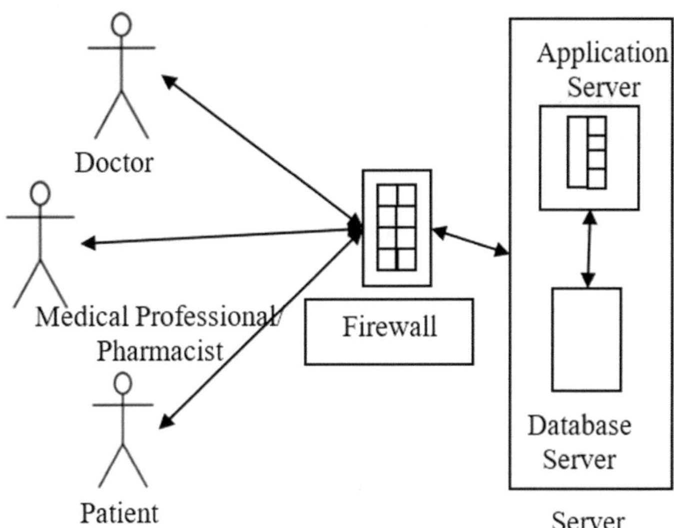

There is no limit for the type of user, it may be any one like-patient, doctor or any health professional or anyone related to patient or doctor. These users can enquire the required information as to the availability of the health care system. This increased the facility to provide information, resources and reduce the gap between people and the information so that a good health service will be produced (Chauhan and Kumar, 2013; Varshney, 2007). The relationship between users and the data or information can be stated as in diagram figure.5.1 given above. The data flow is the responsibility of health service provider, different people related to the health system, through the required technology available (Varshney, 2007; Zhang and Zhou, 2009).

System Environment: Availability of health care information in the remote health care system to a different group of people (Patient, Doctor, and Health care Professional) without delay is the major concern apart from sufficient privacy and security. Initially, the health care information providers used a controlled environment to manage the stored medical records of their patient securely with them. With the increase in technology the remote health care system allowed to increase the uninterrupted availability of information along with privacy, security, and confidentiality. The system tries to focus on the availability of health care information without any interruption at any time (Buyya et al., 2009).

The recent technology provides more flexibility and encourages building the required technology without any hesitation because it reduces not only the cost of the system and system impletion but also increases the availability of health care information system. As the volume, as well as complexity of data, increases day by day, the system must ensure the availability of data with improved service quality and also securely. The system aims to create a cloud-based remote health care system to ensure improved availability of information even-if complexity increases exponentially. Cloud computing is one such technology which provides such facility by reducing the expenditure required in build-up infrastructure, keeping the huge amount of data and providing good quality of service.

The cloud controller in cloud environment manages physical resources, allocates storage, monitor physical machine, and places virtual machine. The cloud controller changes the workload only when there is a new request. Because when there is a new request cloud controller must allocate virtual machine and physical resources. Through network controller the cloud controller identifies the host for placing virtual machine. The application and data are stored somewhere else but not inside the organization. So, availability is one of the major factors because the information must reach on demand. The cloud service provider must provide service to an authorized party.

Figure 4. Basic Architecture of Cloud-Based Remote Healthcare System
Source: Padhi et al., (2012)

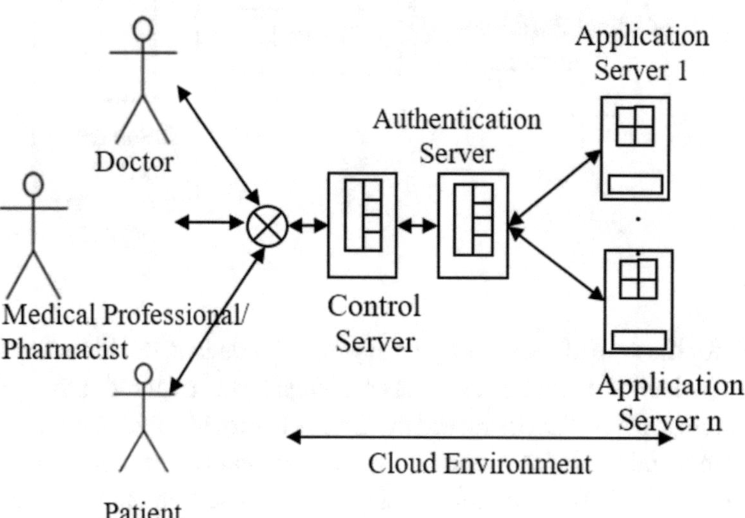

Authentication is a mechanism that checks the identity when a user interacts with the system for health care information which is available in the cloud computing environment.

Cloud computing has been considered as a knowledgeable approach that empowers the enduring information arrangement, record keeping, and gathering the changed data of medical care. The performance of the system is evaluated based on high throughput and high capacity of storing the data characterized by cloud infrastructure. The major worries in the healthcare system is the insurance and protection for the use of cloud-based medical administration. Healthcare systems ought to have digital medical records for utilizing the cloud-based framework for accessing the records, faster accesses to data, and for storing more records. Telemedicine and teleconsultation are the major utilization of the medical services by selecting the cloud advancements (Faridi et al., 2022)

4. SCOPING LITERATURE REVIEW

A large set of data were collected for the purpose of reviewing the cloud computing environment in health care system. After screening of collected data, the final set of topics was grouped and discussed on required topics. Finally, collected articles sorted in an identified and ordered (Figure 3).

Figure 5. Scoping Literature Review Flowchart

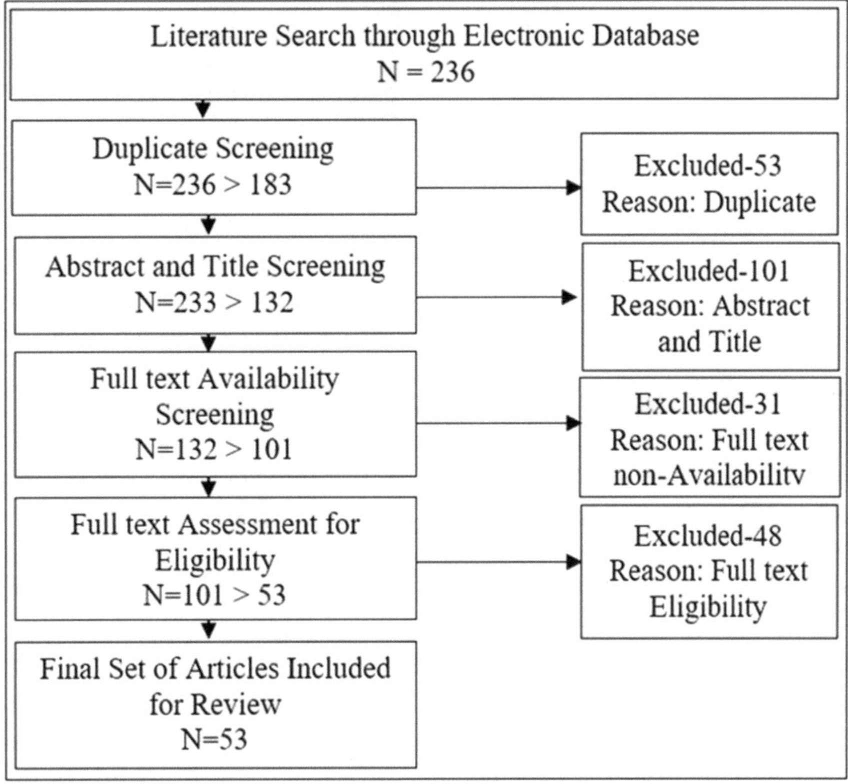

5. RESEARCH TIMELINE

The total number of publications included are taken from different years of publication based on required topic. The selected publications are from the year 2003 to 2022 (Shown in Figure 3).

Figure 6. Time Line of Research Contributions/Publications

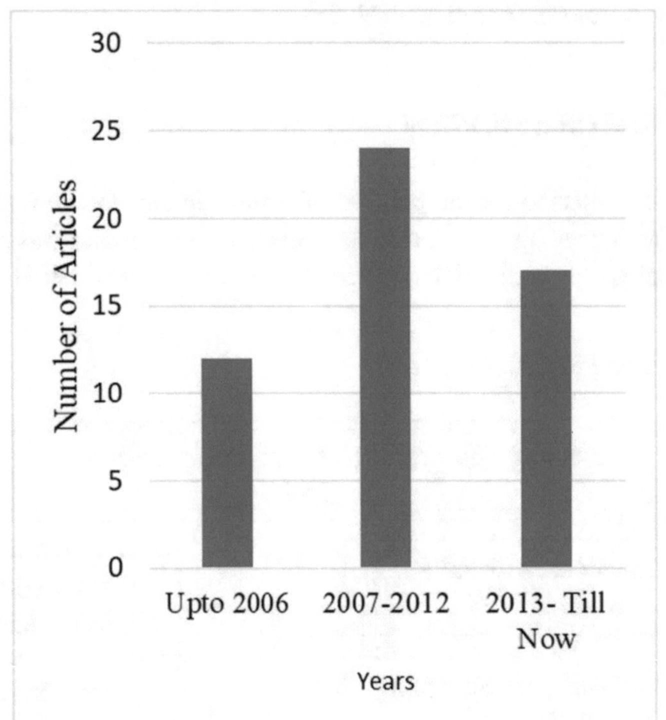

6. HEALTHCARE INFORMATION SYSTEM IN CLOUD COMPUTING

The health care information system has been defined by many but until now there is no such consent on a solitary statement illustrating it because of its vibrant nature. The phrase electronic health and health informatics are frequently applied to depicting various meaning and applications. These two terms are used alternatively as illustrated by International Tele Communication Union (ITU) (ITU, 2008). Mitchell (1999) emphasized the use of new term much needed for depicting implementation of both the technologies (electronic communication and information technology) in the sector of health. The relevance of information technology in depicted by retrieving the electronically stored data and transmitting it for use in the health sector focusing on the area of education, clinical purpose and in administrative work.

Edworthy et al. (2001) illustrated about the definition of e-Health stated by World Health Organization as an implementation of ICT in support of health sector that consists of health care services, surveillance, education, knowledge transmission, and research. WHO with the use of e-Health and health informatics has raised its potentiality by improvising the area of health service, research, and literature in health, and scaling up in delivering the best treatment to thousands of patients in developing countries. Wilson and Lankton (2004) focused the research on information technology (IT) projects that failed even after an investment of a substantial amount of money. The prime reason behind the failure of these services was because of the information system developed that did not respond to the need of their users. WHO (2005) insisted the members to plan out a long term strategy for framing a long term relation with the members and other stack holders and develop infrastructure and center for providing facility to practice electronic health care information system and also national public health information system. Infrastructure established for information and communication technologies.

Gottlied et al. (2005) focused on handling the personal information of the consumers by the law firms and hospitals. The organization that has personal information about their consumers need to be guarded about data security and privacy of the customers. The preference of using online application and storage of data has become frequently used by today's clients. The role of the cloud has started to play a major role in the medical sector by providing easy access to the medical history of the clients for their treatment.

E-Health Resolution (2005) has described it as the most lucrative and safe utilization of concept like ICT in the field of health care system. It may consist of services related to health-care, monitoring, literature, education, and research in health.

Secretariat (2005) describes the increase is the use of e-health services has raised concern on data privacy, security, and discretion of records. Whenever there is an exchange of information, it requires privacy and security of information within the health care information system. The rapid utilization of e-Health needs to be monitored by legal and ethical issues that arise in daily transactions.

National strategy for e-Health (2006) suggested that prior to the implementation of ICT in the area of electronic health care services, it must satisfy certain criteria from National Strategy: (i) In accordance to the development of ICT it is required to be maintained as per legislation and other regulation for full protection of personal information. (ii) The national information structure needs to be created for providing the depth of information and technical structure. (iii) The ICT should be supportive and accessible easily and data transmission should be facilitated across the organization boundaries. (iv) The infrastructure for national technical health care should be a build-up in a view that ECS system will provide a secure linkage between different care units and will be capable of supporting e-Health.

Haux (2006) elaborated on the technology named Electronic medical record (EMR) used as a health care technology. Electronic medical record is a system that stores the details of patients with complete interoperability through the endeavour. The patients' health record stores all the information and services and EMR facilitates in providing a secure and more integrated interface connecting departments. The different functionality of EMR is mentioned as follow: (i) Management system for patients is intended for monitoring bed management, patients record while hospitalization, and for scheduling appointments with doctors. (ii) The prescribed medicines are managed by the pharmacy management system and it advises the possible side effect of medicine prescribed. (iii)The medical test is carried out based on the laboratory request and the reports are stored in the electronic health record. This whole process is maintained by the laboratory management system. (iv) The request made for radiology is maintained by the radiology management system and the report is stored as a record. (v) The cost account of the patient is finalized by issuing the bill and this is handled by the billing and insurance system. (vi) The schedule for the physician and clinical team is managed by the staff management system.

Lee et al. (2007) focused on their article about the advantages of e-Health through e-commerce to medical technology like telemedicine. With the implementation of e-health medical services are being supplied among doctor, nurse, patients, and clinical administrations. E-commerce acts as a blessing to the health sector, patients by making the medical service available in a cost-effective way and saving the time.

Mukherjee and McGinnis (2007) proposed key themes and describe the state of art in the area of e-healthcare. The authors proposed five important themes like electronic records, reduced cost, virtual network, privacy, and credibility of the source. They found the proposed e-healthcare system can maximize the efficiency with minimal cost. But still, the e-healthcare system need access for better patient information system so that patient satisfaction can be increased and a patient outcome.

Majid (2008) illustrated about telemedicine through this technology a physician can offer health care services through a distance by means of advanced electronic communication. The treatment by physician involves a remote examination, automatically providing the results of the examination and reports, executing the operation, and other medical applications. The author in his article mentioned about a multipurpose smart card that stores the health record of the patients. This card is an integrated circuit that stores, recover, and transmit the data. Several countries have been using this multipurpose smart card for accumulating the data collected from the patient's health records. The author illustrated a picture archiving and communication system that examines the digital images better than a physician does through the computer network. The advantage of using this system is that it provides a clear image as compared with the radiological films. The digital system stores the image and reduces the risk of losing the image and also the cost of taking the image the second time. The two main goals for EHR are first is to connect health organizations with data of the patients and the second goal is, to begin with, appropriate communication between patients, doctors, health care providers, and planners.

Jean et al. (2008) emphasized the concept that e-health solutions need coordination within various players who belong to a different culture, intentions, and institutions (UN agencies, educational organizations, research organizations, local health proficient and their relations, customers, benefactors, Institutes may be government or non-government, private sector, media). The cluster of team members whose function, accountability and constrictions will engage in recreation of a field in the area of e-Health so it has to be appreciated, assembled and organized.

Slamanig and Stingl (2008) proposed a concept to prevent disclosure attack and statistical analysis. The authors implemented the concept of pseudonymization to break the link, identity management and obfuscation to prevent an attack. Along with this, privacy can also be maintained with the help of certain other relevant techniques. The authors ensure less effort and elimination of attack.

Hayrinen et al. (2008) focused on defining electronic health record, structure, the context in which it will be used, how to provide access, a different component associated with this system and the purpose. The researchers analyzed a wide range of information system and mainly focused on the content of electronic health care required. They also focused on the documentation of different health care professional with core information for the future scope of research in the field of the electronic health care system.

Maria (2009) pointed out that the definition of cloud computing has been evolving by scholars based on the requirement and efficacy of their dealing. The services offered through cloud computing are delivered just-in-time and it is dynamic in nature. With an increase in the level of productivity, cloud computing is determined to condense the realization, continuance expenditure, and complication.

Peter and Tim (2009) illustrated in their research article about the fact that cloud computing environment that is facilitating network which enables users to access a shared pool of configurable resources like: networks, servers, applications, storage and services. The resources need to be speedily provisioned and unrestricted with nominal management endeavour or cloud service provider interaction.

Nelson (2009) emphasized about defining the technicality, legal, economic and security perspective that remains to be unclear till date. Even though the cloud has made things in such a way that patient could locate and formulate a track record those are related to medical history. The major question raised by the society is about the security, privacy and guarantee with respect to the health information; whereas people of other country have a difference in their opinion about the implication of cloud handling the private information about clients in the medical sector.

Osterhaus (2010) focused on the fact that IT vendors must gain the trust of the population who share their data of medical history by following the standards regulated by HIPPA. In addition to providing security of the data, the structure of the cloud should be designed in such a way that, it will be simple and easy way for user or patient to monitor their medical record.

Guo (2010) mainly intended in their research paper on building up a new smart management structure supported by cloud computing. The paper focused on illustrating the defects in the traditional structure followed in the hospital management system. The research concluded with the fact that the efficiency of cloud computing can be improved by formulating a strong information technology that optimally stored and retrieves the records of the patients.

Ashish (2010) proposed is his research that cloud computing model acts as a better service framework when compared with the traditional computing method thereby reducing the cost. The cloud model will not only provide a big platform for the growth of information technology but ultimately transforms the health care sectors. This transformation will gradually happen. But cloud computing is one of the best options that bring out radical changes in the elevation of service standards provided to citizens in developing countries.

Lohr et al. (2010) conferred in relation to broad-spectrum of setbacks faced by the present e-health system and endow with a technical elucidation for the security of susceptible data and employability in the e-health cloud system. Mostly author focused on shortcomings of current e-health solution and standard or in other word the overall security of e-health care system management. The author showed the way privacy domain can be used to extend the protection of e-health care system and planning to integrate e-health care card system.

Rubin (2010) has discussed six risk factors that need to be addressed seriously for the deployment of IT in the cloud without the intervention of other regulations like government. The first risk factor has been defined as: Regulatory Risk, IP Risk, Enforcement Risk, Performance Risk, Business Continuity Risk and Liability Risk. Regulatory Risk: It consists of data encryption and averting data access, sustaining the data security and confidentiality of the data. It also needs to obey the rules and the requirement fixed by the Health Insurance Portability and Accountability Acts (HIPAA). Each step is supposed to be pursued by HIPAA. IP Risk: Intellectual property risk is the threat of illicit utilization and misuse. The software developed by the IT vendors involved in health sector wanted the possession of the software. It is natural and lawfully right to expand their area of operation by the IT developer but the customer, on the other hand, develop an intention to own the right of the contents that makes its way through the application of the software which creates a controversial situation. The controversy can be resolved by providing cross-licensing and each party is given the control that it owns or its development. Enforcement Risk: Enforcement risk is essential on the part of the vendor to retain harmonization between right and dispute resolution system with termination right. The vendor needs to obey the rights lawfully and create harmony in the system. Performance Risk: The customer needs to be assured that the service provided to them shall be abiding by all pertinent laws and regulation, fault-free operation and materials used during the execution of the system. Likewise, we need to look at other facets where the third-party intellectual property right is not violated. The customer desires to guard their data in opposition to concealed defects. Business Continuity Risk: This issue is basically overlooked by the service provider which emphasizes on customers' point of view. The customer has the right to cancel the agreement prior to the scheduled date mentioned, owing to fear of key disruptions. Correspondingly, the customer can continue with the business-relation with very minimal problem. Liability Risk: Liability risk is aa agreement that ensure zero-violation in the said condition, if such thing will persist then the client will receive the required acquiescence as per law. Simultaneously, in case of the user, no rule shall be broken as per the agreement. The liability risk can be reduced when both the user and the vendor will simultaneously maintain the rule and regulation as per the agreement.

Black et al. (2011) reviewed the e-health to identify accessibility, effectiveness, quality, and safety. The authors developed several strategies, then scrutinized synthesized to find the optimum outcome. Besides the several strategies used, they emphasized to improve quality and safety. The authors also stated that the implementation of technology, quality, safety, and cost-effectiveness needs to be focused further.

Prasad et al. (2011) anticipated intense resemblance connecting standard government execution and the approach of the cloud should be service-oriented. The authors emphasized the issues like implementation, usability, and infrastructure relating to the realization of grid-based e-governance.

Moghaddasi et al. (2011) proposed several factors that influence to improve the service delivery to the peoples. The researchers found three major factors that play a major role in service delivery are economic capacity, strong information, and communication technology. The implementation of e-Health depends upon these factors mostly.

Hsieh and Hsu (2012) focused on challenges to deliver accurate reports for decision making support in emergency telecardiology. Author created a cloud computing and pervasive computing-based electro cardiology service to realize ubiquitous tele diagnosis. And they found the tele-consultation can take-place while the patient is at ambulance and they also found the service is convenient, efficient, and in-expensive. This was also tested, evaluated, and proved by cardiologists.

Meier et al. (2013) reviewed the business model of health care delivery and evaluated past, present, and future to find its potential and impact. In their review, the authors described that e-Health solved it several problems. The problem consisted of capability, expenditure in the developed world, efficiency and optimum result or outcome.

Currie and Seddon (2013) focused on challenges arises for different stack holder like IT industries, health care system and policy makers due to the cross-border exchange of information. They found that, in case of traditional sourcing relationships, the cloud environment providers are act as conduits whereas health data are being superseded by more significant demand to become business associates with shared responsibility and accountability to ensure security and protection of data. Apart from the data protection policies the author found application and interpretation also depends on social norms, culture and values.

Kaur and Chana (2014). advocated the use of the concept of cloud computing for providing efficient and effective cloud health care services. They designed a system "Cloud Based Intelligent Health Care Service" to perform real time monitoring of health care data for diagnosis of several chronic diseases. Author gathered the data through advanced body sensor components and stored in cloud repositories for further analysis and classifications. Most importantly they performed the analysis and found classification accuracy of about 92.59 percentage.

Christoph et al. (2015) focused on providing flexible and scalable infrastructure for providing protection and security to the secondary uses of health care data because it provides large opportunities for health care data and translational results. Authors proposed an architectural design and is evaluated by the data from hundreds of patients from different hospitals and found suitable.

Godinho et al. (2016) discussed services related to the storage, distribution, and visualization of medical data. They found difficulty in establishing communications between multiple geo-distributed locations due to the requirement of managing huge amount of data and bandwidth. They developed a smart routing mechanism to improve the performance of distributed networks. This is a cache system based on splitting and dynamic management of digital imaging and communications. They found the proposed method was better than the conventional approach.

Lian (2017) focused on certain quality related factors that affect cloud computing success of cloud health care because private cloud computing is the major research area. Author advocates the integration of trust in information system model which will have acceptable explanatory power to understand the success of cloud in health care system. Information quality and system quality directly affect cloud computing satisfaction whereas service quality indirectly affects the satisfaction through trust. So, in other way trust act as a mediator between service quality and the satisfaction. The author proposed a model and found 85.7 percentage of respondent have collaborated with third party partners to implement concept of cloud computing in hospital. It is found that the proposed model will help hospitals evaluate success after adapting private cloud health care services and achieve the required value creation purpose.

Ali et al. (2018) presented on different issues, expected opportunities, and also related applications. It also focused on value-added health care towards decision making, privacy, data security and service delivery. Authors found sufficient evidence that the concept of cloud computing bringing significant opportunities to the health care sector irrespective of issues like security and privacy of health care data and loss of control of managing data.

Agarkhed, et. al. (2019) discussed on services by bringing the plenteous resources of health care data in the cloud computing environment to the nearness of portable devices to authorize the performance of the application and preserve the battery life. During the study the author stated that the adoption of the cloud technology in the health care management system for the smart city not only improves the health care services but also provides better public life. In addition to this the author also stated the advantage of concept of mobile cloud computing as the combination of mobile computing and cloud computing which will be beneficial for reduction of energy consumption.

Darwish et al. (2019) presented the breach analysis for different level of integration of required components for the development of Cloud-IoT health care system. Mostly researcher focused on cloud computing environment and integration of IoT components for the development of new health care system. The author also stated the the combination of the concept of cloud computing technology and Internet of Things will provide a storage, scalability, processing, and network capabilities.

Shakil et al. (2020) focused on the problem raised due to ever growing data of health care system because the increase in data will increase the in-security for which author planned to provide security to different users by a cloud based biometric authentication system. After testing of system author found that the proposed system achieved a speedup of 9x which is much better than other systems in recent scenarios. Author also incorporated priority based with existing model and found result in processing of critical records for more secured system.

Kim et al. (2020) stated even if we have automated electronic health record system, it can be used to keep their own record but it cannot be shared on the different health care platform. So, this can be solved by keeping electronic health record in the cloud computing environment. Along with this the storage availability and scalability are two major advantages but at the same time data vulnerability also increases. Author proposed a secure protocol for cloud based electronic health record system using blockchain. It provides data integrity and access control using log transactions and storage, and manages patient electronic health record for the provisioning of secure storage resources. Author found electronic health record system providing secure mutual authentication.

Mehrtak et al. (2021) focused on different issues like encryption, authentication, and classification along with application programming interface (API), with security solution to available cloud infrastructure. Author aimed to focus to provide secure communication even though several challenges.

Javaid et al. (2022) stated different service provider of health care information system. Author described required hardware components, network connections for diverse health care applications. Author also discussed the different applications and stated the way the resources availability and efficiency can be improved.

Pawer (2022) analyzed and concluded that the cloud computing environment can be used to improve the data management procedures in the health care industries. Author also stated that it can aid storage and management of data while also making easily accessible to the organization.

7. POST IMPLEMENTATION

With the implementation of IT in the sector, e-Health has been observed as an added advantage for the physicians. In a survey carried out by the U.S primary care physicians, it was found that 75% of them found that the application of IT has resulted in downsizing the error. Productivity has been observed to have escalated by 70%, over 60% of the population observed that the tools used in IT ensures the huge reduction in cost and facilitate stakeholders by feeling more responsible towards it (Anderson & Balas, 2006).

Electronic-Health information system plays a major role in the sector of health care. Electronic Health Records can be considered as one of the examples. Prior to the application of electronic health records, we used to record the data of patients by the paper-based system. The use of the paper-based system has several errors in the process of entering the details of a patient's personal data, medical records. Whereas, EHRs, stores the data in a very simpler and proficient technique of storing data (Hayrinen, 2008). Grogan acknowledged that there is a fact to sentence that EHRs offer a better and simple method for store the data of patients and it is also error-free (Grogan, 2006). Mullner stated electronic health system that "paper records contain too many errors and inefficiencies, and they hinder the communication between health care providers" (Mullner, 2006).

With reference to the above statement, the researcher found another added advantage that is communication facility. Data from everywhere gathered and stored in one place and physicians have the right to access the data such as health records from the electronic records. In case the patients are shifted from one hospital to a new hospital then these data stored in the electronic health records can be easily transmitted within no time. The e-Health has become a tool for improvising and medium for rapid distribution of health records. The transmission of information may impact to minimize the management of cost for chronic diseases, treatment cost and wellness program costs. With the application of e-Health, there are advantages to doctors, patients, organization, and auxiliary sections (Majid, 2008). Benefits to physicians: The ordering process is totally under the control of physician and this makes it risk-free for the patients. The order placed by the physician is free from the elucidation of hand wrote orders. It is also responsible for reducing the time consumed for reading and locating the patient's health chart by the physician. Benefits for patients: The most benefited section of e-Health. The interdisciplinary communication is improvised by e-health as it avoids error-free prescription that was caused due to handwritten orders e-health plays an imperative function in the safety of the medication. Benefits to subsidiary divisions: The time division between clinical care and order placed by the physician is managed more efficiently with the implementation of e-Health. The ancillary departments such as pharmacists and nurses spend less time in orders placed by the physicians. This results in providing more time free time from the administrative task and diverts that time for providing more value-added service. Benefits to management: The flow of information is done instantaneously within an organization and delivery time for medication is reduced. E-Health facilitates in providing a standardized health care service. On the nationalized level, anyone can coalesce the information related to health care from diverse health associations and recommend protected outcomes for patient.

8. CONCLUSION

During the review, it is observed that application of cloud computing environment in the health care system is disused heavily. It is found that security and privacy are still the major concern for researchers. Most of the work done on the electronic health record was based on different issues like legal, technical, security, privacy, economic and some of the work done on different diseases. Some of the work also done on resource management. Cloud computing need to improve accessibility of health data, ensure efficient management and usage of medical resources, facilitate among health care organizations, and ensure new possibilities attributes like transparency, accessibility, responsibility, remediation, liability, observability, verifiability as non-functional attribute.

REFERENCES

Agarkhed, J., Ashalatha, R., & Patil, S. R. (2019). Smart Healthcare Systems Using Cloud Computing Environments. In R. Bera, S. Sarkar, O. Singh, & H. Saikia (Eds.), *Advances in Communication, Devices and Networking. Lecture Notes in Electrical Engineering* (Vol. 537). Springer. doi:10.1007/978-981-13-3450-4_59

Ali, O., Shrestha, A., Soar, J., & Wamba, S. F. (2018). Cloud computing-enabled healthcare opportunities, issues, and applications: A systematic review. *International Journal of Information Management*, *43*, 146–158. doi:10.1016/j.ijinfomgt.2018.07.009

Anderson, J. G., & Balas, E. A. (2006). Computerization of primary care in the United States. *International Journal of Healthcare Information Systems and Informatics*, *1*(3), 1–23. doi:10.4018/jhisi.2006070101

Ashish, R. (2010). A Model Based Approach to Implement Cloud Computing in E-Governance. *International Journal of Computer Application, 9*(7).

Black, A. D., Car, J., Pagliari, C., Anandan, C., Cresswell, K., Bokun, T., & Sheikh, A. (2011). The Impact of eHealth on the Quality and Safety of Health Care: A Systematic Overview. *PLoS Medicine*, *8*(1), e1000387. Advance online publication. doi:10.1371/journal.pmed.1000387 PMID:21267058

Buyya, R., Yeo, C. S., Venugopal, S., Broberg, J., & Brandic, I. (2009). Cloud computing and emerging IT platforms: Vision, hype, and reality for delivering computing as the 5th utility. *Future Generation Computer Systems*, *25*(6), 599–616. doi:10.1016/j.future.2008.12.001

Chauhan, R., & Kumar, A. (2013). Cloud Computing for Improved Healthcare: Techniques, Potential, and Challenges. *4th IEEE International Conference on E-Health and Bioengineering*, 1-4. 10.1109/EHB.2013.6707234

Christoph, J., Griebel, L., Leb, I., Engel, I., Kopcke, F., Toddenroth, D., Prokosch, H.-U., Laufer, J., Marquardt, K., & Sedlmayr, M. (2015). Secure secondary use of clinical data with cloud-based NLP services: Towards a highly scalable research infrastructure. *Methods of Information in Medicine*, *53*(6), 276–282. doi:10.3414/ME13-01-0133 PMID:25377309

Currie, W., & Seddon, J. (2013). A cross-country study of cloud computing policy and regulation in healthcare. *The European Conference on Information Systems*, 1–16. 10.1016/j.hlpt.2013.09.003

Darwish, A., Hassanien, A. E., Elhoseny, M., Sangaiah, A. K., & Muhammad, K. (2019). The impact of the hybrid platform of internet of things and cloud computing on healthcare systems: Opportunities, challenges, and open problems. *Journal of Ambient Intelligence and Humanized Computing*, *10*(10), 4151–4166. doi:10.1007/s12652-017-0659-1

E-health resolution. (2005). World Health Organization. Retrieved from http://www.who.int/ healthacademy/ media/en/eHealth_EB_Res-en.pdf

Edworthy, S. M. (2001). Telemedicine in developing countries. *British Medical Journal*, *323*(7312), 524–525. doi:10.1136/bmj.323.7312.524 PMID:11546681

Faridi, F., Sarwar, H., Ahtisham, M., Kumar, S., & Jamal, K. (2022). Cloud computing approaches in health care. *Materials Today: Proceedings*, *51*, 1217–1223. doi:10.1016/j.matpr.2021.07.210

Godinho, T. M., Viana-Ferreira, C., Silva, L. B., & Costa, C. (2016). A routing mechanism for cloud outsourcing of medical imaging repositories. *IEEE Journal of Biomedical and Health Informatics*, *20*(1), 367–375. doi:10.1109/JBHI.2014.2361633 PMID:25343773

Gottlieb, L. K., Stone, E. M., Stone, D., Dunbrack, L. A., & Calladine, J. (2005). Regulatory and Policy Barriers to Effective Clinical Data Exchange: Lessons Learned from Meds Info-ED. *Health Affairs*, *24*(5), 1197–1204. doi:10.1377/hlthaff.24.5.1197 PMID:16162563

Grogan, J. (2006). EHRs and information availability: Are you at risk? *Health Management Technology*, *27*(5), 8–16. PMID:16739432

Guo, L., Chen, F., Chen, L., & Tang, X. (2010). The building of cloud computing environment for e-health. *2010 International Conference on E-Health Networking Digital Ecosystems and Technologies (EDT)*. 10.1109/EDT.2010.5496512

Haux, R. (2006). Health information systems – past, present, future. *International Journal of Medical Informatics*, *75*(3-4), 268–281. doi:10.1016/j.ijmedinf.2005.08.002 PMID:16169771

Hayrinen, K., Saranto, K., & Nykanen, P. (2008). Definition, structure, content, use and impacts of electronic health records: A review of the research literature. *International Journal of Medical Informatics*, *77*(5), 291–304. doi:10.1016/j.ijmedinf.2007.09.001 PMID:17951106

Hsieh, J. C., & Hsu, M. W. (2012). A cloud computing based 12-lead ECG telemedicine service. *BMC Medical Informatics and Decision Making*, *12*(77), 1–12. doi:10.1186/1472-6947-12-77 PMID:22838382

ITU. (2008). *International Telecommunication Union Radio Communication Sector*. ITU-R.

Javaid, M., Haleem, A., Singh, R. P., Rab, S., Suman, R., & Khan, I. H. (2022). Evolutionary trends in progressive cloud computing-based healthcare: Ideas, enablers, and barriers. *International Journal of Cognitive Computing in Engineering*, *3*, 124–135. doi:10.1016/j.ijcce.2022.06.001

Jean, C. H. (2008). *Implementing e-Health in developing countries, guidance, and principles*. Retrieved from www.itu.int/ITU-D/cyb/

Kaur, P. D., & Chana, I. (2014). Cloud based intelligent system for delivering health care as a service. *Computer Methods and Programs in Biomedicine, 113*(1), 346-359. doi:10.1016/j.cmpb.2013.09.013

Kim, M., Yu, S., Lee, J., Park, Y., & Park, Y. (2020, May 21). Design of Secure Protocol for Cloud-Assisted Electronic Health Record System Using Blockchain. *Sensors (Basel)*, *20*(10), 2913. doi:10.3390/s20102913 PMID:32455635

Lee, B. W., Min, S. D., Jeong, W., Choo, Y., & Lee, M. (2007). Construction of APEC e-Health Portal Site for e-Health Service Providers and Demanders in APEC area. *2007 9th International Conference on e-Health Networking, Application and Services*. 10.1109/HEALTH.2007.381657

Lian, J. W. (2017). Establishing a cloud computing success model for hospitals in Taiwan. *Inquiry*, *54*(1/6), 1–6. doi:10.1177/0046958016685836 PMID:28112020

Lohr, H., Sadeghi, A. R., & Winandy, M. (2010). Securing the e-health cloud. *Proceedings of the ACM International Conference on Health Informatics - IHI '10*, 220–229. 10.1145/1882992.1883024

Majid, M. A. (2008). *Electronic-health in Saudi Arabia- just around the corner?* College of Public Health and Health Informatics, King Saud bin Abdul-Aziz University for Health Sciences.

Maria, S. (2009). *An Essential Guide to Possibilities and Risks of Cloud Computing*. Whitepaper. Retrieved from http://www.mariaspinola.com/whitepapers/An Essential Guide to Possibilities and Risks of Cloud Computing a Pragmatic Effective and Hype Free Approach for Strategic Enterprise Decision Making.pdf

Mehrtak, M., SeyedAlinaghi, S. A., MohsseniPour, M., Noori, T., Karimi, A., Shamsabadi, A., Heydari, M., Barzegary, A., Mirzapour, P., Soleymanzadeh, M., Vahedi, F., Mehraeen, E., & Dadras, O. (2021). Security challenges and solutions using healthcare cloud computing. *Journal of Medicine and Life*, *14*(4), 448–461. doi:10.25122/jml-2021-0100 PMID:34621367

Meier, C. A., Fitzgerald, M. C., & Smith, J. M. (2013). E-Health: Extending, Enhancing, and Evolving Health Care. *Annual Review of Biomedical Engineering*, *15*(1), 359–382. doi:10.1146/annurev-bioeng-071812-152350 PMID:23683088

Mitchell, J. (1999). *From telehealth to e-health: the unstoppable rise of e-health: Commonwealth Department of Communications*. Information Technology, and the Arts.

Moghaddasi, H., Asadi, F., Hosseini, A., & Ebnehoseini, Z. (2011). E-Health: A Global Approach with Extensive Semantic Variation. *Journal of Medical Systems*, *36*(5), 3173–3176. doi:10.1007/s10916-011-9805-z PMID:22113437

Mukherjee, A., & McGinnis, J. (2007). E-healthcare: An analysis of key themes in research. *International Journal of Pharmaceutical and Healthcare Marketing*, *1*(4), 349–363. doi:10.1108/17506120710840170

Mullner, R. M., & Chung, K. (2006). Current issues in health care informatics. *Journal of Medical Systems, 30*(1), 1–2. doi:10.1007/s10916-006-7390-3 PMID:16548407

National Strategy for e-Health. (2006). Retrieved from www.sweden.gov.se/health

Nayak, B., Padhi, S. K., & Pattnaik, P. K. (2017) Impact of Cloud Accountability on Clinical Architecture and Acceptance of Healthcare System. *6th International Conference on Frontiers of Intelligent Computing: Theory and applications, 701*, 149-157. 10.1007/978-981-10-7563-6_16

Nayak, B., Padhi, S. K., & Pattnaik, P. K. (2019). Cloud-based remote healthcare system environment. *Jour of Adv Research in Dynamical & Control Systems, 11*(5), 1772-1780. https://www.jardcs.org/abstract.php?id=1662

Nelson, M. R. (2009). The cloud, the crowd, and public policy. *Issues in Science and Technology, 25*(4), 71–76.

Osterhaus, L. (2010). Cloud Computing and Health Information. *U of I SLIS Journal*. Retrieved from http://ir.uiowa.edu/bsides/19

Padhy, R. P., Patra, M. R., & Satapathy, S. C. (2012). Design and Implementation of a Cloud based Rural Healthcare Information System Model. *UNIASCIT, 2*(1), 149–157.

Pawer, P. (2022). Implementation Of Cloud Computing in Healthcare. *International Research Journal of Modernization in Engineering Technology and Science, 4*(5). https://www.irjmets.com/uploadedfiles/paper//issue_5_may_2022/24414/final/fin_irjmets1653635314.pdf

Peter, M., & Tim, G. (2009). *The NIST definition of Cloud Computing, Version 15*. Information Technology Laboratory. Retrieved from http://www.hexistor.com/blog/bid/36511/The NIST Definition of Cloud Computing.

Prasad, A., Chaurasia, S., Singh, A., & Gour, D. (2011). Mapping Cloud Computing onto useful E-Governance. *International Journal of Computer Science and Information Security, 8*(5).

Report by secretariat. (2005). *Health – propose tools and services, Executive board, 117th Session 1, Provisional agenda item 4.13*. Retrieved from https://www.who.int/gb/e/e_eb117.html

Rubin, H. (2010). Risk and reward: Health IT SAAS licensing models. *Licensing Journal, 30*(1), 13–15.

Shakil, K. A., Zareen, F. J., Alam, M., & Jabin, S. (2020). BAMHealthCloud: A biometric authentication and data management system for healthcare data in cloud. *Journal of King Saud University. Computer and Information Sciences, 32*(1), 57–64. doi:10.1016/j.jksuci.2017.07.001

Slamanig, D., & Stingl, C. (2008). Privacy Aspects of eHealth. *2008 Third International Conference on Availability, Reliability and Security*.10.1109/ARES.2008.115

Varshney, U. (2007). Pervasive Healthcare and Wireless Health Monitoring. *Mobile Networks and Applications, 12*(2-3), 113–127. doi:10.1007/s11036-007-0017-1

Wilson, E. V., & Lankton, N. K. (2004). Modelling Patients' Acceptance of Provider-delivered E-health. *Journal of the American Medical Informatics Association : JAMIA, 11*(4), 241–248. doi:10.1197/jamia.M1475 PMID:15064290

World Health Organization. (2005). *58th World Health Assembly Report*. WHO.

Zhang, L. J., & Zhou, Q. (2009). CCOA: *Cloud Computing Open Architecture. IEEE International Conference on Web Services.* 10.1109/ICWS.2009.144

Chapter 5
Factors Affecting Digital Healthcare Innovation in India:
A Case Study of Delhi NCR

Pooja Mehra
https://orcid.org/0000-0002-5051-5497
Amity University, Noida, India

Vanshika Verma
Amity University, Noida, India

ABSTRACT

India, recognizing the profound impact of digitization, launched the Digital India campaign in 2015. This study explores the impact of psychological, socio-economic, and demographic factors on awareness and adoption of the available government schemes for digital healthcare. Primary data is collected from both urban and rural areas of Delhi NCR. SPSS is used for structural equation modelling, and it was found that awareness was lacking in rural and marginalised areas which was the reason for the lack of adoption of digital healthcare schemes in rural areas. In urban areas, perception (negative) and level of income play a major role in the lack of awareness and adoption of digital healthcare schemes. To augment awareness and adoption initiatives like mandating digital literacy programmes at the school level, increasing awareness through social media platforms, and tailoring localized and customized awareness campaigns are recommended so that more people can avail the benefits offered by digital healthcare schemes as compared to the traditional healthcare system.

DOI: 10.4018/979-8-3693-1934-5.ch005

1 INTRODUCTION

1.1 Background

Universal Health Coverage (UHC) is a pivotal element of the Sustainable Development Goals), particularly included in SDG3 (Kieny & Bekedam, n.d.). UHC entails ensuring that individuals have access to essential, quality health services without facing financial problems. The UN commitment to 'Leaving No One Behind' is important to UHC, as the term "universal" implies that everyone, regardless of social or economic status, must have the right to health protection (World Health Organization, n.d.).

Countries are actively improving their health financing systems to shift from direct payments to prepayment and pooling mechanisms. This transformation is deemed crucial for guaranteed access to services (Myint & Pavlova, n.d.). Notably, numerous emerging economies are actively working to enhance social health protection by implementing publicly funded health insurance (PFHI) schemes (Lagomarsino & Garabrant, n.d.).

As time has progressed, the internet has brought about revolutionary changes in communication, business, education, and governmental operations. A particularly noteworthy influence is observed in the healthcare domain. Historically, healthcare primarily emphasized improving and maintaining health with the specialized skills of professionals involved in diagnosis, treatment, and prevention. Nevertheless, the incorporation of digital technologies has transformed healthcare delivery, tailoring it to individual needs and streamlining processes, thereby diminishing the dependence on direct engagement with healthcare professionals. (Brenner, 2023)

Digital technologies present tangible opportunities to address challenges within health systems, offering the potential to improve the scope and quality of health practices and services. For instance, digital health interventions can be utilized to facilitate targeted communication to individuals, creating demand and broadening contact coverage. Similarly, these interventions can be directed at health workers, providing them with quick access to decision-support mechanisms or telemedicine consultations.

According to the World Health Organization, digital health is a broad term that includes eHealth. As per a 2021 study by Statista, the global digital health market is expected to grow from $175 billion in 2019 to nearly $660 billion in 2025. This substantial growth underscores both the increasing demand for quality healthcare and the expanding influence of digital technologies. The widespread adoption of digital health solutions has the potential to revolutionize global health standards, granting people improved access to services for the promotion and protection of their well-being. (Perappadan, 2023)

Recognizing the profound impact, the Government of India initiated the Digital India Campaign in 2015, a flagship program that included public health initiatives focused on integrating digital technologies to extend healthcare services into rural areas. Subsequently, in 2017, the National Health Policy aimed at achieving a fully digitized healthcare system in India. The policy proposed a time-bound increase in public health expenditure to 2.5% of the GDP, emphasizing the delivery of a comprehensive primary healthcare package through the establishment of Health and Wellness Centres. This marked a significant shift from a highly selective to a more inclusive primary healthcare approach, encompassing services such as geriatric healthcare, palliative care, and rehabilitative care.

The policy advocated allocating a substantial proportion (up to two-thirds or more) of resources to primary care, followed by secondary and tertiary care. It aspired to provide most secondary care services at the district level, a departure from the current practice primarily concentrated in medical college hospitals. The National Health Policy of 2017 laid the foundation for the commencement of the Digital

Health Mission in India, now known as the Ayushman Bharat Digital Health Mission. Ayushman Bharat represents a move away from a sectoral and segmented approach to healthcare service delivery, aiming to provide comprehensive, need-based healthcare services.

Ayushman Bharat consists of two similar components:

- Health and Wellness Centres (HWCs)
- Pradhan Mantri Jan Arogya Yojana (PM-JAY)

1.1.1 Health and Wellness Centres (HWCs)

In 2018, 1,50,000 Health and Wellness Centres (HWCs) were established by developing existing Sub Centres and Primary Health Centres providing Comprehensive Primary Health Care (CPHC), including maternal and child health services, as well as addressing non-communicable diseases. The services offered encompass free essential drugs and diagnostic services. The goal is to bring healthcare closer to people's homes, ensuring increased access. It works on health promotion and prevention, aiming to make communities to adopt healthy behaviours and make lifestyle changes.

1.1.2 Pradhan Mantri Jan Arogya Yojana (PM-JAY)

On September 23, 2018, the second component i.e., Pradhan Mantri Jan Arogya Yojana (PM-JAY) was launched in Ranchi, Jharkhand, by Shri Narendra Modi Ji and it is one of the world's largest health schemes.

Initially it was named as National Health Protection Scheme (NHPS) and included the existing scheme of Rashtriya Swasthya Bima Yojana (RSBY) that was launched in 2008 and covers all the families included in RSBY. This scheme is completely sponsored by the Government, with the cost shared between the Central and State Governments. One can Access PM-JAY via Ayushman Bharat Health Account (ABHA) cards.

Another digital aspect of Ayushman Bharat Digital Health Mission is eSanjeevani, a telemedicine initiative with two different components in it. The first is eSanjeevani - Health and Wellness Centre, that offers doctor-to-doctor services, in which patients go the centres and connect with doctors. The second is, eSanjeevani OPD, through which patients directly connect to doctors at the comfort of their home. The aim of both the components is to increase accessibility of the people to healthcare.

India, being home to one-sixth of the world's population, improving the healthcare system in the country is necessary on both national and international fronts. To successfully implement and keep such programs going, robust government involvement and support, especially in rural areas, is necessary (Sriwastva, 2023).

Despite technological achievements, challenges persist in accessibility and affordability. The COVID-19 pandemic exposed the strain on India's healthcare infrastructure, revealing issues such as overcrowded hospitals, uneven distribution favouring urban areas, and a shortage of skilled staff. Affordability is a substantial concern, with high medical costs burdening families. While advanced technologies contribute to modern healthcare, the focus should shift to making basic services more economical and accessible. Ensuring quality healthcare for all, regardless of socio-economic status or location, is paramount. Government initiatives like Ayushman Bharat are positive steps, requiring consistent funding, implementation, and public-private collaboration to bridge healthcare gaps. The emphasis should be on people, investing in medical education, training healthcare workers, and implementing quality control measures to guarantee safe and effective treatment. In summary, while technology plays a role, affordable and quality healthcare accessible to all should be the central focus for India's healthcare system (Maheshwari, 2023).

1.2 Digital Healthcare Trends and Policies in India

India is on the verge of transformative changes in healthcare, aligning with the National Health Policy (NHP) 2017. It addresses diverse issues such as the health needs of the young and elderly, the coexistence of communicable and non-communicable diseases, rising mental healthcare demand, and expectations of a growing middle class. The sector anticipates substantial progress driven by technology and increased investments in medicine.

Currently, about 60% of healthcare expenses are paid out of pocket in India, a significant contrast to China and Brazil. The government aims to boost budgetary allocations from 1% to around 2.5% of GDP by 2025. The expansion of private health insurance is expected to lead to industry consolidation and the growth of organized healthcare chains. Experts suggest that up to 85% of primary care can transition to teleconsultations, addressing challenges related to healthcare professional availability in remote areas. Trends in precision surgery and advances in virtual/augmented reality will reshape tertiary healthcare, emphasizing specialized therapy centres. Remote robotic centres will bring tertiary care services closer to citizens. By 2047, the healthcare landscape will undergo significant changes, benefiting consumers with improved access, higher quality care, enhanced service levels, and more affordable healthcare. Policymakers, including government officials, public health experts, and regulatory bodies, will play a pivotal role in shaping India's healthcare transformation, influencing policies, regulations, and key initiatives (Shetty, 2023).

Digital health is termed as using information technology for managing the health and wellness. India's digital health trends focus on transformative technologies, such as expanding telemedicine for remote healthcare access, embracing personalized medicine through genomic insights, and integrating wearables for real-time health monitoring. Advanced technologies like AI, cloud computing, XR, and IoT are important in augmenting diagnostics and facilitating innovative treatments. This digital transformation aims to optimize healthcare delivery, making it more efficient, accessible, and patient-centric (Chowdary, 2023).

Some of the many trends can be seen in the following ways in which Digital Healthcare already exists:

1. eHospital: The eHospital is an online system that helps manage health information in a step-by-step way. It works like a Health Information Management System (HMIS) and can be changed to fit different needs. It's a free system on NIC's National Cloud MeghRaj, using a way of working that's spread out across many places. Right now, over 1000 health places in the country use eHospital, and it follows the rules of Ayushman Bharat Digital Mission (ABDM). eHospital HMIS includes Registration (Casualty Emergency), OPD Clinic, IPD - ADT, Billing, Lab, Radiology, Laundry, Dietary, Operation Theatre, Store & Pharmacy (National Informatics Centre, 2024).
2. e-Shushrut: The e-Sushrut C-DAC's Hospital Management Information System (HMIS) is a significant advancement in healthcare technology, aiming to enhance hospital administration and patient care. This system integrates computerized clinical information, maintaining accurate electronic medical records for patients. The collected data can be used for statistics and research. The real-time HMIS optimizes patient treatment processes, empowering the workforce and improving overall performance while reducing costs. It follows a unique 'patient-centric and medical staff-centric'

approach, benefiting both recipients and providers of healthcare. The system is customizable for various hospitals, including clinics, government hospitals, super-specialty hospitals, and private hospitals. Key features include web-based accessibility, compatibility across different platforms, real-time connectivity across hospitals, customized clinical data, unique patient IDs, cross-consultation capabilities, chart generation, and integration with medical equipment, biometrics, and Aadhar (Ministry of Electronics and Information Technology, 2023).

3. Point-of-Care Diagnostics: Point-of-Care Diagnostics (POCD) is a growing trend in the medical device industry, offering diverse products for accurate diagnostics in resource-limited settings, accessible to both patients and healthcare professionals. This includes biosensors, portable x-rays, hand-held ultrasounds, and smartphone-based POCD applications. Unlike traditional diagnostic methods using expensive equipment, POCD devices are often portable and software-based, enabling on-site use. Particularly beneficial in regions with limited medical facilities like rural areas in India, POCD allows physicians to offer telehealth services post-diagnosis, reducing the need for patients to travel for diagnostic tests at medical facilities (Desai, 2023).
4. e-Pharmacies: In recent years, India has seen a surge in e-pharmacies, which operate over the internet and fulfil orders through mail, courier, or delivery services. These include online-only pharmacies and physical pharmacies with an online presence. E-pharmacies overcome geographical restrictions, allowing pharmacists to serve a broader patient base. Despite the legal status of online pharmacies being uncertain, judicial interpretation may play a role in determining their legal recognition and acceptance (Desai, 2023).

1.3 Research Problem Statement

The health crisis of COVID-19 made way for adoption of telemedicine services, leading to remote and patient-centric care. This shift from traditional to digital healthcare has been important in decentralizing healthcare a big development for both India and the world.

Despite the significant progress in leveraging digital healthcare to address issues of health quality and affordability, the country is only beginning to unlock the vast potential of this approach. Challenges persist, primarily in the form of socio-economic factors that act as barriers to accessibility in smaller cities and rural areas, impacting awareness and the adoption of digital healthcare innovations.

1.4 Scope of the Study

The government introduced the Ayushman Bharat Digital Mission (ABDM) as part of its flagship initiative to establish a better digital healthcare ecosystem.

Through the Ayushman Bharat Health Account (ABHA), patient details and medical records can be digitally accessed, presenting the potential to create population-level health profiles that facilitate a continuum of care and ensure quality healthcare. Since its inception, a total of 23.53 crore ABHA cards have been issued.

The Pradhan Mantri Jan Arogya Yojana (PMJAY), one of the world's largest health assurance schemes, covers approximately 550 people, constituting 40% of India's population. PMJAY uses digital public infrastructure to deliver services, providing people from vulnerable sections quality healthcare services. Combining ABHA cards & health records enhances the efficiency of this process.

Despite the mentioned progress, challenges persist in terms of an awareness and adoption gap in digital health interventions, observed in both rural and urban areas. Many people remain unaware of the available benefits, and even where awareness exists, there is often insufficient incentive for adoption.

1.5 Aim of the Study

The objective of the study is to understand the factors influencing the awareness and adoption of digital health interventions, specifically eSanjeevani under ABDM and the ABHA Card, leading to the adoption of PM-JAY in the NCR region. The aim is to provide valuable information for stakeholders and policymakers. Initially, a pilot study revealed that in rural areas of the Delhi NCR region, the primary deficiency was in awareness, rendering adoption assessment irrelevant. Therefore, the study focused solely on assessing awareness in rural areas and both awareness and adoption in urban areas of Delhi NCR.

The research will explore the current state of digital healthcare in India and analyse various factors affecting its adoption, including smartphone ownership, internet access, and overall digitization. It will also investigate socio-economic factors such as income, education, and knowledge that influence the adoption of digital healthcare in Delhi NCR. Employing a mixed-methods research approach, the study will gather insights from stakeholders. The findings have the potential to contribute to the development of a framework and the formulation of effective policies aimed at promoting the adoption of digital healthcare not only in Delhi NCR but also in other regions of the country.

1.6 Research Gap

When addressing healthcare gaps from both digital and social perspectives, disparities involve uneven access and utilization of technologies in the health sector among different societal segments. This disparity is attributed to factors such as the lack of robust digital infrastructure, including internet and connectivity, varying levels of digital literacy across different populations, geographical disparities, and the affordability of digital technologies. From a social perspective, health equity is influenced by factors like income and social protection, education, unemployment, and job insecurity, conditions in the workplace, food security, housing, basic amenities, and the environment, early childhood development, non-discrimination and social inclusion, structural conflict, and access to affordable health services of decent quality (HealthcareRadius, India, 2021).

The gaps that are identified and will be fulfilled through this research are as follows:

- **Demographic Impact on Healthcare Demand:** Recognition of the role of demographics in boosting healthcare services demand. Lack of research on Indian demographic segmentation and its specific impact on the healthcare industry.
- **Tailor-Made Intervention Plans:** Absence of literature addressing the design of tailor-made intervention plans for patients based on demographic insights.
- **Digital Platforms and Patient Impact:** Scarcity of research on the types of digital platforms, their usage, and their impact on patients.
- **Consumer Feelings, Attitudes, and Perceptions:** Research emphasizes the need to pay attention to consumer feelings, attitudes, and perceptions in healthcare. Limited studies assessing these aspects, calling for more extensive research.

- **Factors Influencing Digital Healthcare Adoption:** Wide research gap in understanding the factors influencing the adoption of digital healthcare. Existence of numerous studies related to adoption, but insufficient focus on key influencing factors.
- **Contextual Analysis in NCR:** Previous research primarily focused on digital healthcare in a general context. Dearth of detailed analyses in the literature on the socioeconomic aspects specifically impacting the adoption of digital healthcare, especially in the National Capital Region (NCR).

Identifying the above gaps in healthcare accessibility holds paramount importance for a diverse array of stakeholders. For policymakers and planners, this insight serves as a crucial tool, allowing them to comprehend the deficiencies in the present healthcare services through the help of digital healthcare and thus strategically allocate resources. Healthcare providers like hospitals benefit by tailoring services to reach vulnerable populations, optimizing delivery through strategic facility placement and adjusting hours, and implementing telemedicine solutions. Public health officials find significance in identifying gaps for focused planning, enabling them to direct attention to areas with the greatest health disparities. Researchers contribute by conducting studies on healthcare access disparities, leading to a deeper understanding of root causes and potential solutions. Communities and advocacy groups gain empowerment to advocate for improved access, engaging policymakers and mobilizing resources. Technology developers can ensure innovations cater to diverse populations, addressing specific accessibility challenges. Lastly, international organizations and donors leverage information about gaps to guide support and funding efforts, making targeted investments that promote global health equity. In essence, identifying these accessibility gaps is pivotal for fostering a more equitable and effective healthcare system on a global scale (Stakeholders In Indian Healthcare Sector 2023: An Overview, 2023).

1.7 Objectives of the Study

This research explores the role of psychological, socio-economic, and demographic factors on Indian consumers' preference for digital healthcare over traditional healthcare. It examines their level of awareness regarding the National Health Policy and Ayushman Bharat Digital Health Mission, aiming to uncover thought process of people and their decisions. To Remove barriers and increase the adoption of digital healthcare in India, it is important to research more.

- To assess the extent of awareness among people in rural areas of Delhi NCR region towards National Health Policy and Ayushman Bharat Digital Health Mission i.e., digital healthcare.
- To determine how the level of awareness of digital healthcare of the people in urban areas of Delhi NCR region influences their intention to adopt it.
- To determine various factors affecting the adoption behaviour of the urban areas of people in Delhi NCR region towards digital healthcare.
- To examines the impact of socio-economic factors on the adoption of digital healthcare in the urban areas of Delhi NCR region.
- To assess the perception/attitude of the people of varying age groups in the urban areas of Delhi NCR region to adopt digital healthcare.
- To assess how level of awareness differs across people of different income category for digital healthcare in both rural and urban areas of Delhi NCR region.

- To assess how level of awareness differs across people of different age category for digital healthcare in both rural and urban areas of Delhi NCR region.

1.8 Significance of the Study

Examining the impact of psychological, socio-economic, and demographic factors on Indian consumers' utilization of digital healthcare is crucial for various reasons. It facilitates the customization of strategies to enhance public access to digital healthcare by comprehensively understanding the factors influencing awareness and adoption. Moreover, the study addresses a research gap and enhances our understanding of how India embraces digital healthcare in comparison to traditional healthcare systems. Overall, the research includes some effective solutions for policy formulation to promote the use of digital healthcare.

2. LITERATURE REVIEW

A survey by Accenture revealed that 26% of respondents in the U.S. reported improved healthcare access since the COVID-19 pandemic and the adoption of digital health. Surprisingly, over a quarter didn't use any digital technologies for health management. Challenges were observed, especially in the decreased use of mobile applications for healthcare. Respondents highlighted the importance of a medical provider explaining the patient's condition and treatment (55%) and a provider who listens, understands needs, and provides emotional support (52%) for a positive healthcare experience (Safavi & Michel, 2021).

Among 800 UK patients surveyed, 42% regularly sought online health information. Physicians and pharmacists were considered more trustworthy than online information. Overall, awareness of quality issues with web health information was insufficient among internet users. Some authors suggested involving healthcare professionals to guide patients in selecting higher-quality online health information (Battineni, 2020).

The success of any health scheme is mainly because of awareness among people regarding the scheme. It is a crucial step in publicly funded health insurance (PFHI) of improving access to healthcare. The absence of knowledge becomes a barrier to access healthcare (Sen, 2008). Not being aware of what you're entitled to under programs for Universal Health Coverage can affect how these programs are adopted and, in the end, how successful they are. (Jacobs, Ir, & Bigdeli, 2012). People in poverty face problem of genuine healthcare again because of awareness, access to information and exclusion (BRAC, 2001; Ahmed et al., 2006).

PM-JAY achieving Universal Health Coverage (UHC) is the world's largest fully government-funded scheme, healthcare services along with financial protection to impoverished and vulnerable Indians (Angell BJ, 2019). The registration process for it is also cashless, in comparison to Publicly Funded Health Insurance (PFHI) schemes. It identifies households based on deprivation and occupational criteria established by the government through the Socio-Economic Caste Census of 2011 (SECC 2011). It is currently operational in 33 out of 36 states and Union Territories in India and allows individuals to undergo the verification process at government centres or when going to a hospital after an illness.

PM-JAY has simplified the process in contrast to the RSBY scheme PM.(Smith O, 2019). Research conducted by Reddy N (2020) discovered that healthcare workers had low awareness and readiness for implementing PM-JAY, with those who had higher awareness showing increased readiness (Kanore L, 2019).

The National Health Authority (NHA), invented communication strategy at both nationally and at the state level (Government of India, 2018) through media channels like radio and TV commercials. They also introduced initiatives and community mobilization through Accredited Social Health Activists (ASHA) (Bakshi, Sharma, & Kumar, 2018).

Digital healthcare holds the promise of preventing diseases, reducing healthcare expenses, and aiding patients in monitoring and managing chronic conditions. Furthermore, it has the potential to customize medicine for individual patients. However, realizing the full potential of digital healthcare in India requires addressing significant challenges. The rural-urban healthcare system disparity in the country is substantial, with over 75% of healthcare infrastructure concentrated in metropolitan cities, where only 27% of the total population resides. The remaining 73% of the Indian population lacks even basic medical facilities. Primary medical centres face a shortage of over 3,000 doctors, a deficit that has increased by over 200% in the last decade. Additionally, India's Out-Of-Pocket Expenditure (OOPE) for health was notably high, reaching 63% in 2018 (Bajaj, 2023).

Rural India continues to grapple with persistent health challenges, including longstanding issues like tuberculosis, malaria, and diarrheal diseases, as well as newer problems related to environmental pollution, especially air and water contamination. This underscores the severe lack of healthcare accessibility in rural areas, contributing to high maternal and infant mortality rates, malnutrition, low life expectancy, and limited vaccination coverage. The COVID-19 pandemic has exacerbated these challenges, posing a dilemma for the Health Ministry as 70% of India's population resides in rural regions, facing scarcity of healthcare facilities and high disease-related mortality. In contrast, the private healthcare sector predominantly focuses on urban areas, despite most of the India's population residing in rural regions. This concentration of urban healthcare has implications for India's pursuit of universal health coverage and the improvement of national health indicators (Rao, 2022).

According to Bouarar et al. (2022), digitalization is not a new requirement for businesses, but the urgency of adopting it has increased with COVID-19. The post-COVID-19 era is anticipated to bring new challenges and opportunities, prompting a swift trend towards digitalization. To sustain their presence in the market during health crises, healthcare services must embrace digitalization (Aigbogun et al., 2023). Factors such as perceived usefulness, perceived ease of use, attitudes, perceived self-efficacy, intention to use, and trust in the digital health system significantly influence the adoption of digital health apps (Mouloudj, Bouarar, & Saadaoui, 2023).

We are currently experiencing a profound technological revolution. In the healthcare sector, where there is a notable integration of digital technologies and health, giving rise to various digital care programs collectively known as "Digital Health.". The availability of online health information (OHI) plays a crucial role in influencing online health practices, providing information about health risks and health-promoting measures. The internet allows individuals, regardless of their medical qualifications, to disseminate health-related information. In the expanding digital ecosystem, health misinformation becomes a significant risk, particularly when it originates from non-evidence-based sources.

Mobile phones are the most frequently used technological devices. Among students' awareness of using digital tools is low. This overlooks the importance of guiding and supporting students, ensuring they get the most benefits (Hassan, 2023).

India's healthcare system needs a fundamental shift, transcending the WHO's doctor-patient ratio metric. Achieving infrastructure parity across regions is crucial. Currently, 75% of the population outside urban areas has limited access to hospitals, leading to neglect in preventive measures. Teleconsultation emerges as a promising solution, addressing infrastructure challenges and reducing consultation times (Jain, 2020).

The 2017 National Health Policy outlines a strategic approach to address gaps in the health system, emphasizing government involvement in creating an integrated public healthcare system. It advocates collaboration with the private sector for initiatives like strategic purchasing and capacity building. The policy aims for a 2.5% GDP allocation for public health expenditure, prioritizing comprehensive primary healthcare with a shift from selective to inclusive services. Specific goals include reducing disease prevalence, improving health system performance, and aligning medical device policies with public health objectives by 2020. Key principles focus on professionalism, ethics, equity, affordability, and patient-cantered care. The policy aims to enhance access to quality care, reduce out-of-pocket expenses, build trust in public healthcare, and guide private sector growth in line with public health goals, emphasizing pre-emptive care for child and adolescent health through school programs and curriculum integration. Overall, the NHP of 2017 seeks to clarify and strengthen the government's role in shaping a holistic and inclusive healthcare system (PIB, A study of awareness about Ayushyaman Bharat Yojana among low income urban families. An exploratory study, 2020).

The National Telemedicine Service, eSanjeevani, has successfully served 3 crore beneficiaries, with 2,26,72,187 using eSanjeevani AB-HWC and 73,77,779 benefiting from eSanjeevani OPD. Over 1,00,000 doctors and specialists have joined the service, demonstrating widespread acceptance in rural India. In line with the Ayushman Bharat scheme's goal of Universal Health Coverage, eSanjeevani provides free, quality healthcare, emphasizing its 'Make in India' origin. Developed by the Health Informatics Group at Mohali's C-DAC branch, the service maintains over 99.5% uptime. Plans to enhance capacity to support over 10 lakhs consultations daily with AI-led interventions are underway. The top states in eSanjeevani adoption are Andhra Pradesh, Karnataka, West Bengal, Tamil Nadu, Uttar Pradesh, Bihar, Maharashtra, Madhya Pradesh, Gujarat, and Assam (PIB, addressing access barriers to health services: an analytical framework for selecting appropriate interventions in low-income Asian countries. Health Policy and Planning, 2022).

India's healthcare landscape reveals significant disparities between urban and rural areas. Urban centres grapple with challenges such as overcrowded facilities, non-communicable diseases, and mental health issues. In contrast, rural regions face obstacles like limited healthcare access, inadequate sanitation, and a higher burden of communicable diseases. Despite the expanding private healthcare sector providing quality services, a substantial part of the population experiences healthcare inequalities, particularly due to insufficient access. Urban challenges involve crowded hospitals, escalating non-communicable diseases, health problems related to air pollution, limited access to clean water, mental health concerns, and healthcare disparities for marginalized groups. Rural areas encounter hurdles like inadequate healthcare infrastructure, deficient transportation, poor sanitation, malnutrition, a notable prevalence of communicable diseases, low awareness, and restricted access to quality healthcare. However, the Indian government has initiated programs like the National Health Mission and the Ayushman Bharat scheme to address these issues and enhance healthcare accessibility and quality. The rise of digital healthcare, expected to reach USD 11.2 billion by 2025, is a transformative trend. Telemedicine, especially during the COVID-19 pandemic, has showcased its potential to improve healthcare access. Nevertheless, challenges, particularly infrastructure limitations in rural areas, hinder the widespread adoption of digital healthcare. As the nation progresses, concerted efforts are expected to address these challenges, ensuring that a larger portion of the population, regardless of location or economic status, can access high-quality healthcare services (Pennep, 2023).

In its fifth year, the AB-PMJAY (Ayushman Bharat Pradhan Mantri Jan Arogya Yojana) has successfully provided health coverage to over 15.5 crore families, 5.39 crore admission events worth Rs 66,284 crore in the last five years. The scheme has proven instrumental in cost savings, preventing a nearly two-fold increase in treatment expenses if availed outside its coverage, leading to savings exceeding Rs 1 lakh crore for beneficiaries. The impact of AB-PMJAY includes a significant reduction of 60% in Out-of-Pocket Expenditure (OOPE) for beneficiaries. Public hospitals have experienced increased bed occupancy rates and revenue generation (Rakheja et al, 2023).

AB-PMJAY faces challenges in rural awareness, uneven healthcare distribution, and reimbursement issues. To improve effectiveness, there's a need for enhanced outreach, addressing infrastructure gaps, and streamlining reimbursement processes (Indian Express, 2023).

Adopting digital solutions in healthcare, covering prevention, diagnosis, and treatment, is India's smartest path toward achieving "health for all." This approach addresses challenges of access, affordability, and quality. The integration of a digital health system aligns with India's strategic vision, reflected in initiatives like Ayushman Bharat and Digital India, aiming to create a healthy and prosperous society. Health technology, a transformative force in the Fourth Industrial Revolution, presents India with an opportunity to influence global health policy and improve its competitiveness in technology development, unlike space technology, where India has already excelled (Ranganathan, 2020).

The 2020 National Digital Health Blueprint (NDHB) outlines essential design principles for the ambitious task of establishing a comprehensive electronic health records database, serving as the authoritative source for individual health data in India. The blueprint emphasizes standards for ensuring the privacy and security of digitized health information. Key prerequisites for the NDHB's success include nationwide internet access, an extensive network of primary healthcare centres, and a trained health workforce, all requiring consistent government support. The integrated national-health database, once in place, will serve as an asset for conducting advanced data analytics, benefiting policy design and implementation control. It enables automated interventions in the health system, such as targeted health messaging, stock-level notifications, and warnings for managing health supplies. Moreover, it provides training content for medical research and education, laying the groundwork for innovation. The operational database is anticipated to streamline India's fragmented health system, representing the initial step toward efficiency and future readiness, even though it won't completely remedy the system (Ranganathan, 2020).

3. RESEARCH METHODOLOGY

3.1. Sampling Design

3.1.1 Target Population

Delhi NCR region is considered as the sample area for the study and analysis for this research. This is because Delhi and Delhi NCR, is one of the most populous cities in terms of both urban and rural population. Delhi is fifth most populous city in the world and the largest city in India area-wise (world population review, 2024). Studying this area can provide large insights in terms of demographics, behaviours and perceptions, people of different cultural and social background. It is also one of the most accessible regions of the country which has further helped in being cost effective and efficient. The above reasons have helped in making the research helpful and point out the actual trends in terms of adoption of digital healthcare.

The districts in Delhi NCR that are taken into consideration for a primary survey are, Delhi NCT, Gautam Budh Nagar, Ghaziabad, Faridabad, Meerut, Gurugram which gives an overall picture of the Delhi NCR region. This research seeks to examine the variables/factors affecting awareness and adoption in the NCR region. The study is furthered by the varied socio-economic terrain of the NCR region, which includes both urban and rural part of the above districts.

Understanding the effects of socioeconomic factors, benefits, perception, and level of awareness on digital healthcare adoption will help identify the challenges and opportunities faced by people from various income brackets, educational backgrounds, vocations, and social classes.

Policymakers, industry stakeholders, and in the NCR, region will find the research's conclusions useful. The goal is to increase knowledge and offer suggestions for encouraging the use of digital based healthcare services in this diverse and heavily populated urban and rural environment of Delhi NCR region.

3.1.2 Sampling Technique

Both probability and non-probability sampling approaches are used to define the sample. Stratified sampling and cluster sampling arc examples of probability sampling procedures. By separating the NCR region into strata according to factors like geography, income, and education, participants are randomly chosen from each stratum using stratified sampling. The NCR region is divided into random geographic clusters, and all the inhabitants of those clusters are included in the sample. Techniques for non-probability sampling are used, including convenience sampling which involves choosing participants who are easily reachable and eager to participate. The validity and generalizability of the research findings will be improved by the employment of a variety of sampling strategies to ensure inclusivity and diversity within the sample.

Sample Size

The determination of an appropriate sample size is crucial in research to ensure that the findings are reliable and representative of the target population. In the study, the sample size will be determined using the Fisher's Formula

The PM-JAY policy considers providing the lowest 40% of the population, which is fulfilling criteria followed by the government in the Socio-Economic Caste Census of 2011. Hence lower 40% of the population is considered as the total amount to derive the sample size from. Accordingly 40% of 1.3 billion equals to 6 crore.

The formula used is as follows:

$$n = \frac{z^2 p(1-p)}{m^2}$$

Where,

n is the sample size,

Z is the z-value,

p is the proportion of population (generally taken as 0.5),

m is the margin of error.

The sample size comes out to be 384, but because of we have boils it down to 150, with 75 primary survey each in urban and rural areas of Delhi NCR.

3.1.3 Collection of Data

Primary and secondary data sources will be used to discover changes caused by socioeconomic factors, benefits, perception, and level of awareness on the adoption of digital healthcare in the NCR region.

Surveys are used for urban and face to face interviews in rural will be used to obtain primary data, with an emphasis on quantitative information such as socioeconomic status, awareness, perception, benefits about and of the schemes, and adoption factors, as well as qualitative insights into socioeconomic drivers and incentive perceptions. Further, secondary data from various publications and available data will be used. This mix of primary and secondary data allows a complete investigation of the subject and specific insights from the target community.

Google forms were used to collect the data from 75 respondents in the urban Delhi NCR regions consisting of Delhi NCR, Gautam Budh Nagar, Ghaziabad, Faridabad, Meerut, Gurugram and 75 respondents were surveyed through.

While Section B & C followed the dichotomous scale of simple Yes/No. Section B tested the awareness in both urban and rural areas and Section C tested the reasons for adoption of digital healthcare and the schemes only in urban areas.

Section A concentrated on demographic and basic information about the respondents. The demographic research and further the analysis on the basis of demographic factors has been done because analysing such factors helps in recognition and of the trends and shifts over time, helping in formulating impactful policies addressing the distinct requirements of diverse age groups, income levels, or cultural backgrounds and also helps in efficient allocation of resources by the government and institutions.

A pre-test with 20 participants was done to face validity of the scale items was established.

3.1.4 Concepts and Variables Used

Benefits of the schemes (Independent Variable): It refers to the benefits provided by the schemes taken into consideration to check the adoption of digital healthcare. The benefits are INR 500 000 per family per year ignoring the family size, age or gender, is fully financed by the government, up to 3 days before getting hospitalised and 15 days after hospitalization expenses are covered in PM-JAY.

Figure 1. Concepts and Variables Used
Source: Author's Analysis

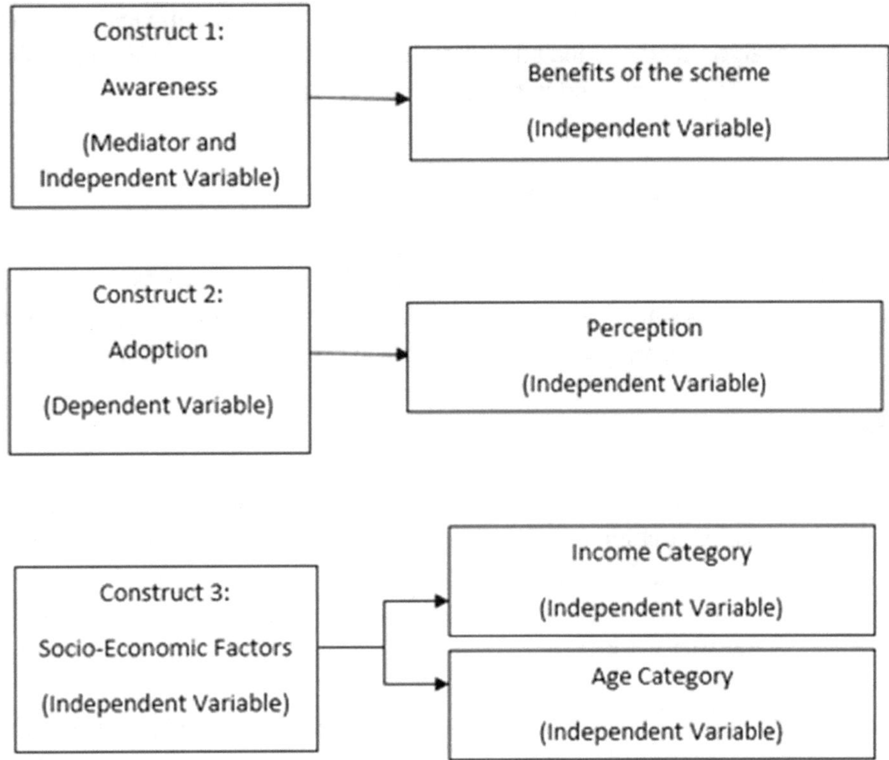

Expected outcome of it, on Adoption of Digital Healthcare based schemes, is positive.

Socio-economic factors (Independent Variable): This includes a variety of social and economic aspects that affect people's choices regarding the use of two-wheel electric vehicles.

Income, education, occupation, age are examples of socioeconomic factors.

Expected outcome of it, on Adoption of Digital Healthcare based schemes, is positive.

Awareness (Mediator & Independent Variable): It examines how well people are informed about the digital healthcare-based schemes rolled out by government for the benefits of the masses.

Expected outcome of it, on Adoption of Digital Healthcare based schemes, is positive.

Perception (Independent Variable): How masses perceive the advantages and disadvantages of digital healthcare-based schemes for adoption. Individuals' attitudes and intentions towards adoption are significantly influenced by their perceptions and level of awareness.

Expected outcome of it, on Adoption of Digital Healthcare based schemes, is positive.

Digital Healthcare Adoption (Dependent Variable): This idea refers to the choice and action taken by people or households to use digital based healthcare platforms as their main means of healthcare check-up which entails considering a few variables, such as benefits, perception, awareness, and the accessibility of these digital based healthcare schemes.

3.1.5 Analytical Tools

The Statistical Package for Social Sciences (SPS) version 23.0 was used to analyse the data that had been gathered. Data analysis methods included descriptive statistics, correlation analysis, Factor and Regression Analyses were performed and interpreted through SPSS.

4. DATA ANALYSIS AND INTERPRETATION

This section presents the analyses starting from correlation analysis, factor analysis and then the application of regression analysis. For this statistical tool of SPSS has been used. Through Regression analysis, the relationship, its direction and degree, between independent and dependent variables has been showcased.

4.1 Correlation

Correlation analysis is used to measure the strength of the linear relationship. It is judged between two variables and their association is computed. In other words, it calculates the level of change in one variable with respect to the change in the other.

4.1.1 Correlation Between Variables

As discussed above, the variables taken into consideration for Socioeconomic factors (Family monthly income, Age), Benefits, perception, Awareness and Adoption.

Hence, firstly collinearity is checked in between the above factors to check for the feasibility of the analysis.

Figure 2. Socioeconomics Correlations
Source: Author's Calculation
Abbreviations used above in the analysis is as follows:
AW – Awareness
B – Benefits
AD – Adoption
P – Perception

Correlations

		Family Income (per month)	Age	AW	B	AD	P
Family Income (per month)	Pearson Correlation	1	-.082	-.618*	-.564*	-.365	.344
	Sig. (2-tailed)		.763	.011	.023	.164	.193
	N	16	16	16	16	16	16
Age	Pearson Correlation	-.082	1	.154	.426	-.288	-.338
	Sig. (2-tailed)	.763		.569	.100	.279	.200
	N	16	16	16	16	16	16
AW	Pearson Correlation	-.618*	.154	1	.801**	-.089	-.635**
	Sig. (2-tailed)	.011	.569		.000	.743	.008
	N	16	16	16	16	16	16
B	Pearson Correlation	-.564*	.426	.801**	1	-.134	-.785**
	Sig. (2-tailed)	.023	.100	.000		.620	.000
	N	16	16	16	16	16	16
AD	Pearson Correlation	-.365	-.288	-.089	-.134	1	.314
	Sig. (2-tailed)	.164	.279	.743	.620		.237
	N	16	16	16	16	16	16
P	Pearson Correlation	.344	-.338	-.635**	-.785**	.314	1
	Sig. (2-tailed)	.193	.200	.008	.000	.237	
	N	16	16	16	16	16	16

*. Correlation is significant at the 0.05 level (2-tailed).
**. Correlation is significant at the 0.01 level (2-tailed).

- Here we can we see that Family income and adoption are negatively correlated which shows a negative relationship between the two i.e., people tend to not adopt schemes like PM-JAY, which offers insurance coverage of Rs. 5,00,000 for the whole family and tend to look for insurance coverages from other sources when family income increases.
- Age and awareness are positively related, having a positive relationship, i.e., awareness is found to augment with age.
- Age and adoption show a negative correlation and relationship which was the case because as the primary survey showed, that people with old age tend to hesitate to use such services and are mostly dependent on their children who again trust on other sources for insurance coverage.
- Adoption and perception are seen to be negatively correlated and having an inverse relationship. People had a lack of faith, trust issues to adopt the digital platforms when it came to their healthcare and hence did not adopt them.

4.1.2 Correlation Among the Factors

By finding the correlation among the actual factors that make up the above variables, we try to better justify the results in correlation shown above amongst the variables. In this correlation analysis we have tried and in-depth relationship between the factors, through the correlation amongst the questions asked in the survey.

Table 1. Correlations Among Factors

Correlations

	Family Income	Age	1	2	3	4	5	6	7	8	9	10	11	12	13	14	15	16	17	18	19	20	21	22	23	24	25	26	27	28	29	30	31
Family Income																																	
Age	-0.08																																
1	-.52**	0.09																															
2	-.52**	0.09	1.00**																														
3	-.60**	0.01	0.03	0.03																													
4	-.52**	0.09	.42**	.42**	.59**																												
5	-.36**	.52**	.59**	.59**	0.16	.59**																											
6	-.68**	.21*	.76**	.76**	.36**	.76**	.78**																										
7	-.59**	.49**	.45**	.45**	.24*	.45**	.76**	.59**																									
8	-.59**	.49**	.45**	.45**	.24*	.45**	.76**	.59**	1.00**																								
9	-.29**	.28**	.32**	.32**	0.04	.32**	.54**	.42**	.71**	.71**																							
10	.33**	-.34**	-0.17	-0.17	-0.2	-0.17	-.29**	-.23*	-.38**	-.38**	0.12																						
11	-1.00**	0.08	.52**	.52**	.60**	.52**	.36**	.68**	.59**	.59**	.29**	-.33**																					
12	b	b	b	b	b	b	b	b	b	b	b	b																					
13	-.77**	0.05	.67**	.67**	.52**	.67**	.63**	.88**	.67**	.67**	.48**	-.26*	.77**	b																			
14	-.59**	.20*	.45**	.45**	.24*	.45**	.49**	.59**	.71**	.71**	.37**	-.38**	.59**	b	.67**																		
15	0.2	0.15	0.17	0.17	-.33**	0.17	.29**	.23*	.38**	.38**	.54**	0.07	-0.2	b	.26*	.38**																	
16	-.59**	.20*	.45**	.45**	.24*	.45**	.49**	.59**	.71**	.71**	.37**	-.38**	.59**	b	.67**	1.00**	.38**																
17	-.49**	.22*	.25*	.25*	.29**	.25*	.43**	.33**	.56**	.56**	.30**	-.68**	.49**	b	.38**	.56**	-0.1	.56**															
18	-.45**	.44**	.39**	.39**	0.15	.39**	.65**	.51**	.86**	.86**	.83**	-.45**	.45**	b	.58**	.54**	.45**	.54**	.65**														
19	-.29**	.52**	.32**	.32**	0.04	.32**	.54**	.42**	.71**	.71**	.59**	-.54**	.29**	b	.48**	.37**	.54**	.37**	.30**	.83**													
20	.73**	-.36**	-.52**	-.52**	-.33**	-.52**	-.62**	-.68**	-.87**	-.87**	-.62**	.33**	-.73**	b	-.77**	-.87**	-.33**	-.87**	-.49**	-.75**	-.62**												
21	b	b	b	b	b	b	b	b	b	b	b	b	b	b	b	b	b	b	b	b	b	b											
22	.59**	-.49**	-.45**	-.45**	-.24*	-.45**	-.76**	-.59**	-1.00**	-1.00**	-.71**	.38**	-.59**	b	-.67**	-.71**	-.38**	-.71**	-.56**	-.86**	-.71**	.87**	b										
23	.59**	-.49**	-.45**	-.45**	-.24*	-.45**	-.76**	-.59**	-1.00**	-1.00**	-.71**	.38**	-.59**	b	-.67**	-.71**	-.38**	-.71**	-.56**	-.86**	-.71**	.87**	b	1.00**									
24	.29**	-0.19	-.56**	-.56**	-.49**	-.56**	-.33**	-.43**	-.25*	-.25*	-0.18	0.1	-.29**	b	-.36**	-.25*	-0.1	-.25*	-0.14	-.22*	-0.18	.29**	b	.25*	.25*								
25	0.1	-0.09	-.25*	-.25*	0.1	-.25*	-.43**	-.33**	-.56**	-.56**	-.79**	-0.1	-0.1	b	-.38**	-.56**	-.68**	-.56**	-.43**	-.65**	-.30**	.49**	b	.56**	.56**	0.14							
26	-.47**	-0.01	.24*	.24*	.33**	.24*	.36**	.42**	.31**	.31**	-0.04	-.33**	.47**	b	.52**	.31**	-0.2	.31**	0.1	0.15	.29**	-.47**	b	-.31*	-.31*	0.1	.29**						
27	-1.00**	0.08	.52**	.52**	.60**	.52**	.36**	.68**	.59**	.59**	.29**	-.33**	1.00**	b	.77**	.59**	-0.2	.59**	.49**	.45**	.29**	-.73**	b	-.59**	-.59**	-.29**	-0.1	.47**					
28	-.24*	-0.1	-0.16	-0.16	.31**	0.13	0.05	.22*	-0.13	-0.13	-.37**	-0.17	.24*	b	0.13	0.16	-.38**	0.16	.25*	-.23*	-.37**	0.03	b	0.13	0.13	.25*	0.15	.24*	.24*				
29	.33**	-0.11	-.31**	-.31**	-0.2	-.31**	-0.16	-0.1	-.52**	-.52**	-.37**	0.2	-.33**	b	-.26*	-.52**	-0.2	-.52**	-.29**	-.45**	-.37**	.60**	b	.52**	.52**	.49**	.29**	-0.07	-.33**	.52**			
30	b	b	b	b	b	b	b	b	b	b	b	b	b	b	b	b	b	b	b	b	b	b	b	b	b	b	b	b	b	b	b		
31	-.29**	0.19	.56**	.56**	.49**	.56**	.33**	.43**	.25*	.25*	0.18	-0.1	.29**	b	.38**	.25*	0.1	.25*	0.14	.22*	0.18	-.29**	b	-.25*	-.25*	-1.00**	-0.14	-0.1	.29**	-.25*	-.49**	b	

** Correlation is significant at the 0.01 level (2-tailed).

* Correlation is significant at the 0.05 level (2-tailed).

b Cannot be computed because at least one of the variables is constant.

Source: Author's Calculation

- Here we can see that family income across 13-19 (questions testing awareness) has a negative correlation, i.e., a negative relationship which shows that even people with high income strata both in urban and rural areas of Delhi NCR do not have awareness towards digital healthcare-based schemes.
- Also, family income and "28" (which shows the faith of the people in these schemes i.e., perception) have a negative correlation, i.e. people of high income strata tend to have less faith in the insurance coverages offered by such schemes and try meet their insurance needs from other sources.

4.2 Factor Analysis

Factor analysis assumes several assumptions: there is linear relationship, there is no multicollinearity, it includes relevant variables into analysis, and there is true correlation between variables and factors. Several methods are available, but principal component analysis is used most commonly.

Figure 3. Factor Analysis
Source: Author's Calculation

Factor Analysis

[DataSet4] /Users/vanshikaverma/Downloads/Untitled2.sav

KMO and Bartlett's Test

Kaiser-Meyer-Olkin Measure of Sampling Adequacy.		.660
Bartlett's Test of Sphericity	Approx. Chi-Square	41.550
	df	15
	Sig.	.000

Communalities

	Initial	Extraction
Family Income (per month)	1.000	.827
Age	1.000	.458
AW	1.000	.797
B	1.000	.905
AD	1.000	.789
P	1.000	.767

Extraction Method: Principal Component Analysis.

For a model to be of a good fit, the Kaiser-Meyer-Olkin Measure of Sampling Adequacy should be more than .5 and in the analysis above we can see that the value of it is coming out to be .660.

For communalities we check for range which should generally be more than .7 and in the above analysis shows the values under extraction column well above .7 which shows that variables considered to be of a good fit and relevant to be considered in the analysis.

Figure 4. Total Variance Explained
Source: Author's Calculation

Total Variance Explained

Component	Initial Eigenvalues			Extraction Sums of Squared Loadings			Rotation Sums of Squared Loadings		
	Total	% of Variance	Cumulative %	Total	% of Variance	Cumulative %	Total	% of Variance	Cumulative %
1	3.049	50.819	50.819	3.049	50.819	50.819	2.906	48.431	48.431
2	1.494	24.896	75.716	1.494	24.896	75.716	1.637	27.284	75.716
3	.756	12.593	88.309						
4	.349	5.812	94.121						
5	.237	3.956	98.077						
6	.115	1.923	100.000						

Extraction Method: Principal Component Analysis.

Component Matrix[a]

	Component	
	1	2
Family Income (per month)	-.654	-.632
Age	.454	-.502
AW	.873	.185
B	.951	-.003
AD	-.177	.870
P	-.847	.224

Extraction Method: Principal Component Analysis.

a. 2 components extracted.

Figure 5. Rotated Component Matrix
Source: Author's Calculation

Rotated Component Matrix[a]

	Component	
	1	2
Family Income (per month)	-.815	.404
Age	.280	.616
AW	.888	.089
B	.905	.292
AD	.095	-.883
P	-.739	-.470

Extraction Method: Principal Component Analysis.
Rotation Method: Varimax with Kaiser Normalization.

a. Rotation converged in 3 iterations.

Component Transformation Matrix

Component	1	2
1	.953	.304
2	.304	-.953

Extraction Method: Principal Component Analysis.
Rotation Method: Varimax with Kaiser Normalization.

4.3 Regression Analysis

Regression analysis tests the relationship between dependent and independent variables to examine multi-level dependence relationships where a dependent variable becomes an independent variable in subsequent relationships within the same analysis, which in this case is the variable of awareness.

In the analysis above, three relationships have been considered to fulfil the objectives enlisted in our analysis. They are as follows:

$$Adoption = b_1 + b_2(Awareness) + \in$$

$$Adoption = b_1 + b_2(other\ factors) + \in$$

$$Awareness = b_1 + b_2(other\ factors) + \in$$

Where ϵ is the error term

Accordingly the hypothesis framed are as follows:

Hypothesis

H1: Awareness significantly impacts the Adoption in both Urban and rural areas of Delhi NCR.

H2: Benefits, Perception, and socio-economic factors significantly impacts the Adoption in urban areas of Delhi NCR.

H3: Benefits, Perception, and socio-economic factors significantly impacts the Awareness in both rural & urban areas of Delhi NCR.

4.3.1 Cases

Figure 6. Case Summary 1
Source: Author's Calculation

Model Summary

Model	R	R Square	Adjusted R Square	Std. Error of the Estimate	Change Statistics: R Square Change	F Change	df1	df2	Sig. F Change
1	.643[a]	.414	.408	.387	.414	66.413	1	94	.000

a. Predictors: (Constant), AW

ANOVA[a]

Model		Sum of Squares	df	Mean Square	F	Sig.
1	Regression	9.932	1	9.932	66.413	.000[b]
	Residual	14.058	94	.150		
	Total	23.990	95			

a. Dependent Variable: AD
b. Predictors: (Constant), AW

Coefficients[a]

Model		Unstandardized Coefficients B	Std. Error	Standardized Coefficients Beta	t	Sig.
1	(Constant)	.339	.149		2.278	.025
	AW	.694	.085	.643	8.149	.000

a. Dependent Variable: AD

Figure 7. Case Summary 2
Source: Author's Calculation

Model Summary

Model	R	R Square	Adjusted R Square	Std. Error of the Estimate	Change Statistics: R Square Change	F Change	df1	df2	Sig. F Change
1	.844[a]	.713	.700	.275	.713	56.482	4	91	.000

a. Predictors: (Constant), Age, P, Family Income (per month), B

ANOVA[a]

Model		Sum of Squares	df	Mean Square	F	Sig.
1	Regression	17.101	4	4.275	56.482	.000[b]
	Residual	6.888	91	.076		
	Total	23.990	95			

a. Dependent Variable: AD
b. Predictors: (Constant), Age, P, Family Income (per month), B

Coefficients[a]

Model		Unstandardized Coefficients B	Std. Error	Standardized Coefficients Beta	t	Sig.
1	(Constant)	2.076	.203		10.242	.000
	B	.129	.082	.100	1.562	.122
	P	-.327	.062	-.327	-5.289	.000
	Family Income (per month)	-.211	.021	-.614	-10.246	.000
	Age	.051	.021	.142	2.412	.018

a. Dependent Variable: AD

Figure 8. Case Summary 3
Source: Author's Calculation

Model Summary

Model	R	R Square	Adjusted R Square	Std. Error of the Estimate	Change Statistics				
					R Square Change	F Change	df1	df2	Sig. F Change
1	.845[a]	.714	.701	.255	.714	56.786	4	91	.000

a. Predictors: (Constant), Age, P, Family Income (per month), B

ANOVA[a]

Model		Sum of Squares	df	Mean Square	F	Sig.
1	Regression	14.726	4	3.681	56.786	.000[b]
	Residual	5.899	91	.065		
	Total	20.625	95			

a. Dependent Variable: AW
b. Predictors: (Constant), Age, P, Family Income (per month), B

Coefficients[a]

Model		Unstandardized Coefficients B	Unstandardized Coefficients Std. Error	Standardized Coefficients Beta	t	Sig.
1	(Constant)	1.140	.188		6.078	.000
	B	.611	.076	.515	8.018	.000
	P	-.214	.057	-.231	-3.739	.000
	Family Income (per month)	-.120	.019	-.376	-6.280	.000
	Age	.006	.020	.019	.323	.748

a. Dependent Variable: AW

In all the cases the independent variables are significantly impacting the dependent variable at 99% level of significance which can be checked in the "sig." column of Coefficients table except:

- In case 2, age and benefits are not significant i.e., not less than .01 and hence we accept the null hypothesis that age and benefits do not significantly impact the adoption.
- Similar is the case in case 3, where Age is not significantly impacting awareness level.

The three regressions under the model are also found to be good fit which can be checked through the value of R square.

4.4. Frequency Analysis

Frequency analysis is a statistical technique used to analyse the distribution of values or events in a dataset. It is commonly applied to predict the likelihood of different values occurring within a variable phenomenon and to assess the reliability of such predictions.

4.4.1 To Assess the Extent of Awareness Among People in Rural Areas of Delhi NCR Region Digital Healthcare-Based Schemes

Figure 9. Frequency Table, Awareness
Source: Author's Calculation

Frequency Table			
Awareness	Yes	No	Total
About ABDHM	12	48	60
About PM-JAY	6	54	60
Have ABHA cards	6	54	60

Majority of the sample did not have awareness about any of the above-mentioned schemes and its features.

4.4.2 To Assess the Extent of Awareness Among People in Urban Areas of Delhi NCR Region Digital Healthcare-Based Schemes

AW1 – Ayushman Bharat digital mission policy
AW2 – PM-JAY
AW3 – ABHA CARD HOLDERS

Figure 10. Frequency Table: AW1, AW2, AW3
Source: Author's Calculation

Frequency Table

AW1

		Frequency	Percent	Valid Percent	Cumulative Percent
Valid	1	36	100.0	100.0	100.0

AW2

		Frequency	Percent	Valid Percent	Cumulative Percent
Valid	1	24	66.7	66.7	66.7
	2	12	33.3	33.3	100.0
	Total	36	100.0	100.0	

AW3

		Frequency	Percent	Valid Percent	Cumulative Percent
Valid	2	36	100.0	100.0	100.0

To judge awareness through frequency table of AW 1, AW 2, AW 3: 1 depicts Yes & 2 depicts No

4.4.3 To Assess How the Level of Awareness Differs Across People of Different Income and Age Category for Digital Healthcare in Both Rural and Urban Areas of Delhi NCR Region

Figure 11. Frequency Table: Family Income Per Month
Source: Author's Calculation

Frequency Table

Family Income (per month)

		Frequency	Percent	Valid Percent	Cumulative Percent
Valid	1	60	62.5	62.5	62.5
	4	36	37.5	37.5	100.0
	Total	96	100.0	100.0	

Age

		Frequency	Percent	Valid Percent	Cumulative Percent
Valid	1	24	25.0	25.0	25.0
	2	18	18.8	18.8	43.8
	3	18	18.8	18.8	62.5
	4	24	25.0	25.0	87.5
	5	12	12.5	12.5	100.0
	Total	96	100.0	100.0	

AW

		Frequency	Percent	Valid Percent	Cumulative Percent
Valid	1	30	31.3	31.3	31.3
	2	66	68.8	68.8	100.0
	Total	96	100.0	100.0	

Figure 12. Family Income Categories
Source: Author's Calculation

Family income categories were as follows (in Rs)	Age categories (in yrs.)
1. 0-30,000	18-25
2. 30,000-60,000	25-30
3. 60,000-90,000	30-40
4. 90,000- 1,20,000	40-60
5. 1,20,000- 1,50,000	60 & above

To judge awareness through frequency table of awareness: 1 depicts Yes & 2 depicts No

- The sample studied was divided in two categories, Category 1 in family income was majorly met by rural people and category 4 by urban.
- Majority of people in age categories belonged to 18-25 & 40-60.

4.5 Interpretation

- Objective 1 i.e. "To assess the extent of awareness among people in rural areas of Delhi NCR region towards Digital Healthcare", was checked through frequency analysis which said that majority and 83.3% of the people in survey said that they didn't know about Digital Healthcare based schemes.
- Objective 2 i.e. "To determine how the level of awareness of digital healthcare of the people in urban areas of Delhi NCR region influences their intention to adopt it", showed that in urban areas, 100% were aware about ABDM but 100% of the people in the sample were ABHA card holders and 66.7% were unaware about PM-JAY and the provisions and benefits offered by it.
- Objective 3 & 4 i.e. "To determine various factors affecting the adoption behaviour of the urban areas of people in Delhi NCR region towards digital healthcare", Feasibility of the factors' determining adoption was checked through correlation and factor analysis methods of statistics. Then the factors that significantly impact adoption was seen through Regression analysis. The factors significantly impacting adoption were family income in socio economic factors and, awareness, and perception of the people for digital healthcare-based schemes. Age in socio-economic factors and benefits of the policies did not have a significant impact on Adoption.
- Objective 5 i.e. "To assess the perception/attitude of the people of varying age groups in the urban areas of Delhi NCR region to adopt digital healthcare" was analysed as, that perception significantly impacted adoption but Adoption and perception are seen to be negatively correlated and having an inverse relationship. People had a lack of faith, trust issues to adopt the digital platforms when it came to their healthcare and hence did not adopt them.
- For Objective 6 & 7 i.e. "To assess how level of awareness differs across people of different income and age category for digital healthcare in both rural and urban areas of Delhi NCR region" the analysis was as follows:
  - i) 31.3% of the people who were aware about the Digital Healthcare based schemes came from the age category of 18-25 & 30-40 and family income ranges from ₹ 0-30,000 which belonged to rural areas.
    - (ii) 68.8% of the people belonging to rest of the age group and income categories taken into consideration and were not aware Digital Healthcare based schemes.

5. CONCLUSION AND RECOMMENDATIONS

5.1 Summary of the Findings

The study aimed to assess public awareness and adoption of Digital Healthcare-based schemes, including ABDM, eSanjeevani, and PM-JAY provisions. The findings revealed significant lack of awareness in both rural and urban areas of Delhi NCR. In rural areas, 83.3% of respondents were unaware of Digital

Healthcare-based schemes. In urban areas, while 100% were aware of ABDM, 66.7% lacked awareness of PM-JAY and its benefits, despite holding ABHA cards.

Awareness varied across family income and age categories. For those aware, 31.3% belonged to the age group of 18-25 & 30-40 with a family income of ₹0-30,000 in rural areas. Factors influencing adoption, determined through correlation and factor analysis, were family income, awareness, and perception of digital healthcare-based schemes. Regression analysis confirmed these factors significantly impacting adoption.

5.2 Implications to the Findings

Awareness was analysed to be lacking in rural areas for Digital Healthcare schemes. Till now, there has also not been a detailed examination of the factors influencing awareness of the schemes and its eligibility in India. Moreover, among those who knew about the mentioned schemes, less than 80% knew they were eligible which implies that the communication channels are not effective. There is a necessity for more effective awareness campaigns, especially for vulnerable groups, to provide clear and detailed information about available benefits. The findings suggest a negative impact of insufficient awareness on the schemes. Education was found to influence the awareness which was further linked to the state of residence. Household wealth impacted eligibility knowledge, consistent with other studies on education and wealth gradients in health insurance awareness.

Lack of awareness in urban areas is possibly because of no proper dissemination of information, digital divide, Technical Jargons of government information and ineffective communication channels. This further leads to wastage of resources, financial strain on people that were targeted but still unaware, Increased burden on healthcare facilities and thus diminished public health impact.

Perception was found to play an active role when it came to adoption of Digital Healthcare schemes of the Government especially in urban areas which implies that this section of the population has somewhat negative perception of the benefits offered by Government for public Healthcare. They find such initiative irrelevant and have a distrust when it comes to their adoption. They always have the availability of private alternative options and want to avoid the Bureaucratic hurdles.

Awareness for public healthcare schemes differing in different ages and income category imply that tailored communication strategies are needed to be used, socio economic disparities are need to be bridged so that individuals are equally informed; educational initiatives focused on specific age groups or income brackets should be introduced; Accessibility challenges are need to be catered to; policy adjustments to address specific challenges faced by different age groups or income categories and to introduce Inclusive outreach programmes.

5.3 Discussion

The lower awareness of government schemes in rural areas as compared to urban areas stems from factors such as limited access to communication channels like television and internet, educational disparities leading to reduced proactive information-seeking, language barriers in official communications, a digital divide hindering online outreach, infrastructure challenges for effective distribution, lesser community engagement and support structures, limited direct government engagement in rural areas, and economic disparities focusing attention on immediate survival needs rather than seeking information about government initiatives (Parisi & Jain, 2022).

The lower adoption of government policies in urban areas, despite awareness, can be attributed to various factors. Firstly, urban residents may perceive the policies as less relevant to their immediate needs or fail to see immediate benefits, leading to a diminished motivation to adopt. Trust issues in government institutions and scepticism about policy effectiveness contribute to a hesitancy among urban populations to embrace these initiatives. Cumbersome bureaucratic processes, red tape, and complicated application procedures further discourage active adoption by urban residents. The presence of diverse and competing priorities in urban lifestyles, coupled with the perceived complexity or inconvenience of policy adoption, may result in a lower uptake. Even if there is awareness, communication gaps regarding the adoption process or benefits may persist, contributing to a lack of motivation. Social and cultural factors influencing decision-making in urban settings may also play a role, and these factors might differ from those in rural areas. Additionally, issues in the effective implementation of policies, such as delays or inefficiencies, pose further barriers to active participation and adoption by urban residents (Parisi & Jain, 2022).

Further, the awareness of government schemes can also vary across income and age categories. Higher-income individuals benefit from superior access to information channels such as television, newspapers, and the internet, enabling them to stay well-informed about government initiatives. Moreover, higher levels of education are linked to increased awareness, as individuals with greater incomes and educational attainment actively seek information about these schemes. A digital divide is observed, with younger age groups leveraging online platforms for information, while older individuals, particularly in lower-income brackets, may experience limited familiarity with digital technologies. Occupational differences also contribute, as higher-income individuals employed in sectors with robust information dissemination tend to be more aware of government initiatives. Conversely, those in lower-income categories, often engaged in informal or rural occupations, may have restricted exposure to such information. Additionally, perceived relevance varies across age groups, with younger individuals prioritizing certain schemes related to education, employment, or technology, while older individuals in lower-income groups may prioritize basic needs, perceiving certain schemes as less relevant to their immediate concerns. Understanding these dynamics is crucial for tailoring effective communication strategies and ensuring equitable awareness of government schemes (Parisi & Jain, 2022).

5.4 Recommendations

Digital literacy programmes should be made mandatory at the school level in both government and private schools and colleges. This programme should aim to increase accessibility of the people as to how to go about the important websites and apps and should work towards increasing their awareness, at least towards important areas like healthcare.

- With so much of spur in social media accounts like Instagram, Facebook etc, the advertisements for digital based healthcare schemes should increase on such platforms.
- Collaborate with private sector entities, non-governmental organizations (NGOs), and community groups to amplify the reach of awareness campaigns.
- In metros, hoardings on buses, the awareness can through them can be highly effective.
- Consider providing financial incentives or rewards for individuals or communities that actively participate in and promote government schemes.
- There should be localised campaigns and Customized awareness campaigns to cater to the specific needs and concerns of different regions or demographics.

- Conduct training programs for government officials involved in implementing and promoting schemes. Ensure they have the necessary knowledge and skills to effectively communicate with the public.
- Establish key performance indicators (KPIs) to measure the success of awareness campaigns and adoption rates and accordingly make improvements.

5.5 Limitations of the Study

- Firstly, the region considered for the primary research was just Delhi NCR which does portray the views of the people residing in other states and union territories of the country.
- Secondly, there was time constraint due to other obligations of the researcher.
- Thirdly, lack of suitable source of access to approach people residing in rural areas.
- Lastly, lack of acceptance at the part of the respondents to fill out the questionnaire because of again, lack of trust.

REFERENCES

Acharya, A., & Vellakal, S. (2012). mpact of national health insurance for the poor and the informal sector in low- and middle-income countries. Evidence for Policy and Practice Information and Co-ordinating Centre (EPPI-Centre).

Angell, B. J., Prinja, S., Gupt, A., Jha, V., & Jan, S. (2019). The Ayushman Bharat Pradhan Mantri Jan Arogya Yojana and the path to universal health coverage in India: overcoming the challenges of stewardship and governance in India: overcoming the challenges of stewardship and governance. *PLoS Medicine*, *16*(3), e1002759. doi:10.1371/journal.pmed.1002759 PMID:30845199

Bajaj, S. (2023). *Digital health for all: Importance of digital healthcare in India.* New Delhi: Times of India.

Bakshi, H., Sharma, R., & Kumar, P. (2018). yushman Bharat Initiative (2018): What we stand to gain or lose! *Indian Journal of Community Medicine*, *43*, 63. PMID:29899601

Battineni, E. (2020). Factors affecting the quality and reliability of online health information. *Digital Health, 6.*

Brenner, S. (2023). Government health insurance and spatial peer effects: New evidence from India. *Social Science & Medicine*, 196.

Chowdary, M. (2023). *The Future of Digital Health in India.* https://www.linkedin.com/pulse/future-digital-health-india-promising-trends-watch-meghana-chowdary-1c/

Desai, N. (2023). *Digital Health in India.* Nishith Desai Associates.

Hassan, R. (2023). Digital Health Usage and Awareness among MedicalStudents: A Survey Study. *Open Access Macedonian Journal of Medical Sciences.*

HealthcareRadius. (2021). *Social determinants of health in India.* Retrieved from HealthcareRadius: https://www.healthcareradius.in/uncategorized/29442-social-determinants-of-health-in-india

Indian Express. (2023). *Achievements and challenges of Ayushman Bharat health scheme.* Indian Express.

Jacobs, B., Ir, P., Bigdeli, M., Annear, P. L., & Van Damme, W. (2012). Addressing access barriers to health services: An analytical framework for selecting appropriate interven- tions in low-income Asian countries. *Health Policy and Planning, 27*(4), 288–300. doi:10.1093/heapol/czr038 PMID:21565939

Jain, S. (2020). Healthcare goes mobile: Evolution of teleconsultation and e-pharmacy in new Normal. *EY, 37*(5).

Kanore L, S. S. (2019). A study of awareness about Ayushyaman Bharat Yojana among low income urban families. An exploratory study. *Remarking an Analisation., 4*(1, part 1).

KienyM.BekedamH. (n.d.). Strengthening health systems for universal health coverage and sustainable development. Bulletin of the World Health Organization*, 537*(9).

Lagomarsino, G., & Garabrant, A. (n.d.). Moving towards universal health coverage: Health insurance reforms in nine developing countries in Africa and Asia. *Lancet*, 380. doi:10.1016/S0140-6736(12)61147-7 PMID:22959390

Maheshwari, T. (2023). *Business outlook and money.* Retrieved from Healthcare In India: Bridging The Gap Between Innovation And Access: https://business.outlookindia.com/news/healthcare-in-india-bridging-the-gap-between-innovation-and-access

Ministry of Electronics and Information Technology. (2023). *e-shushrut.* Retrieved from Ministry of Electronics and Information Technology Government of India: https://apps.gov.in/content/e-shushrut-hospital-management-information-system

Mouloudj, K., Bouarar, A. C., & Saadaoui, L. (2023). *Factors Influencing the Adoption of Digital Health Apps: An Extended Technology Acceptance Model (TAM).* Integrating Digital Health Strategies for Effective Administration. doi:10.4018/978-1-6684-8337-4.ch007

Myint, C.-Y., & Pavlova, M. (n.d.). A systematic review of the health-financing mechanisms in the Association of Southeast Asian Nations countries and the People's Republic of China: Lessons for the move towards universal health coverage. *PLoS One*, 14. doi:10.1371/journal.pone.0217278 PMID:31199815

National Informatics Centre. (2024). *eHospital.* Retrieved from NIC: https://www.nic.in/products/e-hospital/

Parisi, D., & Jain, N. (2022). *Awareness of India's national health insurance scheme (PM-JAY): a cross-sectional study across six states.* Oxford.

Pennep. (2023). *Digital Healthcare in India: Challenges and Opportunities for Transformation.* Retrieved from https://www.linkedin.com/pulse/digital-healthcare-india-challenges-opportunities-transformation/

Perappadan, B. S. (2023). *Digital innovations in healthcare must be for public good: PM Modi.* Retrieved from The Hindu: https://www.thehindu.com/news/national/open-innovations-for-public-good-pm-tells-g-20-health-ministers/article67209733.ece

PIB. (2020). *A study of awareness about Ayushyaman Bharat Yojana among low income urban families. An exploratory study*. Retrieved from PRESS INFO BEUARUE: https://pib.gov.in/newsite/Printrelease.aspx?relid=159376#:~:text=The%20primary%20aim%20of%20the,of%20good%20health%20through%20cross

PIB. (2022). *Addressing access barriers to health services: an analytical framework for selecting appropriate interventions in low-income Asian countries. Health Policy and Planning*. Retrieved from Press Information Beaureu: https://pib.gov.in/PressReleaseIframePage.aspx?PRID=1809569

Rakheja. (2023). *Five Years of AB-PMJAY*. Retrieved from Drishti IAS: https://www.drishtiias.com/daily-updates/daily-news-editorials/five-years-of-ab-pmjay

Ranganathan, S. (2020). *Towards a Holistic Digital Health Ecosystem in India.* Retrieved from ORF ISSUE BRIEF: https://www.orfonline.org/wp-content/uploads/2020/04/ORF_IssueBrief_351_Digital_Health.pdf

Rao, N. (2022). Understanding and information failures: Lessons from a health microinsurance program in India. *Health Policy and Planning*, *38*(3).

Reddy N, B. Y. (2020). Awareness and readiness of health care workers in implementing Pradhan Mantri Jan Arogya Yojana in a tertiary care hospital at Rishikesh. *Nepal Journal of Epidemiology, 32*(4).

Safavi, K., & Michel, B. (2021). *Digital adoption: Reaction or revolution?* Accenture.

Sen, A. (2008). Why and how is health a human right? *Lancet Journal, 372*(9655).

Shetty, D. (2023). Future Of Health Policy. In *India: Trends And Predictions*. Indian School of Public Policy.

Smith, O. D. D. (2019). *PM-JAY across India's states need and utilization PM-JAY policy brief 2*. National Health Authority.

Sriwastva, S. (2023). Implementation of PM-JAY in India: a qualitative study exploring the role of competency, organizational and leadership drivers shaping early roll-out of publicly funded health insurance in three Indian states. *Health Research Policy and Systems, 21*(65).

Stakeholders In Indian Healthcare Sector 2023: An Overview. (2023). Retrieved from Watch doq: https://watchdoq.com/blog/post/stakeholders-in-indian-healthcare-sector-2023:-an-overview

World Health Organization. (n.d.). Leave no one behind: strengthening health systems for UHC and the SDGs in Africa. Brazzaville: WHO Regional Office for Africa.

World Population Review. (2024). Retrieved from world population review: https://worldpopulationreview.com/world-cities/delhi-population

KEY TERMS AND DEFINITIONS

ABHA: The ABHA card, or Ayushman Bharat Health Account card, is a government-issued healthcare ID in India, providing a 14-digit identification number based on mobile and AADHAR numbers.

It serves as a digitalized platform for storing and managing medical history, ensuring easy access to records, consensual sharing with doctors, and maintaining high-security standards. The card enables secure consultations with verified healthcare professionals.

Demographic Factors: It refers to the characteristics of a person/population which are used to describe them. It includes race, age, income, marital status, and education level.

Digital Literacy: It is knowledge and skills required to that enables an individual to effectively and efficiently use digital tools, devices, and platforms.

eHealth: E-Health, also known as electronic health, involves utilizing information and communication technologies (ICT) to enhance and bolster healthcare services. This encompasses a diverse array of applications and services that leverage digital technologies to improve the efficiency and effectiveness of delivering healthcare.

Multicollinearity: It is a situation when independent variables which are used to estimate the dependent variables in a regression model are themselves related to each other. In such a case the analysis or the estimates of the dependent variable are wrong or contains error.

Socioeconomic Factors: It refers to particularly characteristics that tells about the social and economic background of a person. It includes factors such as income, education, employment, community safety and social support.

Universal Health Coverage: It is a situation when all the services related to health, be it checkups, access to medicines, operations related to any kind of disability happened to a person is available to all irrespective of age, caste, gender, race, literacy level.

Chapter 6
Implementation of the Internet of Things (IoT) in Remote Healthcare

Ajay N. Upadhyaya
Department of Computer Engineering, SAL Engineering and Technical Institute, Ahmedabad, India

Asma Saqib
https://orcid.org/0009-0000-0280-5054
Department of Biochemistry, Maharani Cluster University, Bangalore, India

J. Vimala Devi
Department of Computer Science Engineering, Dayananda Sagar College of Engineering, Bengaluru, India

Sreekanth Rallapalli
https://orcid.org/0000-0002-1626-0320
Department of Master of Computer Application, Nitte Meenakshi Institute of Technology, Bengaluru, India

S. Sudha
Department of Master of Computer, Applications Hindustan Institute of Technology and Science, Chennai, India

Sampath Boopathi
https://orcid.org/0000-0002-2065-6539
Muthayammal Engineering College, Namakkal, India

ABSTRACT

Remote patient monitoring is an emerging healthcare technology that uses IoT devices and sensors to monitor patients' health statuses remotely. The healthcare industry holds immense potential for revolutionizing itself through advancements that enhance efficiency, accuracy, and cost-effectiveness in healthcare delivery. These innovations have the power to improve patient outcomes significantly. This conversation discussed the different devices and sensors used in remote patient monitoring, the hardware and software components required for building a remote patient monitoring system, the future developments in IoT technology for remote patient monitoring, and an example programme for remote patient monitoring using an Arduino board. The use of IoT technology in remote patient monitoring has the potential to transform the healthcare industry by providing better healthcare services to patients and healthcare professionals.

DOI: 10.4018/979-8-3693-1934-5.ch006

INTRODUCTION

An Internet of Things (IoT) based remote patient monitoring system can be an effective tool for medical services to remotely monitor patients' health conditions and provide timely interventions. The system can use a combination of sensors, wireless communication technology, and cloud computing to collect, store, and analyze patients' data, and then transmit the information to healthcare professionals.

An IoT-based remote patient monitoring system for home healthcare. The system uses various sensors and a cloud-based platform for data storage and analysis. The authors' evaluation shows the system's reliability and efficiency in remote monitoring, making it a promising approach for improving healthcare delivery (Salunke & Nerkar, 2017). The potential of IoT technology in healthcare management, discussing applications and challenges are explored. It highlights the importance of addressing security, privacy, and interoperability issues, and offers valuable insights for researchers, healthcare professionals, and policymakers (Lv et al., 2021). IoT in healthcare has potential benefits such as improved patient outcomes, but also challenges such as interoperability and security. Systems engineering is suggested to address these challenges (Sharma et al., 2020). The proposed smart lock system uses an ESP8266 Wi-Fi module and an Arduino UNO board to provide secure access control to a room or building. It is able to detect unauthorized access attempts and send real-time notifications to the owner's smartphone. The results show that the proposed system is effective and provides a low-cost solution for secure access control. Overall, the paper provides an interesting application of IoT technology in the field of access control and security (Tao et al., 2019).

The study investigated the association between homocysteine levels and liver fibrosis in a health check-up population. The findings revealed a notable correlation between elevated levels of homocysteine and an increased likelihood of liver fibrosis. This suggests that homocysteine could be a potential biomarker for early detection and prediction of liver fibrosis. The paper provides insight into the role of homocysteine in liver fibrosis and its potential clinical implications for early diagnosis and treatment (Tekeste et al., 2019). This monograph provides a comprehensive account of the Meliaceae family, a group of trees and shrubs found in tropical regions. It is based on extensive fieldwork and botanical research conducted by T.D. Pennington, a renowned botanist and expert on tropical plants. It includes detailed descriptions and illustrations of all known species in the family, as well as information on their distribution, ecology, and economic uses. It also includes sections on the subfamily Swietenioideae and the chemotaxonomy of the family. The monograph is an important reference work for botanists, ecologists, and anyone interested in the flora of tropical regions (Syafa'Ah et al., 2019).

This comprehensive review discusses the advantages and challenges of integrating Internet of Things (IoT) technology in the healthcare industry. It explores the current state-of-the-art technologies and provides an overview of IoT devices used for patient monitoring, including wearable devices, remote patient monitoring systems, and implantable devices. The paper also delves into the latest advancements in IoT-enabled data analytics, machine learning, and artificial intelligence and their applications in healthcare. By examining these topics, the paper offers valuable insights into the future of healthcare IoT and its potential impact on patient care and clinical outcomes. It sheds light on the transformative potential of IoT in improving healthcare delivery, enhancing patient outcomes, and revolutionizing the healthcare industry as a whole (Kassem et al., 2016). The paper titled "An Application of IoT to Develop Concept of Smart Remote Monitoring System" is likely related to the development of a remote monitoring system for patients using IoT technology. It may discuss the features and benefits of the system, as well as its potential applications in healthcare, and provide an overview of the IoT technology used in the system and the challenges associated with its implementation (Solà et al., 2006). This paper presents the design and implementation of a SpO2 sensor embedded in a finger ring. It discusses its advantages and potential applications in medical monitoring and diagnosis, and evaluates its performance in measuring oxygen saturation levels in the blood. The results suggest that the finger ring SpO2 sensor has the potential to provide accurate and continuous monitoring of vital signs in a non-invasive and convenient manner (Bajdor & Starostka-Patyk, 2021). This paper presents a practical implementation of a smart home system using ESP 8266, a low-cost Wi-Fi chip. The system includes an ESP 8266-based NodeMCU microcontroller, sensors, actuators, and an Android application for user interface and control. It can monitor and control various home appliances and provide remote access through a smartphone application. The paper provides detailed information on the hardware and software components and includes experimental results and analysis of the system's performance. It can be useful for researchers and practitioners interested in the development of similar systems (Qadri et al., 2020). The use of hardware-based ciphers to secure data collection in IoT-based healthcare systems illustrated. The authors propose a system that uses a hardware security module to encrypt patient data before transmitting it to a remote server. The results show that the proposed system provides high levels of security while maintaining low latency and energy consumption. Overall, this article provides valuable insights into how hardware-based security solutions can be used to secure healthcare IoT systems (Fernandez & Pallis, 2015). An ultra-low power architecture for detecting the QRS complex, a characteristic waveform of the electrocardiogram (ECG) was done. It is designed to be used in IoT healthcare devices for real-time monitoring of heart health. The system is designed to detect the QRS complex with high accuracy while consuming very little power, enabling long-term monitoring without requiring frequent battery replacement. It is also capable of compressing the ECG signal to reduce the amount of data that needs to be transmitted, enabling efficient data transfer over wireless networks. The proposed architecture was assessed using actual ECG data, and the findings demonstrated its remarkable accuracy, coupled with low power consumption and minimal data transmission rates (Akkaş et al., 2020).

Aforementioned literature survey, there is research activities for implementation of IoT technology for remote health care system. In this chapter, the implementation procedures for Arduino and IoT integrated remote health care system have been elaborately explained. The hardware, and software requirements, logical coding and working principles and challenges and future directions to extend the present research have been elaborated.

IOT DEVICES FOR REMOTE MONITORING PROCESS

There are various devices that can be used in a remote patient monitoring system. Here is a list of some common devices (Salunke & Nerkar, 2017):

A blood pressure monitor is used to measure the force of blood against the walls of arteries, which can help monitor and manage hypertension, heart disease, and other conditions. A glucose monitor is used to measure the level of glucose (sugar) in the blood, a pulse oximeter measures the oxygen saturation level in the blood, an ECG monitor measures the electrical activity of the heart, a temperature monitor measures body temperature, an activity tracker measures physical activity, a remote camera can be used to monitor patients in their home or care facility, a medication dispenser can be used to remind patients to take their medication, a smart pillbox can be used to manage medication schedules and remind patients to take their medication, and a weight scale is used to measure body weight (Boopathi, 2019; Sathish et al., 2023). By connecting these devices to a centralized monitoring system, healthcare providers can receive real-time data, allowing them to remotely monitor and manage patients' health conditions. This setup enables timely interventions to be provided as needed, ensuring effective healthcare delivery and improved patient outcomes. These devices include spirometers, fall detection sensors, blood oxygen monitors, continuous glucose monitoring systems, heart rate monitors, body composition analyzers, blood coagulation monitors, and telehealth platforms. Spirometers measure lung function by measuring the amount of air a patient can exhale and the speed at which they can exhale it (Boopathi, 2023c; Karthik et al., 2023).

Various types of medical devices and sensors play a crucial role in monitoring and assessing patients' health. Fall detection sensors are designed to detect falls in elderly or vulnerable individuals, ensuring prompt assistance is provided. Blood oxygen monitors measure the oxygen saturation levels in the blood, helping to monitor respiratory health. Continuous glucose monitoring systems enable the continuous monitoring of glucose levels, offering valuable insights for diabetes management. Heart rate monitors track the heart rate, providing information about cardiovascular health (Reddy et al., 2023a; Subha, Inbamalar, Komala, et al., 2023). Body composition analyzers help determine the proportion of body fat, muscle mass, and water content, aiding in assessing overall body composition. Lastly, blood coagulation monitors measure the clotting time of blood, assisting in monitoring coagulation disorders. These devices collectively contribute to comprehensive health monitoring and facilitate timely interventions when necessary. Telehealth platforms enable remote consultations between healthcare providers and patients, providing advice, and prescribing medication.

The selection of devices for a remote patient monitoring system depends on various factors, including the patient's health condition, the specific requirements of healthcare providers, and the availability of different devices. The choice of devices is tailored to meet the unique needs of each patient and to ensure effective monitoring and management of their health remotely.

List Various Health Check-Up Parameters

Health check-up parameters can vary depending on the type and purpose of the check-up, the patient's age and gender, and their medical history(Lv et al., 2021). However, some common health check-up parameters are illustrated in Figure 1 and discussed below:

Figure 1. Various Health-Check Parameters

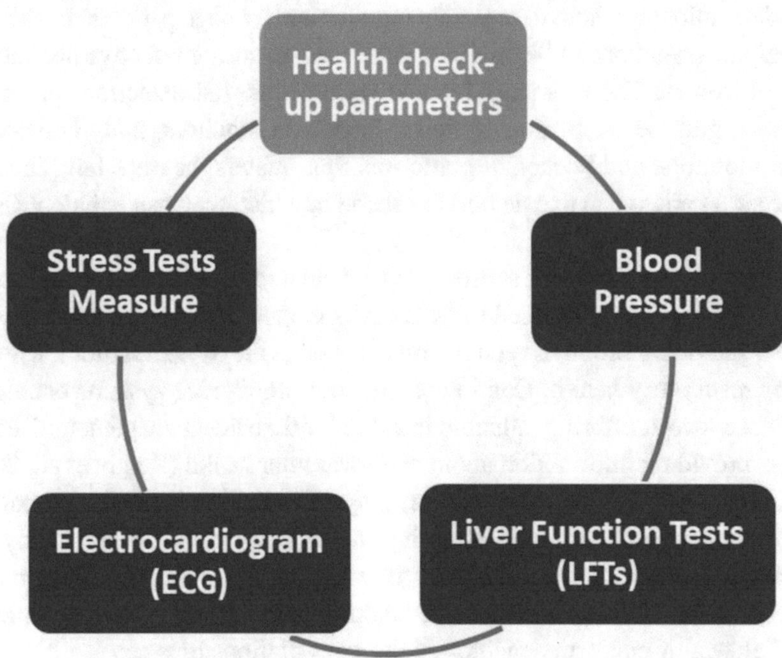

Blood pressure plays a vital role in assessing cardiovascular health, while body mass index (BMI) quantifies body fat based on height and weight. Blood sugar levels serve as significant indicators of diabetes and metabolic health. Lipid profile measurements provide insights into cholesterol, triglyceride, and other fat levels in the bloodstream. Additionally, a complete blood count (CBC) determines the quantities of various blood components, including red blood cells, white blood cells, and platelets.

Liver function tests (LFTs) measure the levels of various enzymes and proteins produced by the liver. These tests can be used to diagnose and monitor liver disease, such as hepatitis, cirrhosis, and liver cancer. Kidney function tests measure the levels of various substances, such as creatinine and urea, in the blood. These tests can be used to diagnose and monitor kidney disease, such as chronic kidney disease and acute kidney injury. Thyroid function tests measure the levels of thyroid hormones and other substances produced by the thyroid gland. These tests can be used to diagnose and monitor thyroid disorders, such as hypothyroidism and hyperthyroidism. Bone density tests measure the density of bones and can be used to diagnose and monitor osteoporosis and other bone-related conditions. These tests can also be used to assess the risk of fracture. Cancer screening tests can be used to detect early signs of cancer and improve treatment outcomes. These tests include mammograms, colonoscopies, and Pap tests (Boopathi, Khare, et al., 2023; Pramila et al., 2023).

An electrocardiogram (ECG) is a diagnostic tool that records the electrical activity of the heart, enabling the diagnosis and monitoring of heart conditions. Pulmonary function tests (PFTs) measure lung function and help assess respiratory health. Blood tests are utilized to diagnose and monitor a wide range of medical conditions. They can assess vitamin and mineral levels, detect sexually transmitted infections (STIs), evaluate cognitive function, conduct stress tests, perform genetic testing, analyze sleep patterns, assess mental health, evaluate physical fitness, determine vaccination status, conduct hearing and vision tests, assess dental health, examine bone and joint health, determine blood type and Rh factor, and facilitate transfusion procedures. These tests measure the levels of various vitamins and minerals in the body, such as vitamin D, B12, and iron. STI tests can be used to detect infections, such as chlamydia, gonorrhea, and HIV, and improve treatment outcomes. Cognitive function tests can be used to assess memory, attention, and other cognitive abilities and detect early signs of cognitive decline (Anitha, Komala, et al., 2023; Subha, Inbamalar, Komala, et al., 2023).

Stress tests measure the heart's response to physical stress and can be used to diagnose and monitor heart conditions. Genetic tests can be used to detect inherited genetic mutations and assess the risk of developing certain medical conditions. Sleep studies can be used to assess the quality and quantity of sleep and diagnose sleep-related disorders. Mental health assessments can be used to assess symptoms of mental health conditions and develop treatment plans.

IoT Devices for Remote Monitoring System

There are several IoT devices that can be used in a remote patient monitoring system, including (Sharma et al., 2020): Wearable sensors encompass a range of devices, including fitness trackers, smartwatches, and health monitors, which are capable of gathering data on vital signs, activity levels, and other health-related metrics. Vital sign monitors are designed to measure essential signs such as blood pressure, heart rate, oxygen saturation, and respiratory rate. These monitors can transmit the collected data to healthcare providers, enabling remote monitoring of patients' health. Glucose monitors, specifically tailored for individuals with diabetes, measure blood sugar levels and transmit the data to healthcare providers for remote monitoring and effective management of the condition. Medication trackers serve as reminders for patients to take their medications and help track adherence to medication regimens. Telehealth equipment can enable remote consultations with healthcare providers and specialists.

Remote monitoring systems can track patients' health metrics, such as weight, blood pressure, and blood glucose levels, and alert healthcare providers when values fall outside of acceptable ranges. Smart pill bottles can track medication usage and alert patients and healthcare providers when medications need to be refilled or doses are missed. Activity trackers can measure physical activity and provide insights into daily exercise and movement patterns. ECG monitors can measure electrical activity in the heart and detect abnormalities, such as arrhythmias and heart blockages. Body temperature monitors can measure The use of IoT devices in a remote patient monitoring system can provide real-time data on patients' health metrics, medication adherence, and activity levels.

Wearable devices, such as fall detection sensors, smart blood pressure monitors, smart thermometers, and smart inhalers, have the potential to revolutionize healthcare delivery. These devices enable more personalized and effective care, reducing the need for in-person visits while improving patient outcomes. Fall detection sensors promptly detect falls or accidents and alert healthcare providers or caregivers for immediate assistance. Smart blood pressure monitors provide real-time data for remote monitoring and management of hypertension or other heart conditions. Smart thermometers measure body temperature, providing insights into fever or signs of infection. Smart inhalers for asthma monitor usage patterns, aiding in the management of the condition. Overall, these devices enhance healthcare accessibility, enable remote monitoring, and contribute to improved patient care.

Smart glucose meters can measure blood sugar levels and provide real-time data to healthcare providers for remote monitoring and management of diabetes. Smart pacemakers can measure heart activity and provide real-time data to healthcare providers for remote monitoring and management of heart conditions. Smart hearing aids can adjust to ambient sound levels and improve hearing quality. Smart contact lenses can measure glucose levels in tears and provide real-time data to healthcare providers for remote monitoring and management of diabetes.

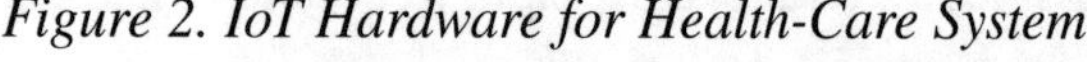

Figure 2. IoT Hardware for Health-Care System

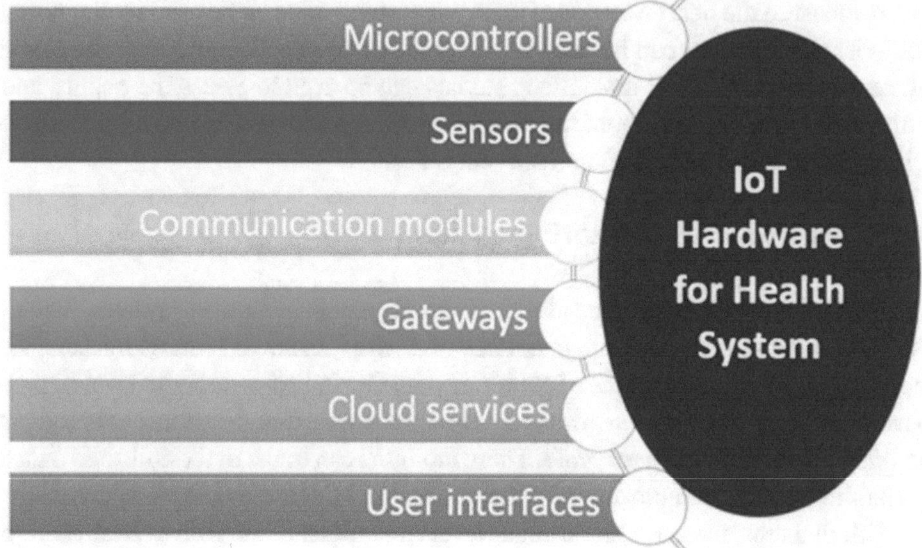

IoT HARDWARE

There are several types of IoT hardware that can be used for remote monitoring of health parameters (Lv et al., 2021; Sharma et al., 2020): The various IOT hardware used in the health care applications are shown in Figure 2.

Microcontrollers: Microcontrollers are small, low-power devices that can control and process data from sensors, communicate with other devices, and interact with cloud services. They are commonly used in IoT systems to collect data from sensors and transmit it to the cloud for processing and storage (Boopathi, 2023c; Samikannu et al., 2023; Syamala et al., 2023).

Sensors: Sensors are devices that can measure physical or environmental parameters, such as temperature, humidity, light, sound, or motion. They can be integrated with microcontrollers to provide real-time data for remote monitoring and analysis (Chandra Saha et al., n.d.).

Communication modules: Communication modules, such as Wi-Fi, Bluetooth, or cellular modules, can be integrated with microcontrollers to enable data transmission and remote control. They can also be used to receive commands and alerts from cloud services or other devices (Koshariya et al., 2023).

Gateways: Gateways are devices that can collect data from multiple sensors or devices and send it to the cloud for processing and storage. They can also perform local processing and analysis of data before transmitting it to the cloud.

Cloud services: Cloud services provide a platform for data storage, processing, and analysis. They can receive data from IoT devices and perform analytics to provide insights and alerts to healthcare providers or patients (Rahamathunnisa et al., 2023; Venkateswaran, Vidhya, Ayyannan, et al., 2023).

User interfaces: User interfaces, such as mobile apps, web portals, or dashboards, can be used to display data and insights from IoT devices and cloud services. They can provide real-time monitoring and alerts to healthcare providers or patients, as well as enable remote control of devices and treatment plans.

Overall, the use of IoT hardware for remote monitoring of health parameters can enable real-time data collection and analysis, remote control and treatment, and improve patient outcomes and engagement. By leveraging the power of microcontrollers, sensors, communication modules, gateways, cloud services, and user interfaces, healthcare providers can develop personalized and effective treatment plans for their patients.

Various Remote Patient Testing's

Remote patient testing refers to the collection of medical data or biological samples from patients in a remote location, which can then be analyzed by healthcare providers for diagnosis, monitoring, or treatment (Boopathi, 2022; Darshan & Anandakumar, 2015; Tao et al., 2019; Thibaud et al., 2018; Xu, 2020). The significant remote patients' testing are illustrated in Figure 3.

Remote blood tests: Home test kits or wearable devices empower patients to collect blood samples for various tests, including blood glucose, cholesterol, or hemoglobin A1C. These samples can be conveniently sent to a laboratory for analysis, and the results can then be shared with healthcare providers. This facilitates the monitoring and management of chronic conditions like diabetes, allowing for proactive healthcare interventions based on accurate and up-to-date information (Boopathi, 2023b).

Figure 3. Various Tests for the Remote Patients

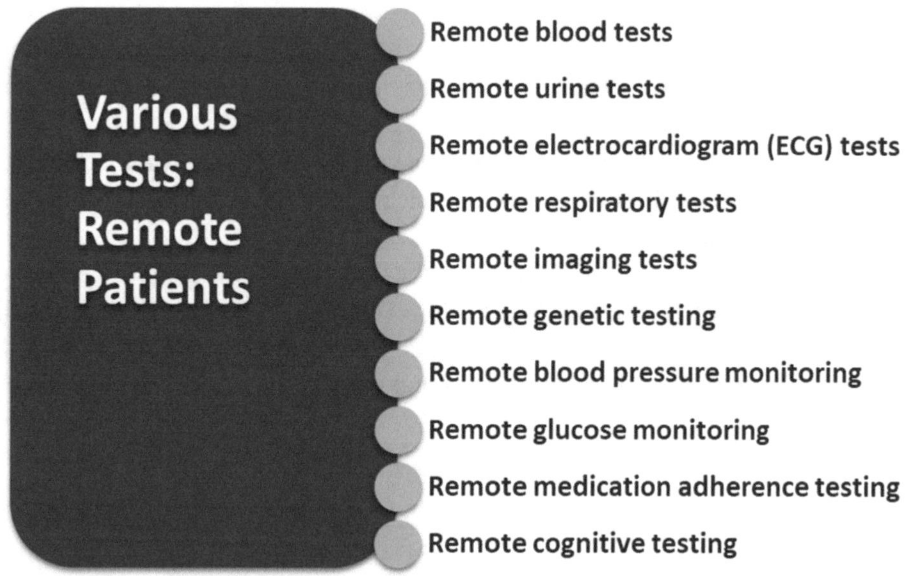

Remote urine tests: Home test kits enable patients to collect urine samples for a variety of tests, including pregnancy, urinary tract infections, or kidney function. These samples can be conveniently sent to a laboratory for thorough analysis, and the resulting findings can be provided to healthcare providers. This facilitates accurate diagnosis and appropriate treatment of various conditions based on reliable test results.

Remote respiratory tests: By utilizing home test kits or wearable devices, patients have the capability to collect data on respiratory parameters like lung capacity, oxygen saturation, or respiratory rate. This collected data can then be transmitted to healthcare providers, enabling them to monitor and effectively manage conditions such as asthma or chronic obstructive pulmonary disease (COPD). This remote monitoring approach allows for proactive interventions and personalized care to optimize respiratory health.

Remote electrocardiogram (ecg) tests: Patients can use wearable devices or smartphone apps to collect ECG data, which can be transmitted to healthcare providers for monitoring and management of heart conditions such as arrhythmias.

Remote imaging tests: Patients can use telemedicine platforms or mobile apps to transmit images such as X-rays, CT scans, or ultrasounds to healthcare providers for diagnosis and treatment.

Remote patient testing can provide several benefits, including increased patient convenience, reduced healthcare costs, and improved access to care, especially for patients who live in rural or remote areas. However, it is important to ensure that the testing devices or kits are accurate and reliable, and that the data is transmitted securely to protect patient privacy.

Remote genetic testing: Patients can use home test kits to collect DNA samples, which can be sent to a laboratory for analysis. Genetic testing can help identify the risk of inherited conditions, provide personalized treatment options, or inform lifestyle and preventive measures.

Remote blood pressure monitoring: Patients can use wearable devices or home monitors to collect blood pressure data, which can be transmitted to healthcare providers for monitoring and management of hypertension.

Remote glucose monitoring: Patients with diabetes can use wearable devices or continuous glucose monitors to collect glucose data, which can be transmitted to healthcare providers for monitoring and management of blood sugar levels.

Remote medication adherence testing: Patients can use electronic pill dispensers or smart medication bottles to track medication adherence, which can be transmitted to healthcare providers for monitoring and management of chronic conditions.

Remote cognitive testing: Patients can use smartphone apps or computer-based tests to assess cognitive function, which can be used for diagnosis and management of conditions such as Alzheimer's disease or traumatic brain injury.

Remote patient testing can help reduce the burden on healthcare facilities, improve patient outcomes, and increase patient engagement in their own care. However, it is important to ensure that the testing devices or kits are reliable and accurate, and that the data is transmitted securely to protect patient privacy. It is also important to provide clear instructions and support for patients to ensure proper use of the testing devices or kits.

Figure 4. Hardware and Software Components for the Health-Care Applications

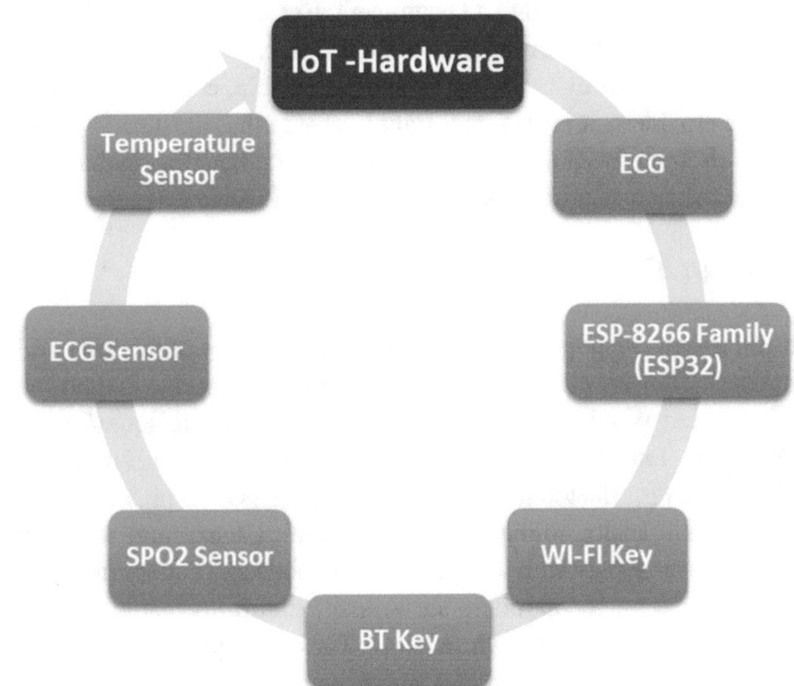

IoT: HARDWARE FOR THE HEALTH-CARE APPLICATIONS

The primary components and their functions of IoT-hardware are explained as given below and depicted in the Figure 4.

ECG

Various hardware options can be employed for remote ECG testing, depending on the specific system or device being utilized. Here are some examples of hardware commonly used for remote ECG testing (Tekeste et al., 2019):

Wearable ecg monitors: These devices are worn on the body and can continuously monitor heart activity, providing data on heart rate, rhythm, and other parameters. Examples of wearable ECG monitors include wrist-worn devices like the Apple Watch or chest strap monitors like the Polar H10.

Portable ECG machines: These devices are small and portable and can be used to take ECG readings in a remote location. Examples of portable ECG machines include the AliveCor Kardia Mobile or the Omron Heart Guide.

Smartphone apps: Some smartphone apps can use the phone's camera and flash to take ECG readings by placing a finger on the camera lens. Examples of smartphone apps include the AliveCor Kardia app or the Instant Heart Rate app.

Telemedicine platforms: Some telemedicine platforms allow healthcare providers to remotely access ECG data from patients using specialized ECG equipment. Examples of telemedicine platforms include the Philips ECG Management System or the BioTelemetry ePatch.

The hardware used for remote ECG testing should be reliable, accurate, and easy to use for both patients and healthcare providers. It is also important to ensure that the data is transmitted securely to protect patient privacy. Remote ECG testing can provide several benefits, including early detection of heart conditions, better management of chronic conditions, and increased patient convenience.

Esp-8266 Family (esp32)

The ESP8266 and ESP32 are two popular members of the ESP family of microcontrollers and wireless communication modules. They are commonly used in IoT applications due to their low cost, low power consumption, and integrated Wi-Fi and Bluetooth capabilities. Here are some hardware details of the ESP8266 and ESP32: The Tensilica LX6 is a 32-bit RISC processor with up to 240 MHz memory, 802.11 b/g/n Wi-Fi transceiver, Bluetooth v4.2 and BLE support, GPIO pins with PWM, I2C, SPI, and UART interfaces, two 12-bit analog-to-digital converters with a maximum sampling rate of 2 Msps, and a 2.2V to 3.6V DC power supply with low-power sleep mode and battery management capabilities.

The ESP8266 and ESP32 microcontrollers are versatile platforms that can be programmed using the Arduino IDE or other development environments. These platforms have extensive support from open-source libraries and projects, enabling developers to explore various IoT applications. They find applications in diverse areas such as remote monitoring, home automation, and robotics, showcasing their flexibility and potential for innovative projects.

WI-FI Key

A Wi-Fi key is a sequence of characters used to secure a wireless network. It is set by the network administrator and can be between 8 and 63 characters long. To connect to a Wi-Fi network, the user must enter the key when prompted. It is important to keep the Wi-Fi key secure and not share it with unauthorized users, and to change it periodically to maintain the security of the network.

BT Key

A BT key is a security feature used to authenticate and encrypt communications between Bluetooth-enabled devices. It is generated by one device and shared with the other during the pairing process. The key is usually a string of random characters that is difficult to guess or predict. It is important to keep the BT key secure and not share it with unauthorized users, as if it is compromised, an attacker may be able to intercept or manipulate the communication between the devices (Abouelmehdi et al., 2018).

SPO2 Sensor

An SPO2 sensor is a medical device designed to measure the oxygen saturation level in an individual's blood. It operates by emitting light into the body and analyzing the absorption of light by the hemoglobin present in the blood. This allows for the accurate assessment of oxygen saturation levels, providing critical insights into a person's respiratory and circulatory health. The sensor is non-invasive and painless, and can be attached to a patient's finger, toe, or earlobe using a clip or adhesive. It is an important tool for monitoring the respiratory status of patients with respiratory conditions, as well as during surgery or other medical procedures (Syafa'Ah et al., 2019).

ECG Sensor

An ECG sensor, short for electrocardiogram sensor, is a medical device that records and measures the electrical activity of the heart. It consists of electrodes that are placed on specific areas of the body to detect and capture the electrical signals generated by the heart muscle. These signals are then amplified and converted into visual representations called electrocardiograms. ECG sensors are commonly used for diagnosing various heart conditions, assessing heart rate and rhythm, monitoring cardiac health during exercise or physical activity, and evaluating the effectiveness of heart medications or interventions.

Health Temperature Sensor

A health temperature sensor is a medical device that measures a person's body temperature. It can be used to monitor a person's body temperature continuously or periodically over a period of time, and is commonly used in hospitals, clinics, and home healthcare settings to monitor the temperature of patients with fever, infection, or other medical conditions. It is non-invasive and painless, and can provide accurate and reliable temperature readings.

IoT SOFTWARE

Eagle

Eagle is a PCB (Printed Circuit Board) design software that is used to create schematics and layouts for electronic circuits. It is a popular software tool among electronics engineers and hobbyists for designing and prototyping IoT (Internet of Things) devices and other electronic projects (Kassem et al., 2016). Eagle offers users a user-friendly interface that simplifies the process of creating and modifying schematics and PCB layouts. The software includes a vast library of electronic components, including sensors, microcontrollers, and wireless modules, which can be easily added to a project. Eagle also includes features such as Design Rule Checking (DRC), which helps ensure that the circuit design meets manufacturing specifications and can be fabricated correctly. It also includes a 3D visualization tool that allows users to visualize their designs in a three-dimensional view3D (Boopathi, Khare, et al., 2023; Senthil et al., 2023).

Eagle supports a range of file formats, including Gerber files, which are used for manufacturing PCBs, and BOM (Bill of Materials) files, which are used to generate a list of components needed for a project. It also supports integration with other software tools, such as SPICE (Simulation Program with Integrated Circuit Emphasis) simulators and firmware development tools.

Arduino IDE

The Arduino Integrated Development Environment (IDE) has found valuable applications in the healthcare sector. With its user-friendly interface and extensive library support, the Arduino IDE enables developers to create innovative healthcare solutions. It can be utilized for prototyping and developing various medical devices and systems, such as patient monitoring devices, biomedical sensors, assistive technologies, and remote health monitoring systems. The Arduino IDE's flexibility and compatibility with Arduino microcontrollers make it accessible for healthcare professionals and researchers to design and implement cost-effective and customized solutions that improve patient care, enhance diagnostics, and facilitate medical research in diverse healthcare settings (Anitha, R, et al., 2023; Babu et al., 2023; Boopathi, Arigela, et al., 2023; Jeevanantham et al., 2023; Subha, Inbamalar, R, et al., 2023).

Thing Speak (Web API Platform)

ThingSpeak, an IoT platform, can be leveraged in healthcare to collect, analyze, and visualize patient data, enabling remote monitoring, personalized care, and data-driven healthcare interventions (Solà et al., 2006). ThingSpeak provides a range of features, including data logging, data visualization, and real-time analytics. Users can create custom dashboards and charts to visualize data, and can use the platform's built-in analytics tools to gain insights into patterns and trends in the data. ThingSpeak also provides integration with other software tools, including MATLAB, which allows users to perform advanced analysis and modeling on the data. It also provides integration with other IoT platforms, such as IFTTT (If This Then That), which allows users to automate actions based on data from connected devices. Thus, ThingSpeak is a powerful and versatile platform for IoT applications (Reddy et al., 2023b).

Bulk SMS Service

Bulk SMS Service allows businesses and organizations to send text messages in bulk.

i. Bulk SMS Service typically works by integrating with an SMS gateway provider, which provides the infrastructure for sending and receiving text messages. The software allows users to upload a list of phone numbers and a message to be sent, and then sends the message to each recipient on the list.
ii. Bulk SMS Service allows users to schedule messages and personalize them.
iii. The service may also include analytics and reporting features, which allow users to track the performance of their SMS campaigns, including delivery rates, open rates, and click-through rates.

Thus, Bulk SMS Service is a powerful tool for businesses and organizations that need to send text messages in bulk. It can help improve communication with customers and clients, increase engagement and conversions, and streamline the process of sending important updates and notifications (Bajdor & Starostka-Patyk, 2021).

Figure 5. Working Flow of IoT integrated Remote Monitoring System

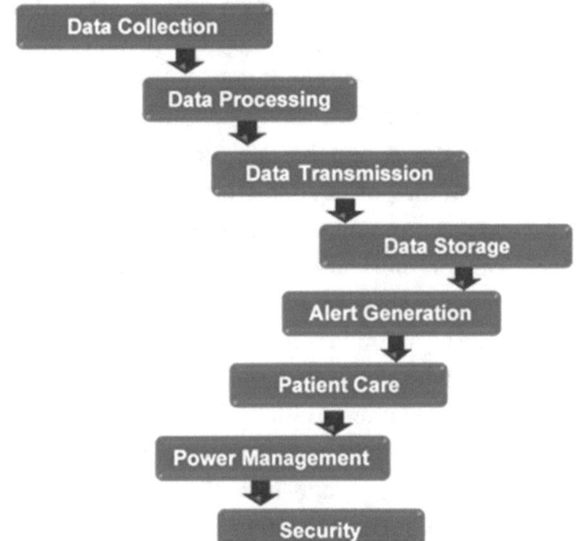

Working Principle

The working procedure of the IoT integrated remote monitoring system is illustrated in Figure 5 and elaborated as below (Anitha, R, et al., 2023; Jeevanantham et al., 2023; Saravanan et al., 2022; Subha, Inbamalar, R, et al., 2023).

Data collection: Data collection is the process of gathering health-related information from a patient's body using sensors and devices. This data is then sent to a microcontroller or microprocessor, which acts as the central hub of the system.

Data processing: Once the data is collected, it needs to be processed in order to be useful. This involves performing various tasks, such as filtering out noise and other unwanted signals, amplifying the signal, and digitizing the data so that it can be transmitted and stored more easily. The microcontroller or microprocessor is responsible for performing these tasks.

Data transmission: Data is transmitted to a cloud server or centralized database using various communication protocols, depending on the distance between the patient and the server, the amount of data being transmitted, and the level of security required.

Data storage: Remote monitoring data is stored in a cloud server or centralized database, allowing healthcare professionals and caregivers to access it from anywhere, at any time, using a computer or mobile device.

Data analysis: Data analytics tools and techniques can be used to identify patterns and trends, and predict potential health risks and issues. For example, if a patient's heart rate is higher than normal, this could indicate an underlying health problem.

Alert generation: If any health parameter falls outside the normal range, an alert is generated, and healthcare professionals and caregivers are notified through various means, such as SMS, email, or mobile application notifications. This allows for timely intervention and treatment, which can help prevent serious health problems from developing.

Patient care: Based on the data collected, healthcare professionals and caregivers can provide personalized care to the patient, such as adjusting medication dosage, scheduling follow-up appointments, or providing advice on lifestyle changes. This helps to improve patient outcomes and reduce healthcare costs, by preventing unnecessary hospitalizations and interventions.

Power management: The sensors and devices used in a remote monitoring system require a power source in order to function. This can be provided through various means, such as batteries or AC power. However, it is important to ensure that the power supply is reliable and can last for extended periods of time, as the system may need to operate continuously for days or even weeks at a time.

Security: Remote monitoring systems must be secure and protected from unauthorized access through encryption, authentication, and access control, as well as regular software updates and maintenance.

User interface: The user interface of a remote monitoring system is the means by which healthcare professionals and caregivers interact with the system and access the collected data. This can take the form of a mobile application, a web-based interface, or a dashboard. The user interface should be intuitive and easy to use, and should provide relevant and actionable information to the user.

Thus, IoT-integrated remote monitoring systems have the potential to revolutionize healthcare, but must be designed and implemented with reliability, security, and user experience in mind.

Arduino Code for Temperature and ECG Testing

Here is an example program for an IoT-Arduino integrated remote monitoring system that measures temperature and ECG data from a patient and transmits the data to a web server for remote access by healthcare professionals (Deshpande & Kulkarni, 2017; Tekeste et al., 2019; Yang et al., 2016):

- Including Header Functions
- WiFi credentials user name and passwords
- ThingSpeak API credentials: API Key and server information.
- Temperature sensor details
- ECG sensor details Gains, resolution scale factors.
- Setup the programs
- Main Program
    - Read temperature data
    - Read ECG data
    - Send data to ThingSpeak
    - Data sent to ThingSpeak"
    - Error connecting to ThingSpeak"
    - Wait for 10 seconds before sending the next set of data.

Figure 6. Flow Chart for IoT: Program for Remote Health-Care Monitoring

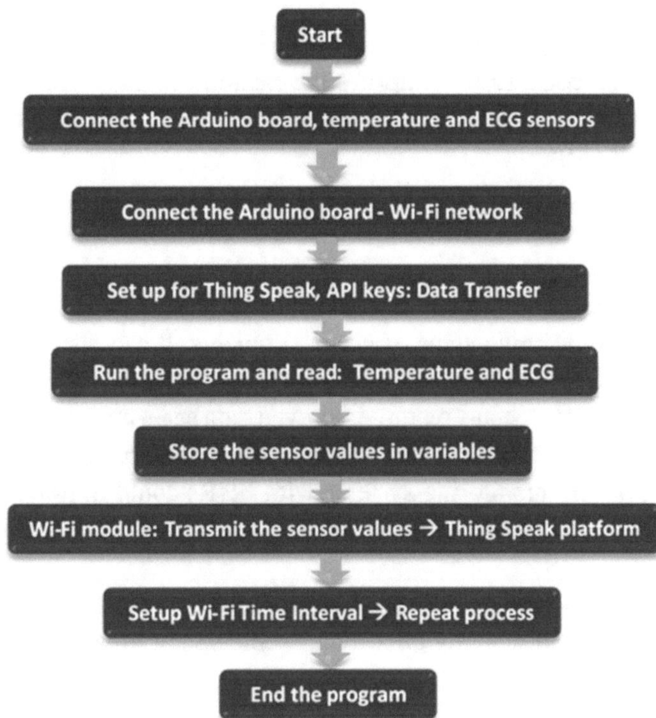

Flow chart for IoT – Program for Remote Health care Monitoring is illustrated in Figure 6. In this program, the ESP32 board is connected to a temperature sensor and an ECG sensor. The temperature sensor uses the Dallas Temperature library to read temperature data from a DS18B20 sensor. The ECG sensor uses the Adafruit_ADS1015 library to read analog voltage data from an ADS1015 analog-to-digital converter.

The program then connects to a Wi-Fi network using the provided credentials, and initializes the sensors. In the loop function, it reads temperature and ECG data from the sensors, and sends the data to ThingSpeak using an HTTP POST request.

Results Obtained From Above Program

The program uses IoT and Arduino to measure and transmit temperature and ECG readings of a patient to a remote location for monitoring and analysis. It uses an Arduino board to read the sensor values and transmit them to a remote server via Wi-Fi. The ThingSpeak platform stores temperature and ECG sensor readings in a channel for remote monitoring and analysis. The results of this program demonstrate the potential of IoT and remote patient monitoring systems for improving healthcare delivery by enabling real-time monitoring and analysis of patient health status. This data can be used for diagnosis and treatment planning.

FUTURE DEVELOPMENTS

The field of IoT technology for remote patient monitoring is rapidly evolving, and there are many potential future developments that could further improve the capabilities and effectiveness of these systems. Some of the most promising areas for future development include (Akkaş et al., 2020; Fernandez & Pallis, 2015; Qadri et al., 2020):

- Wearable devices such as smartwatches and fitness trackers offer a wealth of health-related data, and future developments could include more advanced sensors and improved algorithms.
- AI is becoming increasingly important in healthcare, as it can be used to analyze large quantities of data and detect early warning signs of health problems. It can also alert healthcare providers accordingly (S. et al., 2022; Vanitha et al., 2023).
- Remote patient monitoring systems require improved data security, which could include improved encryption algorithms and more advanced authentication and access control mechanisms.
- Integrating remote patient monitoring systems with EHRs could improve healthcare quality, reduce errors, and improve efficiency by providing a more complete picture of a patient's health status.
- 5G networks offer faster data transfer rates and lower latency, enabling real-time monitoring of patients' health parameters, particularly important in emergency situations (Koshariya et al., 2023).
- Edge computing reduces latency and improves system performance for remote patient monitoring (Boopathi, 2023a; Venkateswaran, Vidhya, Naik, et al., 2023).
- Remote patient monitoring systems can empower patients by providing them with greater control over their own health, with user-friendly interfaces and personalized advice.
- Remote sensing technologies such as satellite imagery and drones can be used to provide additional data for remote patient monitoring systems, such as monitoring changes in the environment and transporting medical supplies.

CONCLUSION

Remote patient monitoring using IoT technology involves collecting, transmitting, analyzing, and notifying healthcare professionals through bulk SMS services. Remote patient monitoring is a revolutionary healthcare technology using IoT devices and sensors to improve efficiency, accuracy, and cost-effectiveness in healthcare services.

Remote patient monitoring utilizes devices and sensors for real-time data collection, providing better insights into patients' conditions. This data-driven approach empowers healthcare professionals to make informed decisions and improve patient outcomes. It reduces the need for in-person visits and offers convenience and comfort for patients with chronic conditions or living in remote areas.

A successful remote patient monitoring system requires a combination of hardware and software components, including IoT devices and sensors, data transmission, storage, and analysis platforms. This integration promotes efficient care management and seamless communication between patients and healthcare providers.

IoT technology advancements in remote patient monitoring offer significant potential. Sensor technology, miniaturization, and connectivity will lead to more sophisticated devices. Artificial intelligence and machine learning algorithms will improve remote monitoring systems, enabling accurate prediction and early detection of health issues. This will result in reduced healthcare costs, improved patient engagement, and proactive interventions in the healthcare industry.

An Arduino-based patient monitoring program demonstrates IoT's versatility in healthcare. It securely transmits vital signs like heart rate, blood pressure, and body temperature to a central database, enabling remote access by healthcare professionals. Alert systems can be set up for critical readings, enabling timely intervention.

Thus, IoT technology in remote patient monitoring has the potential to transform the healthcare industry by offering better services, enhancing patient outcomes, and supporting healthcare professionals in informed decisions. This innovation will lead to improved health outcomes and quality of life for patients worldwide.

REFERENCES

Abouelmehdi, K., Beni-Hessane, A., & Khaloufi, H. (2018). Big healthcare data: Preserving security and privacy. *Journal of Big Data*, *5*(1), 1–18. doi:10.1186/s40537-017-0110-7

Akkaş, M. A., Sokullu, R., & Ertürk Çetin, H. (2020). Healthcare and patient monitoring using IoT. *Internet of Things : Engineering Cyber Physical Human Systems*, *11*, 100173. doi:10.1016/j.iot.2020.100173

Anitha, C., R, K. C., Vivekanand, C. V., Lalitha, S. D., Boopathi, S., & R, Revathi. (2023, February). Artificial Intelligence driven security model for Internet of Medical Things (IoMT). *IEEE Explore*. doi:10.1109/ICIPTM57143.2023.10117713

Anitha, C., Komala, C. R., Vivekanand, C. V., Lalitha, S. D., Boopathi, S., & Revathi, R. (2023). Artificial Intelligence driven security model for Internet of Medical Things (IoMT). *Proceedings of 2023 3rd International Conference on Innovative Practices in Technology and Management, ICIPTM 2023*. 10.1109/ICIPTM57143.2023.10117713

Babu, B. S., Kamalakannan, J., Meenatchi, N., M, S. K. S., S, K., & Boopathi, S. (2023). Economic impacts and reliability evaluation of battery by adopting Electric Vehicle. *IEEE Explore*, 1–6. doi:10.1109/ICPECTS56089.2022.10046786

Bajdor, P., & Starostka-Patyk, M. (2021). The internet of things in healthcare management: Potential applications and challenges. *Smart Healthcare Monitoring Using IoT with 5G. Challenges, Directions, and Future Predictions*, *18*(3), 1–21. doi:10.1201/9781003171829-1

Boopathi, S. (2019). Experimental investigation and parameter analysis of LPG refrigeration system using Taguchi method. *SN Applied Sciences*, *1*(8), 892. Advance online publication. doi:10.1007/s42452-019-0925-2

Boopathi, S. (2022). An Extensive Review on Sustainable Developments of Dry and Near-Dry Electrical Discharge Machining Processes. *Journal of Manufacturing Science and Engineering*, *144*(5), 50801. doi:10.1115/1.4052527

Boopathi, S. (2023a). *Deep Learning Techniques Applied for Automatic Sentence Generation*. doi:10.4018/978-1-6684-3632-5.ch016

Boopathi, S. (2023b). *Internet of Things-Integrated Remote Patient Monitoring System*. doi:10.4018/978-1-6684-6894-4.ch008

Boopathi, S. (2023c). *Securing Healthcare Systems Integrated With IoT*. doi:10.4018/978-1-6684-6894-4.ch010

Boopathi, S., Arigela, S. H., Raman, R., Indhumathi, C., Kavitha, V., & Bhatt, B. C. (2023). Prominent Rule Control-based Internet of Things: Poultry Farm Management System. *IEEE Explore*, 1–6. doi:10.1109/ICPECTS56089.2022.10047039

Boopathi, S., Khare, R., Jaya Christiyan, K. G., Muni, T. V., & Khare, S. (2023). Additive manufacturing developments in the medical engineering field. In Development, Properties, and Industrial Applications of 3D Printed Polymer Composites (pp. 86–106). IGI Global. doi:10.4018/978-1-6684-6009-2.ch006

Chandra Saha, B., Sai Thrinath, B. V., Boopathi, S., Ramya, J., & Sudhakar, M. (n.d.). IOT BASED SMART ENERGY METER FOR. *Smart Grid*.

Darshan, K. R., & Anandakumar, K. R. (2015). A comprehensive review on usage of Internet of Things (IoT) in healthcare system. *2015 International Conference on Emerging Research in Electronics, Computer Science and Technology (ICERECT)*, 132–136. 10.1109/ERECT.2015.7499001

Deshpande, U. U., & Kulkarni, M. A. (2017). IoT based Real Time ECG Monitoring System using Cypress WICED. *International Journal of Advanced Research in Electrical*, *6*(2), 710–720.

Fernandez, F., & Pallis, G. C. (2015). Opportunities and challenges of the Internet of Things for healthcare: Systems engineering perspective. *Proceedings of the 2014 4th International Conference on Wireless Mobile Communication and Healthcare - "Transforming Healthcare Through Innovations in Mobile and Wireless Technologies", MOBIHEALTH 2014*, 263–266. https://doi.org/10.1109/MOBIHEALTH.2014.7015961

Jeevanantham, Y. A., A, S., V, V., J, S. Isaac., Boopathi, S., & Kumar, D. P. (2023). Implementation of Internet-of Things (IoT) in Soil Irrigation System. *IEEE Explore*, 1–5. doi:10.1109/ICPECTS56089.2022.10047185

Karthik, S. A., Hemalatha, R., Aruna, R., Deivakani, M., Reddy, R. V. K., & Boopathi, S. (2023). Study on Healthcare Security System-Integrated Internet of Things (IoT). doi:10.4018/978-1-6684-7684-0.ch013

Kassem, A., El Murr, S., Jamous, G., Saad, E., & Geagea, M. (2016). A smart lock system using Wi-Fi security. *2016 3rd International Conference on Advances in Computational Tools for Engineering Applications, ACTEA 2016*, 222–225. 10.1109/ACTEA.2016.7560143

Koshariya, A. K., Kalaiyarasi, D., Jovith, A. A., Sivakami, T., Hasan, D. S., & Boopathi, S. (2023). AI-Enabled IoT and WSN-Integrated Smart. *Practice, Progress, and Proficiency in Sustainability*, 200–218. doi:10.4018/978-1-6684-8516-3.ch011

Lv, D., Wang, Z., Ji, S., Wang, X., & Hou, H. (2021). Plasma levels of homocysteine is associated with liver fibrosis in health check-up population. *International Journal of General Medicine*, *14*, 5175–5181. doi:10.2147/IJGM.S329863 PMID:34512000

Pramila, P. V., Amudha, S., Saravanan, T. R., Sankar, S. R., Poongothai, E., & Boopathi, S. (2023). *Design and Development of Robots for Medical Assistance*. doi:10.4018/978-1-6684-8913-0.ch011

Qadri, Y. A., Nauman, A., Zikria, Y., Vasilakos, A. V., & Kim, S. W. (2020). The Future of Healthcare Internet of Things: A Survey of Emerging Technologies. *IEEE Communications Surveys and Tutorials*, *22*(2), 1121–1167. doi:10.1109/COMST.2020.2973314

Rahamathunnisa, U., Sudhakar, K., Murugan, T. K., Thivaharan, S., Rajkumar, M., & Boopathi, S. (2023). *Cloud Computing Principles for Optimizing Robot Task Offloading Processes*. doi:10.4018/978-1-6684-8171-4.ch007

Reddy, M. A., Reddy, B. M., Mukund, C. S., Venneti, K., Preethi, D. M. D., & Boopathi, S. (2023a). Social health protection during the COVID-pandemic using IoT. In *The COVID-19 Pandemic and the Digitalization of Diplomacy* (pp. 204–235). IGI Global. doi:10.4018/978-1-7998-8394-4.ch009

Reddy, M. A., Reddy, B. M., Mukund, C. S., Venneti, K., Preethi, D. M. D., & Boopathi, S. (2023b). Social Health Protection During the COVID-Pandemic Using IoT. In *The COVID-19 Pandemic and the Digitalization of Diplomacy* (pp. 204–235). IGI Global. doi:10.4018/978-1-7998-8394-4.ch009

S., P. K., Sampath, B., R., S. K., Babu, B. H., & N., A. (2022). Hydroponics, Aeroponics, and Aquaponics Technologies in Modern Agricultural Cultivation. In *Trends, Paradigms, and Advances in Mechatronics Engineering* (pp. 223–241). IGI Global. doi:10.4018/978-1-6684-5887-7.ch012

Salunke, P., & Nerkar, R. (2017). IoT Driven Healthcare System for Remote Monitoring of Patients. *International Journal for Modern Trends in Science and Technology*, *03*(June), 100–103.

Samikannu, R., Koshariya, A. K., Poornima, E., Ramesh, S., Kumar, A., & Boopathi, S. (2023). *Sustainable Development in Modern Aquaponics Cultivation Systems Using IoT Technologies*. doi:10.4018/978-1-6684-4118-3.ch006

Saravanan, A., Venkatasubramanian, R., Khare, R., Surakasi, R., Boopathi, S., Ray, S., & Sudhakar, M. (2022). *Policy Trends of Renewable Energy and Non Renewable Energy*. Academic Press.

Sathish, T., Sunagar, P., Singh, V., Boopathi, S., Sathyamurthy, R., Al-Enizi, A. M., Pandit, B., Gupta, M., & Sehgal, S. S. (2023). *Characteristics estimation of natural fibre reinforced plastic composites using deep multi-layer perceptron (MLP) technique*. Elsevier. doi:10.1016/j.chemosphere.2023.139346

Senthil, T. S., Ohmsakthivel, R., Puviyarasan, M., Babu, S. R., Surakasi, R., & Sampath, B. (2023). Industrial robot-integrated fused deposition modelling for the 3D printing process. In Development, Properties, and Industrial Applications of 3D Printed Polymer Composites (pp. 188–210). IGI Global. doi:10.4018/978-1-6684-6009-2.ch011

Sharma, M., Singla, M. K., Nijhawan, P., Ganguli, S., & Rajest, S. S. (2020). An Application of IoT to Develop Concept of Smart Remote Monitoring System. *EAI/Springer Innovations in Communication and Computing*, 233–239. doi:10.1007/978-3-030-44407-5_15

Solà, J., Castoldi, S., Chételat, O., Correvon, M., Dasen, S., Droz, S., Jacob, N., Kormann, R., Neumann, V., Perrenoud, A., Pilloud, P., Verjus, C., & Viardot, G. (2006). SpO2 sensor embedded in a finger ring: Design and implementation. *Annual International Conference of the IEEE Engineering in Medicine and Biology - Proceedings*, 4295–4298. 10.1109/IEMBS.2006.260820

Subha, S., Inbamalar, T. M., R, K. C., Suresh, L. R., Boopathi, S., & Alaskar, K. (2023, February). A Remote Health Care Monitoring system using internet of medical things (IoMT). *IEEE Explore*. doi:10.1109/ICIPTM57143.2023.10118103

Subha, S., Inbamalar, T. M., Komala, C. R., Suresh, L. R., Boopathi, S., & Alaskar, K. (2023). A Remote Health Care Monitoring system using internet of medical things (IoMT). *Proceedings of 2023 3rd International Conference on Innovative Practices in Technology and Management, ICIPTM 2023*. 10.1109/ICIPTM57143.2023.10118103

Syafa'Ah, L., Minarno, A. E., Sumadi, F. D. S., & Rahayu, D. A. P. (2019). ESP 8266 for Control and Monitoring in Smart Home Application. *Proceedings - 2019 International Conference on Computer Science, Information Technology, and Electrical Engineering, ICOMITEE 2019*, 123–128. 10.1109/ICOMITEE.2019.8921287

Syamala, M. (2023). Machine Learning-Integrated IoT-Based Smart Home Energy Management System. doi:10.4018/978-1-6684-8098-4.ch013

Tao, H., Bhuiyan, M. Z. A., Abdalla, A. N., Hassan, M. M., Zain, J. M., & Hayajneh, T. (2019). Secured Data Collection with Hardware-Based Ciphers for IoT-Based Healthcare. *IEEE Internet of Things Journal*, *6*(1), 410–420. doi:10.1109/JIOT.2018.2854714

Tekeste, T., Saleh, H., Mohammad, B., & Ismail, M. (2019). Ultra-Low Power QRS Detection and ECG Compression Architecture for IoT Healthcare Devices. *IEEE Transactions on Circuits and Systems. I, Regular Papers*, *66*(2), 669–679. doi:10.1109/TCSI.2018.2867746

Thibaud, M., Chi, H., Zhou, W., & Piramuthu, S. (2018). Internet of Things (IoT) in high-risk Environment, Health and Safety (EHS) industries: A comprehensive review. *Decision Support Systems*, *108*, 79–95. doi:10.1016/j.dss.2018.02.005

Vanitha, S. K. R., & Boopathi, S. (2023). Artificial Intelligence Techniques in Water Purification and Utilization. In *Human Agro-Energy Optimization for Business and Industry* (pp. 202–218). IGI Global. doi:10.4018/978-1-6684-4118-3.ch010

Venkateswaran, N., Vidhya, K., Ayyannan, M., Chavan, S. M., Sekar, K., & Boopathi, S. (2023). *A Study on Smart Energy Management Framework Using Cloud Computing*. doi:10.4018/978-1-6684-8634-4.ch009

Venkateswaran, N., Vidhya, R., Naik, D. A., Michael Raj, T. F., Munjal, N., & Boopathi, S. (2023). *Study on Sentence and Question Formation Using Deep Learning Techniques*. doi:10.4018/978-1-6684-6782-4.ch015

Xu, G. (2020). IoT-Assisted ECG Monitoring Framework with Secure Data Transmission for Health Care Applications. *IEEE Access : Practical Innovations, Open Solutions*, *8*, 74586–74594. doi:10.1109/ACCESS.2020.2988059

Yang, Z., Zhou, Q., Lei, L., Zheng, K., & Xiang, W. (2016). An IoT-cloud Based Wearable ECG Monitoring System for Smart Healthcare. *Journal of Medical Systems*, *40*(12), 1–11. doi:10.1007/s10916-016-0644-9 PMID:27796840

Chapter 7
Innovations in Robotic-Assisted Physiotherapy:
Enhancing Rehabilitation and Recovery

Rabia Aziz
https://orcid.org/0009-0009-7462-9251
Jamia Hamdard University, India

Anam Siddiqui
Jamia Hamdard University, India

Habiba Sundus
Jamia Hamdard University, India

Firdaus Jawed
Jamia Millia Islamia, India

Sohrab Ahmad Khan
Jamia Hamdard University, India

ABSTRACT

Earlier robotic physiotherapy was constricted to specifically gait and movement training, but with recent advancement, it is expanded to dexterous hand and robotic limbs, which are not only improving patient recovery outcomes but also building maximum functional ability. Paradigm shift to incorporating robot assisted physiotherapy in practice requires a comprehensive and detailed knowledge about the same. This chapter embarks on an expedition into the convergence of robotics and physiotherapy, meticulously navigating through the avant-garde technologies and methodologies that are orchestrating a paradigmatic shift in patient care, thereby fostering a person's enhanced outcomes. By illuminating the dynamic interplay of these two domains, this chapter elucidates the transformative potential they hold in revolutionizing patient care, invigorating the trajectory of recovery, and sculpting a landscape of holistic wellness.

DOI: 10.4018/979-8-3693-1934-5.ch007

1. INTRODUCTION TO ROBOTIC-ASSISTED PHYSIOTHERAPY

Robotic-assisted gait training (RAGT), a new rehabilitation technology, has been introduced in an effort to enhance stability, balance, and posture. Because the brain and spinal cord are malleable, RAGT may use forced, high-intensity walking to activate neural pathways and improve gait. According to some publications, RAGT can help adults with neurological problems regain their balance. It also appears to aid in the rehabilitation of young children with physical disabilities. However, the precise function and implications of this therapy were yet unknown (Calabrò et al., 2021).

Exoskeletons or end-effector robots combined with virtual reality (VR) serious games have shown benefits for the neuromotor rehabilitation of the upper limbs, including higher intensity of the training, higher level of motor control of the joints, longer duration, and more sessions with the ability to give variable assistance or resistance force feedback and possibly provide kinesiology information of the patient performance that facilitates the evaluation during the treatment (Molteni et al., 2018).

Robotic-assisted gait training is often employed for patients with other neurological illnesses, such as Parkinson's syndrome or post-stroke conditions as shown in figure 1.1, but there are still questions about this training. The methods by which robotically assisted training enhances gait as well as the gait metrics that may be in charge of the changes are of interest (Calabrò et al., 2021).

Over-ground robotic-assisted gait training devices (O-RAGT) allow the patient to walk in a real-world environment, allowing for significant kinematic flexibility while assuring task success. Because people can use O-RAGT at home in a comfortable environment, it may help people build habits that result in long-term behaviour modification. in the form of a wearable robotic knee orthosis for patients with recurrent stroke. In addition, there was an increase in PA (steps taken) after completing the O-RAGT program that persisted for an additional three months. It is known that O-RAGT improved PA and physical function over time, but it is not known if these effects extend to measures of cardiovascular health like blood pressure and arterial stiffness. This is significant in light of the significant independent risk that arterial stiffness poses for cardiovascular disease (Wright et al., 2021).

Unfortunately, the use of robotics for orthopaedic rehabilitation remains largely unexplored and the research in this area is quite sparse, compared to neurorehabilitation systems, despite the potential advantages, the high incidence of musculoskeletal injuries, and the current demand for faster and better physical therapies (Padilla-Castañeda et al., 2018).

Figure 1. Gait Training Using Robotics
Source: Riener et al. (2006)

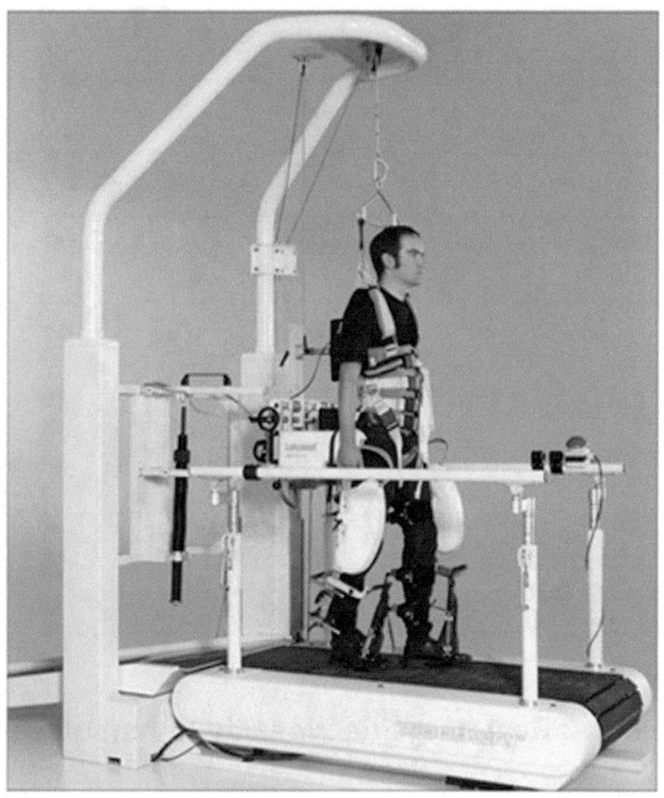

2. TYPES OF ROBOTIC DEVICES IN PHYSIOTHERAPY

2.1 Exoskeletons: Enhancing Mobility and Motor Control

A stiff exterior body covering for the body of some creatures, such the tough chitinous cuticle of arthropods, is known as an exoskeleton. In contrast to the endoskeleton, which is entirely contained within the animal body, an exoskeleton protects, supports, and offers points of attachment for muscles. Humans are endoskeleton animals and lack the capabilities of exoskeletons. Exoskeletons, which primarily refer to wearable technologies that can support, defend, and improve particular human skills, have been developed in response to the growing desire for self-protection, support, strength, and rehabilitation. Prosthetics, which are used to repair structural damage to the human skeletal system, as well as the armor of ancient armies and the Extra Vehicular Activity (EVA) suits of modern astronauts, can all be considered forms of exoskeletons (Sawicki et al., 2020).

Exoskeletons have proven to be helpful instruments for assisting with the execution of neuromotor rehabilitation sessions. Exoskeleton illustrated in Figure 2.1 helps assist the patient while rehabilitation. Hospitals still lack them in great numbers, though. This form of technology is often shunned by therapists, which lowers its acceptance and, consequently, its regular use in clinical practice (Linder M. Susan (Department of Biomedical Engineering, 2014).

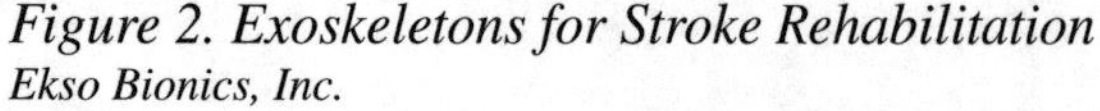

Figure 2. Exoskeletons for Stroke Rehabilitation
Ekso Bionics, Inc.

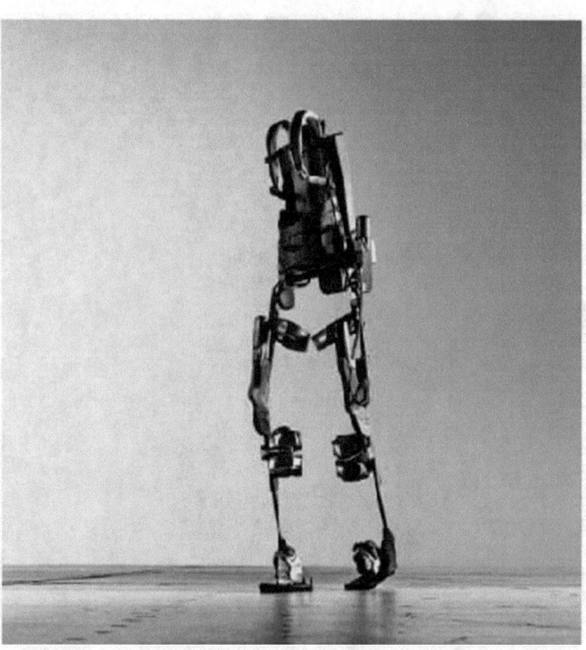

2.2 Robotic Prosthetics: Restoring Functionality to Amputees

Commercially available lower-limb prostheses do not offer the user either voluntary active control or sensory feedback. As a result, amputees using these systems frequently lament the necessity for visual signals when operating their prostheses on a daily basis. Recently, systems that give users active control over their prostheses have been proposed by research teams and prosthetic manufacturers. From the viewpoints of neural control and biomechanics, the control of gait necessitates multisensory fusion, strong control mechanisms, and kinematic and dynamic coordination of the limbs and muscles. Adapting the pattern of locomotion to the needs of the environment is dynamically influenced by sensory feedback from muscle and skin afferents as well as other sensory modalities (Valle et al., 2021).

An exoskeleton-based prosthesis is one that uses motors to provide more strength and endurance than a conventional prosthesis. In order to provide a more individualized experience, these exoskeletons can also be modified to meet the needs of the user. Exoskeleton-based prostheses are employed in many different fields today, from industrial automation to medical rehabilitation. These exoskeletons' powers will develop along with technology, giving users even more mobility and dexterity (Sawicki et al., 2020).

2.3 Robot-Assisted Training Systems: Enhancing Strength and Coordination

Robotic therapy's efficacy is still being investigated, and its usage in clinical settings is yet relatively undeveloped. The practicality of using these devices may be one of the causes. In reality, individuals for whom usage of the robot is recommended are typically quite incapacitated and need support from a caregiver to travel to appointments and therapeutic sessions (Calabrò et al., 2021). The use of robotic devices for at-home rehabilitation may be the answer to this issue. Most modern robotic rehabilitation devices are made to be brought to the patient's home, where they can be used their multiple times each day. Using gadgets like tablets and cellphones, as well as webcams, home treatments can also be given. According to recent research, telerehabilitation appears to produce similar outcomes to clinical rehabilitation in terms of motor recovery following stroke. This review suggests that technological rehabilitation programs should be incorporated into conventional therapy for patients who are both subacute and chronic (Wright et al., 2021).

2.4 Assistive Robots: Aiding Therapists and Patients During Sessions

The majority of robotic devices rely solely on the clinical judgment of the therapist to manually adjust the robotic support to the patient's ability. This may result in a robotic support that is not ideal for the patient and a failure to effectively challenge the patient. An assist-as-needed robotic controller can be utilized to solve these issues. Based on an ongoing evaluation of each patient's capabilities, the required level of robotic help is regulated. Such assist-as-needed (AAN) controllers for robotic gait rehabilitation devices have been developed (Laut et al., 2016)

Since the early 2000s, the Lokomat, a robotic exoskeleton that runs on a treadmill, has been widely applied in clinical settings across the world. Several patient populations (including those with stroke, spinal cord injury (SCI), and multiple sclerosis, to name a few) have had the effects of Lokomat therapy extensively examined. This study evaluated the adaptive gait support (AGS), an intelligent algorithm that was recently included to the Lokomat®Pro (Sensation exercise package, Hocoma AG, Volketswil, Switzerland) program. A training exercise called AGS has been put into place and is accessible from the Lokomat user interface. Based on the patient's capacity to follow a physiological gait pattern, which ought to be correlated with the patient's level of impairment, AGS automatically and continually modifies the robotic support of the Lokomat orthosis (Laszlo et al., 2023).

3. BENEFITS AND CHALLENGES

3.1 Benefits of Robotic-Assisted Physiotherapy for Patients and Therapists

There has been a long-standing search for efficient ways based on virtual reality, biofeedback, or assistive robotic technologies to supplement the traditional neuro-rehabilitation process in gait and mobility impairments in stroke patients. Numerous earlier papers have discussed the advantages of adopting robotic-assisted gait training (RAGT) in the re-education of gait in stroke patients. Masiero et al. noted that robots effectively enhance conventional post-stroke rehabilitation by enabling numerous repetitions of movement in the same pattern and without showing signs of tiredness. Static robots such as Lokomat or Gait Trainer and dynamic robots as wearable exoskeletons or soft exoskeletons are now available, allowing the patient to move more independently, depending on their functional state and the severity of their motor impairments (Schwartz et al., 2009).

Table 1. Applications of Robotic-Assisted Physiotherapy

STUDY	ROBOTIC DEVICE	NO. OF SUBJECTS	DURATION	CONCOMITANT THERAPY	SUMMARY
Buesing et al. (2015)	SMA Honda Stride Management Assist	50	45 min, 3 times per week for 6-8 weeks, 18 session total	No	No difference
Ochi et al. (2015)	Gait-assistance robot	26	60 min, maximum 10 sessions	No	More effective
Stein et al. (2014)	Bionic Leg (robotic leg brace)	24	50 min, 3 times per week for 6 weeks	No	More effective
Watanabe et al. (2014)	Hybrid Assistive Limb	32	20 min, for 4 weeks, total 12 sessions	No	More effective
Lo et al. (2010)	InMotion2	21	1 hour, 3 times per week for 6 weeks	No	No difference
Burgar et al. (2011)	MIT-MANUS	127	A maximum of 36 sessions over 12 weeks	No	More effective
Conroy et al. (2011)	MIME	54	1 hour, 5 times per week for 3 weeks	No	No difference

(Gassert et al., 2018)

3.2 Addressing Challenges Such as Cost, Accessibility, and Patient Adaptability

The use of rehabilitation robots in clinical and home-based settings has been significantly hampered by the high expense of such devices and the difficulty in convincing hospitals to commit funds to pay for them. Currently available rehabilitation robotics range in price from $75,000 to $350,000, all of which are included in the price and excluding taxes, installation, training, maintenance, and shipping. The "World Health Organization Choosing Interventions that are Cost-Effective" initiative states that a health intervention will be deemed cost-effective if its price is less than three times the country's yearly GDP (GDP) per capita. If the overall cost of a robotically assisted therapy in the UK is less than $120,852 (update from the World Bank in December), it is deemed to be cost-effective or low-cost (Akbari et al., 2021).

Regarding the kinds of patients for whom robot treatment would not be appropriate, participants voiced a number of worries and challenges. This includes patients with stroke-related non-motor disabilities, such as behavioral, cognitive, perceptual, communicative, or visual challenges that would prevent them from using or comprehending the robot. However, one participant pointed out that some of these disabilities, as well as motor issues, would benefit from employing rehabilitation robots, which might, for instance, encourage visual scanning and practice memory and problem-solving activities. Pain, weariness, skin integrity, spasticity, or a limited range of motion, particularly in fixed joint contractures, were additional issues that would restrict the patient's capacity to engage in robot therapy or jeopardize their safety. These issues should be carefully evaluated before usage (Padilla-Castañeda et al., 2018).

4. TECHNOLOGICAL INNOVATIONS

4.1 Sensors and AI in Adaptive Therapy Planning

In terms of effectiveness, efficiency, and cost, industrial robots have matured. The necessity to use robotic technology in dangerous, safety-sensitive, and labor-intensive fields like space exploration and interventional medicine is what is causing today's robotics issues. The latter is very demanding regarding safety, precision, miniaturization, working area, minimal encumbrance, and interaction needs for carrying out important and exhausting activities in risky circumstances and unknown locations. The intraoperative ultrasound (US) probe, the intraoperative Doppler US probe, the robot encoders, the force sensor, and the sensor manager (SM) are among the field sensors that the SM combines. The SM collects data (Akbari et al., 2021; Lubner et al., 2021)

The potential cost reductions connected with the usage of wearable sensors and AI in healthcare were examined in research titled "A Systematic Review of Wearable Patient Monitoring Systems - Current Challenges and Opportunities for Clinical Adoption". These technological advancements can aid in lowering healthcare costs by streamlining treatment programs and minimizing the need for in-person appointments.

According to these researches and other data, including sensors and AI into adaptive therapy planning may improve the efficiency, effectiveness, and personalization of rehabilitation and treatment outcomes across a variety of healthcare settings. However, to further validate these results and improve AI-driven adaptive therapeutic techniques, research and clinical trials must be conducted. IA methods provide for task execution and successful human-machine interaction (path planning and negotiation, uncertainty management, and intelligent interface), To improve the robot's fundamental accuracy and dependability through a feedback control loop and sensor-robot-robot collaboration (Lubner et al., 2021).

In healthcare, especially physiotherapy, adaptive therapy planning entails modifying treatment schedules in response to feedback from patients and real-time data. Artificial intelligence (AI) and sensors are essential to this process. Intelligent route planning relies on more data than an end user can manage in real time, making it potentially faster and more accurate. It may also save time during surgery, which would help the system as a whole be more well-liked (Laszlo et al., 2023).

4.2 Virtual Reality Integration for Immersive Rehabilitation

A useful tool for making the treatment process more effective is a method based on rehabilitation robots and physiotherapy games. In contrast, the majority of current research in rehabilitation robotics is focused on neurorehabilitation for patients with lesions at the central nervous system (CNS), with a greater emphasis on stroke patients and a lesser extent on patients with other neural ailments, such as in the spinal cord (Jacofsky & Allen, 2016) .

The interface for collaborative human-machine or robot interaction and communication is crucial because it allows the human operator to give directions and monitor the task's performance. Examples of this interface include input through a keyboard, voice, gestures, etc. However, the user receives visual feedback on a screen and an external monitor using conventional interfaces, such as a mouse and keyboard. The majority of these visualizations are not intuitive enough, call for excellent hand-eye coordination, and may be distracting (Laszlo et al., 2023)

4.3 Gamification for Enhancing Patient Engagement.

Gamification strategies can boost patients' motivation and involvement in their recovery. Patients may adhere to treatment regimens and advance toward their recovery objectives by using game-like aspects in the rehab process. The effects of gamification on customized post-stroke rehabilitation training and its use in recommendation systems, however, are not well understood. Recommending post-stroke rehabilitation training using a data mining and gamification technique is somewhat restricted and was not inclusive owing to data location. Furthermore, healthcare professionals can gain a better understanding of patient progress and outcomes by integrating data mining and gamification approaches. Additionally, this combination may aid in treatment plan optimization and enhanced patient results (Jacofsky & Allen, 2016; Ozgur et al., 2022).

5. HUMAN-ROBOT INTERACTION

5.1 Importance of Maintaining a Human Touch in Therapy

Touch is a versatile sense that may be employed for emotive, exploratory, and communicative goals. By exploring its physiological and somatic components, neuroaffective and cognitive sciences approach touch. In welcoming and farewell meetings, this chapter explains how body contact, language, and other modalities are arranged. It shows how caring, compassionate touch is employed during comforting, empathic intertwinings, and how touch achieves guiding and instruction across various age cohorts (Langer et al., 2019).

Even when employing robotics for physiotherapy, it is crucial to keep a human touch in the treatment since a human physiotherapist can give patients the emotional support, empathy, and motivation that are critical for their wellbeing and recovery. Robots can help with physical training, but they lack human capabilities such as emotional intelligence and compassion. Human therapists are able to modify their methods in accordance with each patient's requirements, preferences, and development. They can determine the emotional condition of the patient and modify the therapy as necessary. Robots might not be able to offer such individualized treatment (Vignais et al., 2013).

An effective therapist-patient relationship depends on effective communication. Human therapists are capable of having in-depth discussions with patients, comprehending their problems, and answering their queries. Robots may have trouble comprehending the subtleties of human connection even though they are capable of fundamental communication. Therapy requires a lot of trust. When dealing with physical difficulties or discomfort, patients are more likely to trust a human therapist. For an accurate diagnosis and treatment planning, patients must feel comfortable enough to be candid about their pain, limits, and worries. Complex decisions that are based on a patient's progress, amount of discomfort, and responses to treatment are frequently made during therapy. Robotic therapists may follow pre-programmed patterns without taking into account the patient's particular circumstances, whereas human therapists can modify therapy programs in real-time (Langer et al., 2019).

Individual attitudes and cultural influences can have an impact on therapy. In order to respect the patient's cultural background and preferences, human therapists can negotiate these cultural nuances and modify their approach. Nonverbal cues such as body language, tone of voice, and facial emotions make up the majority of human communication. These cues can elicit emotions like empathy, comprehension, and assurance that are difficult for robots to successfully mimic.

Dynamic assessments, which may involve manually examining joint mobility, muscle tone, or other physical features, can be carried out by human therapists during therapy sessions. This practical evaluation can help guide treatment choices and guarantee the best possible outcome.

Sometimes, therapy involves more than just physical activity and also includes advice on how to live your life. A patient's illness can be treated holistically by human therapists by addressing both the physical and psychological components of their disease (Ozgur et al., 2022)..

Robotics in physiotherapy can provide advantages including constant workout support, measurable progress tracking, and the capacity to provide therapy in off-the-grid or underserved places. But it should be carried out in a way that enhances rather than substitutes the invaluable human touch and knowledge that physiotherapists offer. The most efficient and kind treatment for patients can be achieved through a balanced strategy that integrates the advantages of both humans and machines.

Maintaining a human touch in therapy is of the utmost importance, as it entails a multidimensional approach to communication and connection that goes beyond words. When we contemplate the numerous roles that touch performs in the therapeutic process, human contact is an effective method for establishing an emotional connection between the clinician and the client. It communicates tangible sympathy, understanding, and support. A hand on the shoulder or a comforting embrace can convey care and concern in a way that words alone cannot match (Ozgur et al., 2022).

Additionally, in therapy, contact can serve as a tool for exploration. For instance, a therapist may help a client become more aware of their emotions and physical reactions by guiding them through an exploration of bodily sensations. Moreover, contact can provide a sense of security and reassurance to individuals experiencing distress or anxiety, bringing them solace.

Occasionally, clients may find it difficult to verbally express their emotions and thoughts. Touch can function as an alternative mode of communication in such circumstances. Creating a secure space for nonverbal expression, it enables clients to express their emotions, anxieties, and vulnerabilities without the need for extensive verbalization (Vignais et al., 2013).

Touch can also be used as an instrument for guidance and instruction in the context of therapy. Touch may be utilized in certain therapeutic modalities, such as somatic experiencing and body-oriented therapies, to assist clients in releasing physical tension, processing trauma, and developing body awareness. This tactile guidance can aid in promoting healing and personal development (Altimier & Phillips, 2016). The importance of maintaining a human contact in therapy transcends age groups. The therapeutic use of touch encompasses the entire human lifespan, from neonates who require physical contact for healthy development to the elderly who may benefit from touch's calming effects (McParlin et al., 2023).

Moreover, compassionate touch conveys sincere concern and comprehension, fostering a sense of safety and trust between the therapist and the client. It can be especially beneficial in situations where clients are experiencing trauma, bereavement, or emotional suffering, as it can provide comfort and support. The significance of maintaining a human contact in therapy is highlighted by its ability to strengthen the therapeutic relationship, foster emotional connection, and promote healing. It is a versatile and potent tool that therapists can use to address the emotional, physical, and psychological requirements of their clients, leading to more effective and holistic therapeutic outcomes (Altimier & Phillips, 2016).

5.2 Ethical Considerations and Patient Preferences

Ethical considerations and patient preferences play pivotal roles in shaping the landscape of Human-Robot Interaction (HRI), an emerging field with profound implications for healthcare and various other domains. These considerations encompass a range of complex issues that involve ensuring the welfare and autonomy of individuals while leveraging the benefits of advanced robotics and artificial intelligence (Varkey, 2021).

One of the primary ethical concerns in HRI is the preservation of patient privacy and data security. Robots equipped with sensors and cameras can collect sensitive information about individuals, raising concerns about data breaches and misuse. Ensuring robust data encryption and strict access controls is essential to maintain patient trust and confidentiality. Moreover, respecting informed consent and allowing patients to control the extent of data sharing is crucial (Ferrer et al., 2018).

Respecting patient autonomy and preferences is another fundamental ethical consideration. Robots must be programmed to adapt to individual preferences regarding care, communication, and personal boundaries. Some patients may prefer a robotic caregiver for certain tasks, while others may find it discomforting. HRI systems should provide options for patients to customize their interactions with robots, ensuring that they feel respected and empowered in their care decisions (Rueben et al., 2019).

Transparency and accountability are key ethical principles in HRI. Patients should be informed when they are interacting with a robot rather than a human caregiver, and there should be clear lines of responsibility in case of errors or adverse events. Manufacturers and developers must also be transparent about the capabilities and limitations of their robots, avoiding overpromising and misleading patients or healthcare providers (Varkey, 2021)

Additionally, considerations of fairness and equity must guide the development and deployment of robotic systems in healthcare. Ensuring that HRI technologies are accessible and affordable to all segments of society, regardless of socioeconomic status, is essential to prevent exacerbating existing healthcare disparities (Varkey, 2021).

6. DATA COLLECTION AND ANALYSIS

6.1 Utilizing Robotic Systems to Gather Biomechanical Data

Utilizing robotic systems to gather biomechanical data has revolutionized the field of biomechanics, providing researchers with unprecedented insights into the intricacies of human movement and the biomechanics of various organisms. These advanced systems are equipped with sensors, cameras, and precise control mechanisms that allow for the collection of highly accurate and detailed data (Ozgur et al., 2022).

One of the primary advantages of employing robotic systems in biomechanical research is their ability to replicate and control movements with remarkable precision. Researchers can program these robots to mimic specific actions, such as walking, running, or even the fluttering of a bird's wings, enabling them to isolate and study the biomechanical factors involved in these motions. This level of control is virtually impossible to achieve with human subjects alone, as it eliminates the variability introduced by individual differences in anatomy and coordination (Jacofsky & Allen, 2016). Furthermore, robotic systems can capture biomechanical data in real-time, providing researchers with immediate feedback. This capability is invaluable in sports science, rehabilitation medicine, and ergonomics, as it allows for on-the-fly adjustments and optimizations to enhance performance or aid in injury recovery (Vignais et al., 2013).

Robotic systems are also essential tools in biomechanical studies involving dangerous or extreme environments, such as space exploration or deep-sea research. They can be remotely operated in environments where human presence is impractical or hazardous, offering a safe and effective means of collecting crucial biomechanical data. In addition to their precision and adaptability, robotic systems can collect data continuously for extended periods, which is particularly advantageous when studying long-duration activities or monitoring biological processes over time. This extended data collection capability helps researchers uncover trends and patterns that might be missed with limited data samples (Hribernik et al., 2022).

6.2 Applying Machine Learning for Personalized Treatment Plans

Applying machine learning for personalized treatment plans within the realm of robotics in physiotherapy represents a revolutionary stride towards optimizing patient care and rehabilitation outcomes. In this cutting-edge approach, data-driven algorithms harness the power of artificial intelligence to tailor treatment strategies to the unique needs of each individual, heralding a new era of precision medicine (Yagi et al., 2023).

Traditionally, physiotherapy has relied on standardized treatment protocols, often neglecting the inherent diversity among patients. However, the integration of robotics and machine learning changes the game. These smart robotic systems can collect an extensive array of data points, including a patient's range of motion, muscle strength, pain levels, and even biometric data. This wealth of information is then processed and analyzed by machine learning algorithms, which can recognize subtle patterns and trends that might elude human clinicians (Cunha et al., 2023; Yagi et al., 2023).

Through continuous monitoring and adjustment of therapy sessions, machine learning algorithms adapt treatment plans in real-time. For example, if a patient exhibits faster-than-expected progress in a specific area, the system can intensify exercises in that particular domain while easing off in areas requiring more time. Conversely, if a patient experiences discomfort or struggles with a particular exercise, the system can swiftly modify the regimen to ensure both safety and effectiveness. Moreover, machine learning models can consider a patient's medical history, lifestyle, and even psychological factors to tailor treatment plans further. This holistic approach not only enhances physical rehabilitation but also addresses the psychological and emotional aspects of recovery, thereby improving overall patient well-being (Yagi et al., 2023).

7. FUTURE SCOPE

7.1 Predicting the Trajectory of Robotic-Assisted Physiotherapy

Predicting the trajectory of robotic-assisted physiotherapy is a pivotal endeavor in the realm of healthcare and rehabilitation. This innovative approach combines the precision and repeatability of robotic systems with the expertise of physiotherapists, promising enhanced outcomes for patients. The trajectory prediction in this context involves a multifaceted process that integrates cutting-edge technologies and data analytics (Pérez et al., 2010).

At the heart of this predictive framework is the utilization of advanced sensors and motion capture devices. These sensors are strategically placed on both the robotic system and the patient's body, allowing for the real-time tracking of movements and biomechanical data. This continuous stream of information forms the foundation for trajectory prediction. Machine learning algorithms, particularly deep learning models, play a crucial role in processing this data. These algorithms are trained on vast datasets of patient profiles, physiotherapy protocols, and movement patterns to discern patterns and trends (Basiratzadeh et al., 2022; Taati et al., 2012).

The prediction process encompasses several key aspects. First, it anticipates the patient's range of motion during each session, ensuring that the robotic-assisted therapy aligns with the patient's individualized treatment plan. Second, it factors in the patient's progress over time, adapting the therapy trajectory as the individual's condition evolves. Moreover, these predictive models can estimate the duration required for rehabilitation, providing patients and healthcare providers with a clearer roadmap towards recovery (Taati et al., 2012).

A critical advantage of trajectory prediction in robotic-assisted physiotherapy is its ability to minimize the risk of injury. By anticipating potential deviations from the desired trajectory, the system can make real-time adjustments to prevent undue strain or discomfort for the patient. This predictive capability enhances the safety and effectiveness of the therapy.

7.2 Potential for Home-Based Robotic Rehabilitation Solutions

The potential for home-based robotic rehabilitation solutions represents a groundbreaking frontier in the field of healthcare and physical therapy. This innovative approach leverages the power of robotics and technology to provide individuals with personalized and convenient rehabilitation options within the comfort of their own homes (McParlin et al., 2023).

First and foremost, home-based robotic rehabilitation solutions address the pressing issue of accessibility. Many patients, particularly those living in remote or underserved areas, face significant challenges when it comes to accessing rehabilitation centers. By bringing the rehabilitation process to their homes, these individuals can receive timely care without the need for extensive travel, reducing both physical and financial barriers to treatment. Moreover, home-based solutions are especially relevant in situations like the COVID-19 pandemic, where in-person visits to healthcare facilities are limited (Radanliev et al., 2020).

Furthermore, these systems offer personalized rehabilitation plans. Modern robotics and artificial intelligence can assess an individual's specific needs and adapt exercises and routines accordingly. This tailoring ensures that each patient receives treatment that is optimized for their condition, promoting more effective outcomes and faster recovery times. It also allows for continuous progress monitoring, enabling healthcare professionals to make real-time adjustments to the rehabilitation program (Aceto et al., 2020).

The convenience factor cannot be overstated. Home-based robotic rehabilitation solutions provide patients with the flexibility to schedule their sessions at their own convenience, making it easier to integrate rehabilitation into their daily lives. This fosters greater patient compliance and adherence to prescribed exercises, ultimately contributing to better results.

In addition to benefiting patients, these solutions also alleviate the burden on healthcare systems. With an aging population and an increasing prevalence of chronic conditions, the demand for rehabilitation services is growing rapidly. Home-based robotics can help healthcare providers meet this demand efficiently while also reducing the strain on already overstretched resources (Aceto et al., 2020; Zuccon et al., 2022).

7.3 Collaborations Between Engineers, Therapists, and Patients

Collaborations between engineers, therapists, and patients have ushered in a new era of innovation and effectiveness in the field of physiotherapy, thanks to the integration of robotics. This interdisciplinary synergy harnesses the strengths of each stakeholder, ultimately benefiting the patients' recovery and overall well-being (Aceto & Persico, 2018).

Engineers play a pivotal role in this collaboration by designing and developing cutting-edge robotic devices tailored for physiotherapy. These devices, often powered by advanced artificial intelligence algorithms, offer precise and personalized rehabilitation exercises. Engineers work closely with therapists to understand the specific needs of patients, ensuring that the technology aligns seamlessly with therapeutic goals. The result is a range of robotic solutions that assist therapists in providing highly customized treatment plans, from stroke rehabilitation to mobility enhancement (Proffitt & Lange, 2015).

Therapists, on the other hand, bring their clinical expertise and patient-centered care to the collaboration. They guide engineers in defining the therapeutic objectives and tailoring robotic interventions to the unique requirements of each patient. Therapists also play a crucial role in monitoring patients' progress and adjusting treatment plans accordingly. This close interaction with engineers empowers therapists to provide more effective and engaging rehabilitation experiences, promoting quicker recovery and improved outcomes (McEwen & Cassimally, 2014).

Patients are at the heart of this collaboration, benefiting from the synergistic efforts of engineers and therapists. Robotic devices not only facilitate rehabilitation but also make it engaging and motivating. Patients often find themselves more committed to their treatment plans, as the technology offers real-time feedback and data tracking. This transparency empowers patients to take an active role in their recovery, leading to better adherence to therapy and enhanced long-term results (McEwen & Cassimally, 2014).

8. INTEGRATION INTO HEALTHCARE SYSTEMS

8.1 Overcoming Regulatory Hurdles and Integrating Robotics Into Medical Practice

Overcoming regulatory hurdles and integrating robotics into medical practice represents a pivotal advancement in the healthcare industry. The integration of robotics in medicine holds immense potential to enhance patient care, streamline procedures, and improve overall outcomes. However, this transformative journey is not without its challenges, primarily stemming from stringent regulatory frameworks that govern medical devices and procedures.

One of the foremost regulatory hurdles in adopting medical robotics is ensuring safety and efficacy. Regulatory bodies like the FDA in the United States demand rigorous testing and validation of robotic systems to guarantee patient safety. Manufacturers must meticulously demonstrate that their robots are not only technologically advanced but also meet strict medical standards, ensuring they do not compromise patient well-being. This rigorous evaluation process often requires substantial resources and time (M. Boyd & W. Chaffee, 2019).

The diverse array of medical robotics, from surgical assistants to rehabilitation devices, necessitates cohesive standards to ensure seamless integration into existing healthcare infrastructures. Achieving interoperability ensures that robotic systems can work harmoniously with various medical instruments, databases, and electronic health records, facilitating efficient data sharing and analysis (Radanliev et al., 2020).

Moreover, reimbursement policies are a critical concern for healthcare providers. For widespread adoption, medical robotics must prove their cost-effectiveness, which can be challenging given the initial investment required. Convincing insurers to cover robotic-assisted procedures can be a protracted process, delaying the integration of these technologies into medical practice (Proffitt & Lange, 2015).

Despite these challenges, the medical community recognizes the transformative potential of robotics. Advances in technology continue to drive innovation, pushing the boundaries of what robots can achieve in healthcare settings. Furthermore, collaborations between regulatory agencies, healthcare institutions, and technology developers are paving the way for a more streamlined regulatory process (McEwen & Cassimally, 2014).

8.2 Training Healthcare Professionals to Effectively Use Robotic Devices

Training healthcare professionals to effectively use robotic devices is a critical component of modern healthcare. Robotic devices have become increasingly prevalent in medical settings, assisting in surgeries, rehabilitation, and patient care. To harness the full potential of these advanced technologies and ensure patient safety, healthcare providers must undergo comprehensive training programs (Baker et al., 2006).

These training programs encompass various aspects, starting with the fundamentals of robotics and their applications in healthcare. Healthcare professionals learn about the different types of robotic devices, their capabilities, and how they can enhance medical procedures and patient outcomes. They also gain insights into the latest advancements in robotic technology, ensuring they stay up-to-date with the rapidly evolving field (Ferrer et al., 2018).

Additionally, healthcare professionals are trained in the practical operation of robotic devices, including hands-on experience with simulation systems and real-life scenarios. This allows them to develop the necessary skills to control and manipulate the robots effectively, whether in surgical procedures, diagnostic imaging, or physical therapy sessions (Dwivedi et al., 2008; Nishimura, 2022).

Safety is paramount in robotic-assisted healthcare, and professionals receive training on protocols and precautions to minimize risks and avoid potential complications. They learn how to troubleshoot technical issues and respond to emergencies, ensuring patient well-being at all times.

CONCLUSION

Integration of robotics into physiotherapy provides a vast array of advantages, which is one of the most important outcomes from our investigation. These advantages include improved precision and consistency in treatment, the ability to tailor interventions to the specific requirements of each patient, and the facilitation of earlier and more effective rehabilitation. Moreover, the potential for remote monitoring and tele-rehabilitation opens up new avenues for increasing patient compliance and expanding access to care, particularly in an increasingly digital era.

Nevertheless, it is essential to recognize that the road to maximizing the potential of robotics in physiotherapy is not without obstacles. Among the obstacles that must be overcome to ensure responsible and effective integration are ethical considerations, cost implications, and the need for rigorous clinical validation. In addition, maintaining a human-centered approach in the design and implementation of these technologies is crucial for preventing dehumanization of the therapeutic process and fostering patient trust.

The future prospects for this interdisciplinary collaboration are undeniably promising. As technology continues to advance at an unprecedented rate, we anticipate increasingly sophisticated autonomous systems that are capable of adapting to the diverse requirements of patients, integrating seamlessly with electronic health records, and collaborating with other healthcare technologies. These innovations have the potential to significantly improve patient outcomes and redefine rehabilitation's boundaries.

This chapter serves as a valuable resource for a broad audience, including researchers, clinicians, engineers, and anyone with an interest in the ever-changing intersection of healthcare and technology. In addition to informing future research, collaboration, and innovation in the burgeoning field of robotics-enhanced physiotherapy, it is our intention that the insights presented in this paper will also inspire such endeavors. Together, we can create a future in which these innovative technologies are integral to advancing the practice of rehabilitation and enhancing the lives of patients.

REFERENCES

Aceto, G., & Persico, V. (2018). The role of Information and Communication Technologies in Healthcare : The role of Information and Communication Technologies in Healthcare. *Taxonomies, Perspectives, and Challenges.*, (February). Advance online publication. doi:10.1016/j.jnca.2018.02.008

Aceto, G., Persico, V., & Pescapé, A. (2020). Industry 4.0 and Health: Internet of Things, Big Data, and Cloud Computing for Healthcare 4.0. *Journal of Industrial Information Integration*, *18*, 1–14. doi:10.1016/j.jii.2020.100129

Akbari, A., Haghverd, F., & Behbahani, S. (2021). Robotic Home-Based Rehabilitation Systems Design: From a Literature Review to a Conceptual Framework for Community-Based Remote Therapy During COVID-19 Pandemic. *Frontiers in Robotics and AI*, *8*(June), 1–34. doi:10.3389/frobt.2021.612331 PMID:34239898

Altimier, L., & Phillips, R. (2016). The Neonatal Integrative Developmental Care Model: Advanced Clinical Applications of the Seven Core Measures for Neuroprotective Family-centered Developmental Care. *Newborn and Infant Nursing Reviews; NAINR*, *16*(4), 230–244. doi:10.1053/j.nainr.2016.09.030

Baker, D. P., Salas, E., & Barach, P. (2006). *E Vidence -B Ased R Elation*. Academic Press.

Basiratzadeh, S., Lemaire, E. D., & Baddour, N. (2022). A Novel Augmented Reality Mobile-Based Application for Biomechanical Measurement. *BioMed*, *2*(2), 255–269. doi:10.3390/biomed2020021

Boyd, A., & Chaffee, B. (2019). Critical Evaluation of Pharmacy Automation and Robotic Systems: A Call to Action. *Hospital Pharmacy*, *54*(1), 4–11. doi:10.1177/0018578718786942 PMID:30718928

Calabrò, R. S., Sorrentino, G., Cassio, A., Mazzoli, D., Andrenelli, E., Bizzarini, E., Campanini, I., Carmignano, S. M., Cerulli, S., Chisari, C., Colombo, V., Dalise, S., Fundarò, C., Gazzotti, V., Mazzoleni, D., Mazzucchelli, M., Melegari, C., Merlo, A., Stampacchia, G., ... Bonaiuti, D. (2021). robotic-assisted gait rehabilitation following stroke: A systematic review of current guidelines and practical clinical recommendations. *European Journal of Physical and Rehabilitation Medicine*, *57*(3), 460–471. doi:10.23736/S1973-9087.21.06887-8 PMID:33947828

Cunha, B., Ferreira, R., & Sousa, A. S. P. (2023). Home-Based Rehabilitation of the Shoulder Using Auxiliary Systems and Artificial Intelligence: An Overview. *Sensors (Basel)*, *23*(16), 1–22. doi:10.3390/s23167100 PMID:37631637

Dwivedi, A., Wickramasinghe, N., Bali, R. K., & Naguib, R. N. G. (2008). Designing intelligent healthcare organisations with KM and ICT. *International Journal of Knowledge Management Studies*, *2*(2), 198–213. doi:10.1504/IJKMS.2008.018321

Ekso Bionics. (n.d.). *Robotic exoskeleton used during 4 weeks of inpatient gait training*. Ekso-GTWebsite: https://www.eksobionics.com/ekso

FerrerE. C.RudovicO.HardjonoT.PentlandA. (2018). *RoboChain: A Secure Data-Sharing Framework for Human-Robot Interaction*. http://arxiv.org/abs/1802.04480

Gassert, R., & Dietz, V. (2018). Rehabilitation robots for the treatment of sensorimotor deficits: A neurophysiological perspective. *Journal of Neuroengineering and Rehabilitation*, *15*(1), 46. doi:10.1186/s12984-018-0383-x PMID:29866106

Hribernik, M., Umek, A., Tomažic, S., & Kos, A. (2022). Review of Real-Time Biomechanical Feedback Systems in Sport and Rehabilitation. *Sensors (Basel)*, *22*(8), 3006. Advance online publication. doi:10.3390/s22083006 PMID:35458991

Jacofsky, D. J., & Allen, M. (2016). Robotics in Arthroplasty: A Comprehensive Review. *The Journal of Arthroplasty*, *31*(10), 2353–2363. doi:10.1016/j.arth.2016.05.026 PMID:27325369

Langer, A., Feingold-Polak, R., Mueller, O., Kellmeyer, P., & Levy-Tzedek, S. (2019). Trust in socially assistive robots: Considerations for use in rehabilitation. *Neuroscience and Biobehavioral Reviews*, *104*(July), 231–239. doi:10.1016/j.neubiorev.2019.07.014 PMID:31348963

Laszlo, C., Munari, D., Maggioni, S., Knechtle, D., Wolf, P., & De Bon, D. (2023). Feasibility of an Intelligent Algorithm Based on an Assist-as-Needed Controller for a Robot-Aided Gait Trainer (Lokomat) in Neurological Disorders: A Longitudinal Pilot Study. *Brain Sciences*, *13*(4), 612. Advance online publication. doi:10.3390/brainsci13040612 PMID:37190576

Laut, J., Porfiri, M., & Raghavan, P. (2016). The Present and Future of Robotic Technology in Rehabilitation. *Current Physical Medicine and Rehabilitation Reports*, *4*(4), 312–319. doi:10.1007/s40141-016-0139-0 PMID:28603663

Linder,, M. (2014). Program To Improve Arm Function Following Stroke : A Case Study. *Journal of Neurologic Physical Therapy; JNPT*, *37*(3), 125–132. doi:10.1097/NPT.0b013e31829fa808 PMID:23872687

Lubner, M. G., Gettle, L. M., Kim, D. H., Ziemlewicz, T. J., Dahiya, N., & Pickhardt, P. (2021). Diagnostic and procedural intraoperative ultrasound: Technique, tips and tricks for optimizing results. *The British Journal of Radiology*, *94*(1121), 20201406. Advance online publication. doi:10.1259/bjr.20201406 PMID:33684305

McEwen, A., & Cassimally, H. (2014). *Designing the Internet of things*. https://ebookcentral-proquest-com.pxz.iubh.de:8443/lib/badhonnef/detail.action?docID=1471865

McParlin, Z., Cerritelli, F., Manzotti, A., Friston, K. J., & Esteves, J. E. (2023). Therapeutic touch and therapeutic alliance in pediatric care and neonatology: An active inference framework. *Frontiers in Pediatrics*, *11*(February), 1–15. doi:10.3389/fped.2023.961075 PMID:36923275

Molteni, F., Gasperini, G., Cannaviello, G., & Guanziroli, E. (2018). Exoskeleton and End-Effector Robots for Upper and Lower Limbs Rehabilitation: Narrative Review. *PM & R*, *10*(9), S174–S188. doi:10.1016/j.pmrj.2018.06.005 PMID:30269804

Nishimura, Y. (2022). Primary Care, Burnout, and Patient Safety: Way to Eliminate Avoidable Harm. *International Journal of Environmental Research and Public Health*, *19*(16), 10–12. doi:10.3390/ijerph191610112 PMID:36011747

Ozgur, A. G., Wessel, M. J., Olsen, J. K., Cadic-Melchior, A. G., Zufferey, V., Johal, W., Dominijanni, G., Turlan, J. L., Mühl, A., Bruno, B., Vuadens, P., Dillenbourg, P., & Hummel, F. C. (2022). The effect of gamified robot-enhanced training on motor performance in chronic stroke survivors. *Heliyon*, *8*(11), e11764. Advance online publication. doi:10.1016/j.heliyon.2022.e11764 PMID:36468121

Padilla-Castañeda, M. A., Sotgiu, E., Barsotti, M., Frisoli, A., Orsini, P., Martiradonna, A., Laddaga, C., & Bergamasco, M. (2018). An Orthopaedic Robotic-Assisted Rehabilitation Method of the Forearm in Virtual Reality Physiotherapy. *Journal of Healthcare Engineering*, *2018*, 1–20. Advance online publication. doi:10.1155/2018/7438609 PMID:30154992

Pérez, R., Costa, Ú., Torrent, M., Solana, J., Opisso, E., Cáceres, C., Tormos, J. M., Medina, J., & Gómez, E. J. (2010). Upper limb portable motion analysis system based on inertial technology for neurorehabilitation purposes. *Sensors (Basel)*, *10*(12), 10733–10751. doi:10.3390/s101210733 PMID:22163496

Proffitt, R., & Lange, B. (2015). Considerations in the efficacy and effectiveness of virtual reality interventions for stroke rehabilitation: Moving the field forward. *Physical Therapy*, *95*(3), 441–448. doi:10.2522/ptj.20130571 PMID:25343960

Radanliev, P., De Roure, D. C., Walton, R., Van Kleek, M., Montalvo, R. M., Santos, O., Maddox, L., & Cannady, S. (2020). COVID-19 What Have We Learned? The Rise of Social Machines and Connected Devices in Pandemic Management Following the Concepts of Predictive, Preventive and Personalised Medicine. SSRN *Electronic Journal*, 311–332. doi:10.2139/ssrn.3692585

Riener, R., Lünenburger, L., & Colombo, G. (2006). Human-centered robotics applied to gait training and assessment. *Journal of Rehabilitation Research and Development*, *43*(5), 679. doi:10.1682/JRRD.2005.02.0046 PMID:17123208

Rueben, M., Aroyo, A. M., Lutz, C., Schmolz, J., Van Cleynenbreugel, P., Corti, A., Agrawal, S., & Smart, W. D. (2019). Themes and Research Directions in Privacy-Sensitive Robotics. *Proceedings of IEEE Workshop on Advanced Robotics and Its Social Impacts, ARSO,* 77–84. 10.1109/ARSO.2018.8625758

Sawicki, G. S., Beck, O. N., Kang, I., & Young, A. J. (2020). The exoskeleton expansion: Improving walking and running economy. *Journal of Neuroengineering and Rehabilitation*, *17*(1), 1–9. doi:10.1186/s12984-020-00663-9 PMID:32075669

Schwartz, I., Sajin, A., Fisher, I., Neeb, M., Shochina, M., Katz-Leurer, M., & Meiner, Z. (2009). The Effectiveness of Locomotor Therapy Using Robotic-Assisted Gait Training in Subacute Stroke Patients: A Randomized Controlled Trial. *PM & R*, *1*(6), 516–523. doi:10.1016/j.pmrj.2009.03.009 PMID:19627940

Taati, B., Wang, R., Huq, R., Snoek, J., & Mihailidis, A. (2012). Vision-based posture assessment to detect and categorize compensation during robotic rehabilitation therapy. *Proceedings of the IEEE RAS and EMBS International Conference on Biomedical Robotics and Biomechatronics*, 1607–1613. 10.1109/BioRob.2012.6290668

Valle, G., Saliji, A., Fogle, E., Cimolato, A., Petrini, F. M., & Raspopovic, S. (2021). Mechanisms of neuro-robotic prosthesis operation in leg amputees. *Science Advances*, *7*(17), eabd8354. Advance online publication. doi:10.1126/sciadv.abd8354 PMID:33883127

Varkey, B. (2021). Principles of Clinical Ethics and Their Application to Practice. *Medical Principles and Practice*, *30*(1), 17–28. doi:10.1159/000509119 PMID:32498071

Vignais, N., Miezal, M., Bleser, G., Mura, K., Gorecky, D., & Marin, F. (2013). Innovative system for real-time ergonomic feedback in industrial manufacturing. *Applied Ergonomics*, *44*(4), 566–574. doi:10.1016/j.apergo.2012.11.008 PMID:23261177

Wright, A., Stone, K., Martinelli, L., Fryer, S., Smith, G., Lambrick, D., Stoner, L., Jobson, S., & Faulkner, J. (2021). Effect of combined home-based, overground robotic-assisted gait training and usual physiotherapy on clinical functional outcomes in people with chronic stroke: A randomized controlled trial. *Clinical Rehabilitation*, *35*(6), 882–893. doi:10.1177/0269215520984133 PMID:33356519

Yagi, M., Yamanouchi, K., Fujita, N., Funao, H., & Ebata, S. (2023). Revolutionizing Spinal Care: Current Applications and Future Directions of Artificial Intelligence and Machine Learning. *Journal of Clinical Medicine*, *12*(13), 4188. Advance online publication. doi:10.3390/jcm12134188 PMID:37445222

Zuccon, G., Lenzo, B., Bottin, M., & Rosati, G. (2022). Rehabilitation robotics after stroke: A bibliometric literature review. *Expert Review of Medical Devices*, *19*(5), 405–421. doi:10.1080/17434440.2022.2096438 PMID:35786139

Chapter 8
IoT Networks for Real-Time Healthcare Monitoring Systems

T. Venkat Narayana Rao
Sreenidhi Institute of Science and Technology, India

Lahari Mothukuri
Sreenidhi Institute of Science and Technology, India

Sangers Bhavana
Sreenidhi Institute of Science and Technology, India

ABSTRACT

In overpopulated nations, the need for medical treatment is increasing along with the population; healthcare difficulties are becoming more common. The population's need for high-quality care is growing despite decreasing treatment costs. An internet of things (IoT) network is a group of hardware and software components, including sensors, gadgets, appliances, and software, that can share data and information among themselves without the assistance of a human. IoT benefits healthcare by enabling remote patient monitoring, telemedicine, medication management, resource optimization, infection control, and more. IoT is crucial in healthcare for remote monitoring, timely interventions, cost reduction, and data-driven care, ultimately improving patient outcomes and healthcare system efficiency. Nowadays, much advancement is taking place in the field of IoT especially in healthcare monitoring. Some of them are wearable IoT-enabled real-time health monitoring system, real-time remote health monitoring system driven by 5G MEC-IoT, which are further discussed in this chapter.

DOI: 10.4018/979-8-3693-1934-5.ch008

1. INTRODUCTION

Real-time monitoring made possible by IoT networks revolutionises healthcare by changing the way we treat patients. These networks provide a smooth web of data interchange by connecting systems, sensors, and devices. IoT makes it easier to continuously monitor a patient's vital signs, adherence to medicine, and general wellbeing in the healthcare industry. The quality of treatment is improved, quick interventions are possible, and patient outcomes are eventually improved by this real-time data transfer. IoT networks are influencing a future where proactive and individualised medical care becomes the standard by fusing technology and healthcare. A revolutionary age in patient care has been ushered in by the recent integration of Internet of Things (IoT) networks into healthcare systems. The ability to track, collect, and evaluate real-time data from a range of medical equipment and sensors has transformed the healthcare environment, particularly in the field of proactive and continuous patient monitoring. The significant influence of IoT networks on real-time healthcare monitoring is examined in this chapter, with a focus on how these networks may transform patient care delivery, improve diagnostic capabilities, and enhance overall healthcare outcomes (Zhang et al., 2020; Prodhan et al., 2017).

2. THE FOUNDATION OF IOT NETWORKS IN HEALTHCARE

With the use of technology to improve monitoring, diagnosis, and treatment, the introduction of IoT networks into the healthcare industry represents a significant change in patient care. This section explores the fundamental components that form the foundation of IoT networks in the medical field (Birje et al., 2020).

2.1 IoT Development in Healthcare

The Internet of Things (IoT) was first introduced in the healthcare industry as a result of the convergence of rapidly advancing technology and the urgent need for more thorough, proactive patient care. The foundation for the networked environment we see today was initially established by simple remote monitoring systems. IoT networks in healthcare have grown quickly as a result of the confluence of wireless connection, data analytics, and miniature sensors (Shanmugasundaram et al., 2018).

2.2 Key Components of IoT Networks

IoT networks in healthcare encompass a diverse array of components:

1. Sensors and Devices: These form the frontline of IoT, capturing real-time data such as vital signs, movement, glucose levels, and more. Wearable devices, implantable sensors, and monitoring equipment constitute this category.
2. Connectivity Protocols: Wireless protocols like Bluetooth, Wi-Fi, Zigbee, and cellular networks facilitate seamless communication between devices and central databases or monitoring stations.
3. Data Transmission and Storage: The collected data is transmitted securely to centralized servers or cloud platforms, enabling storage, analysis, and accessibility for healthcare professionals.

4. Analytics and Interpretation: Advanced analytics and machine learning algorithms process the incoming data, providing insights, predictive analysis, and actionable information for healthcare practitioners.
5. User Interfaces and Applications: User-friendly interfaces and applications enable both healthcare providers and patients to access and interpret the monitored data, fostering informed decision-making and patient engagement.

2.3 Inter-Connectivity and Data Integration

The ability of IoT networks to seamlessly integrate disparate systems and devices is what makes them stand out in the healthcare industry. Standards and integration protocols make it easier to combine data from different sources while maintaining coherence and compatibility. Because of their interconnectedness, patients' health can be viewed holistically, allowing for thorough analysis and prompt interventions. A unified ecosystem is created through the integration of data from wearables, medical devices, electronic health records (EHRs), and other sources. Interoperability standards are essential for maintaining data coherence because they facilitate efficient information sharing and communication between various systems and devices. Thus, the core of IoT networks in healthcare is their capacity to combine, evaluate, and extract valuable information from various sources of health-related data, ultimately transforming the way that healthcare is provided and received (Babakerhell et al., 2019).

3. REAL TIME HEALTH MONITORING USING IOT

The use of IoT (Internet of Things) for real-time monitoring in healthcare has revolutionised patient care and administration. IoT devices gather patient data in real time, allowing healthcare providers to provide prompt interventions and individualised care. Examples of these devices include wearable sensors, linked medical devices, and health monitoring systems. This is the impact that IoT is having:

1.Continuous Patient Monitoring: Health bands and smartwatches are examples of wearable technology that monitors a patient's arterial pressure, temperature, pulse, and blood sugar levels. Rapid detection of irregularities or modifications in a patient's status is made feasible by the constant flow of data (Yu et al., 2018).

2.Remote Patient Management: Through the Internet of Things, patients may be watched over from a distance by healthcare institutions. Doctors can track the health of a patient in the moment from a distance, doing away with the need for licences and frequent hospital visits.

3.Improved Data Accuracy: The Internet of Things allows medical professionals to obtain precise, up-to-date data straight from the patient's body. This facilitates the process of making better decisions without depending exclusively on data reported by patients or on sporadic check-ups.

4.Timely Alerts and Notifications: When specific health parameters surpass predetermined thresholds, IoT systems have the ability to produce alerts and notifications for patients as well as healthcare providers. This makes it possible to take quick action and possibly avoid health issues.

5.Enhanced Patient Engagement and Compliance: By giving patients immediate feedback, Internet of Things (IoT) devices motivate patients to take a more active role in their own health. Actively tracking their health metrics can help patients stay motivated to adhere to treatment regimens and lead healthier lifestyles. IoT systems can perform predictive analytics and early detection by continuously gathering and evaluating streams of health data. Simplified Processes for Healthcare Practitioners: Healthcare practitioners' workflow is streamlined by real-time data transmission via Internet of Things devices. They are able to swiftly and more intelligently make decisions and rank patient care according to urgency. IoT implementation in healthcare is still fraught with difficulties, though, including managing the massive amount of data generated, interoperability between devices and systems, and privacy and data security concerns. In spite of these obstacles, IoT integration in healthcare is still developing and offers potential ways to enhance patient outcomes and healthcare delivery via data-driven interventions and real-time monitoring (Nie et al., 2019).

4. IOT MEDICAL DEVICE CONNECTIVITY

Narrowband-IoT: A standards-based low power wide area (LPWA) technology called NB-IoT was created to make a variety of new IoT devices and services feasible. It uses a spectrum in the lower MHz range with a bandwidth of 200kHz, offering more channels than LTE or Wi-Fi. All of the security and privacy capabilities of mobile networks, such as entity authentication, secrecy, integrity of data, and mobile equipment identification, are advantageous to this NB-IoT network design.

Bluetooth Low Power: This choice is a Bluetooth personal area network (PAN) variation that uses less power and is intended for use by internet-connected devices. The Bluetooth 4.0 specification included Bluetooth Low Energy (BLE) as a replacement for conventional Bluetooth. It uses frequency-hopping wireless technology, which operates in the unlicensed 2.4 GHz radio band, to link neighbouring devices. With 0.01 to 0.5 watts of power consumption, BLE can reach a maximum speed of 1 Mbps. This amounts to almost half of what traditional Bluetooth uses for power.BLE is intended to cover a limited area, often between 30 and 100 metres within a small structure. It offers open access to the necessary specs, a very simple development procedure, and widespread use in smartphones. Some of the disadvantages of this technology include the requirement for a gateway device in order to connect the end devices to the internet and interference from other users of the 2.4 GHz protocol.

IEEE 802.11ax: The most recent version of LANs, IEEE 802.11ax (Wi-Fi 6), gives healthcare facilities a notable boost in coverage, capacity, and efficiency without compromising key capabilities like interoperability, security, and user-friendliness. When thousands or even hundreds of devices need connectivity at the same time, these networks can manage dense environments with efficiency. With Wi-Fi-enabled devices, nurses and doctors may access imaging findings, patient information, and real-time patient monitoring data. IEEE 802.11ax offers improved functionality for more client gadgets per access point, efficient utilisation of airtime, and lower power consumption. Medical gadgets can run on batteries for longer periods of time thanks to Wi-Fi 6 networks, which also improve user experience overall. IEEE 802.11ax's improved data processing capabilities allow medical staff members to access digital data and images from radiography, ultrasound, and MRI devices from anywhere in the hospital. It used to be difficult to transport and operate with these sorts of very big files fast. IEEE 802.11ax's target wake time function prolongs a device's battery life and sleep time.

Zigbee: The Zigbee (IEEE 802.15.4) technical standard specifies how a low-rate wireless PAN should function. It details media access as well as the physical layer. With secure, dependable wireless network architectures at its core, Zigbee is an open global standard for wireless radio networks that was created to offer a user-friendly wireless data solution.The flexible network structure, long battery life support, and simplicity of installation of Zigbee are among its benefits. Its limited range, high maintenance costs, and lack of a complete solution are some of its drawbacks. Furthermore, unlike Wi-Fi-based secured systems, Zigbee is not secure.

5G cellular: 5G technologies are widely used for smartphone connectivity and offer dependable, global access to Internet of Things devices that are designed to be mobile. Because 5G supports both high and low data rates, it can be used for a wide range of purposes. However, there is a fee associated with subscribing to a 5G network provider through an integrated network.

Many connection methods need to be employed in order to interface and connect IoT devices in a major healthcare application. An overlay architecture that integrates cloud computing resources for distant device connectivity, edge computing at the hospital, and occasionally local communication via Bluetooth from an IoT device to a smartphone functioning as a relay should be in place for administrators. The degree of heterogeneity of the wireless technologies included determines how complicated the architecture will ultimately be (Young et al., 2003).

5.A REAL-TIME HEALTH MONITORING SYSTEM ENABLED BY WEARABLE IOT

5.1. Overview of IoT-Enabled Healthcare Architecture

When modern information and communication technologies (ICT) are incorporated into the healthcare system, it is expected that patients who are elderly and/or have chronic conditions would obtain more effective and efficient healthcare services as shown in figure 1. In the meanwhile, other phenomena have surfaced, such as ambient assisted living (AAL), IoT for healthcare, and ubiquitous healthcare. These words are not interchangeable, despite their relationship. The Internet of Things (IoT) emphasises how everything is connected, both digitally and physically. This covers a wide range of products, including as sensors, smart gadgets, cyber sensors, and more. Data exchange and transmission can be done automatically and efficiently thanks to the Internet of Things. Therefore, it is believed that utilising networked medical sensors to improve the use of IoT in healthcarespecially wearable or implantable onescan provide intelligent, accurate, and fairly cost customised healthcare services. Fig. 1 depicts the whole architecture of IoT-enabled healthcare. The sensing layer's job is to keep an eye on users' emotional, mental, and physical health. Numerous sensors, including wearable ones for collecting biological parameters (such blood pressure and ECG), GPS sensors for localization and tracking, and RFID readers for identification, may be included to achieve this goal. Moreover, smart homes are often utilised to gather data on the user's immediate environment, such as the condition of the house and the items in use. The network layer, secondarily, facilitates efficient and secure data transmission to corresponding data processing units. Numerous short-range communication protocols, such as ZigBee, are widely in use. Many new methods have recently been introduced, such as 6LowPAN, NB-IOT, and LoRa. Then, the third-layer Data Processing module is responsible for deriving meaningful insights from the sensor data that was obtained from the first layer. As of right now, the most promising strategy for data mining is learning-based. Ultimately, the conduction of the top three layers may be used to deliver intelligent services and applications, such as smart help, behaviour identification, and illness detection (Lv et al., 2020; Perez et al., 2016).

Figure 1. IoT-Enabled Healthcare Architecture

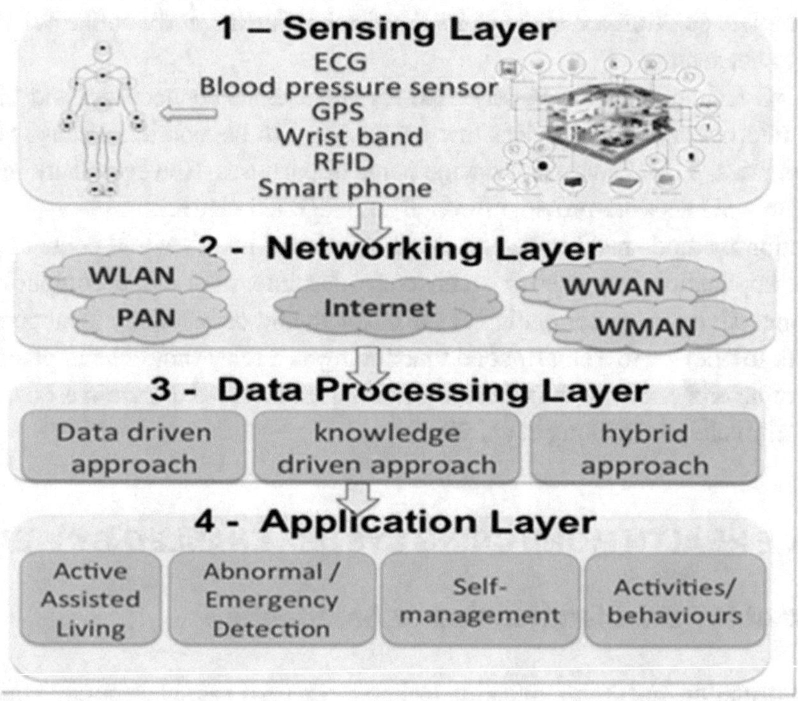

5.2. The Way the WISE System is Designed

A variety of networked wearable sensors are used by the wearable IoT-cloud-based wellness tracking system (WISE) to monitor the subject's health. One can acquire a range of biological signals, such as body temperature, heart rate, and blood pressure. The sensor data acquired from those wearable sensors will be sent straight to the cloud server due to the sensor nodes' low memory and computing power as well as to prevent using a smartphone as a processing unit. Figure 2 shows the general layout of the WISE system. The WISE body area network (W-BAN), the WISE cloud (W-Cloud), and the WISE Users are the three main parts of the WISE system.

Figure 2.

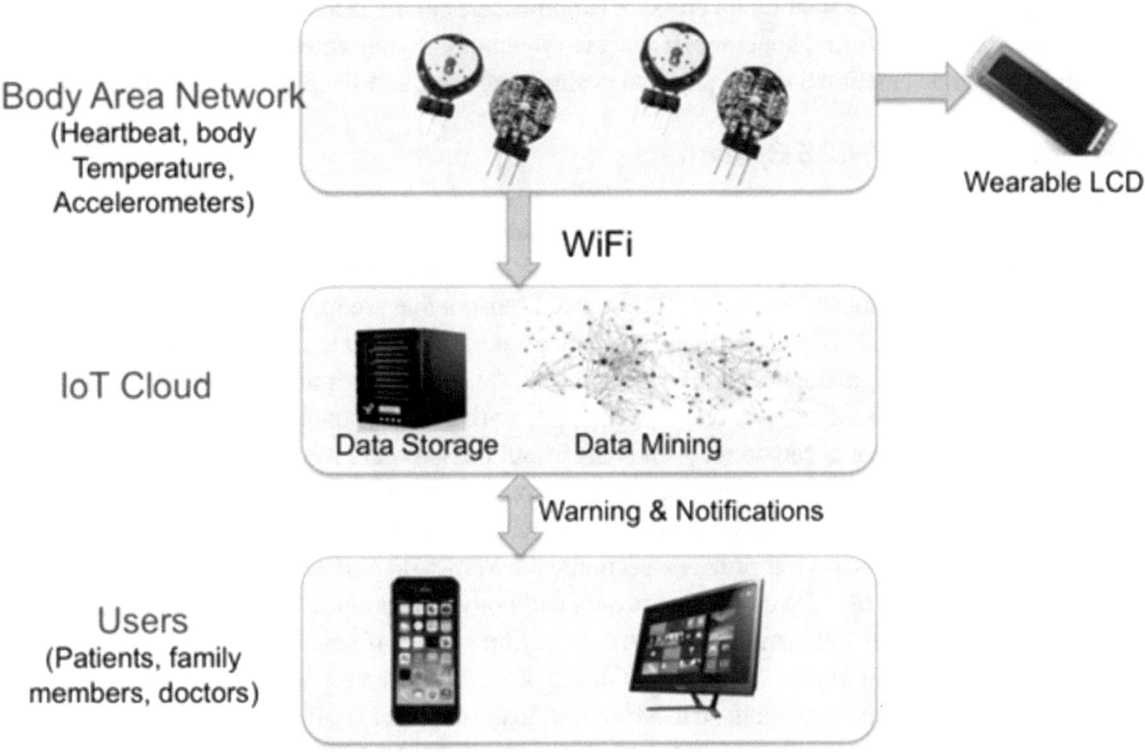

The W-BAN consists of three categories of sensing devices, which are the heartbeat sensors, the body temperature sensors and the blood pressure sensor which are depicted as below Figure 3.

Figure 3.

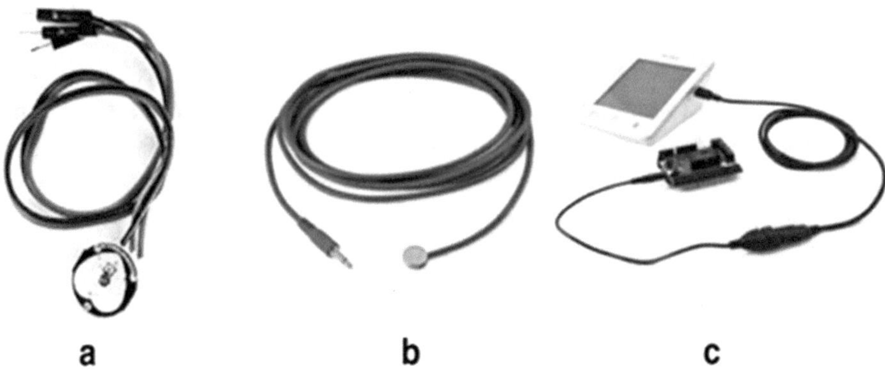

The circuit's temperature sensor will measure the ambient temperature and display the result in Celsius (degrees). The low-voltage integrated circuit (IC) LM35 requires power of about +5VDC. The non-invasive blood pressure sensor is intended to measure an individual's blood pressure. It makes use of the oscillometric technique to measure the systolic, diastolic, and mean arterial pressure. Many people find that it's crucial to check their blood pressure at home, particularly if they have high blood pressure. Blood pressure fluctuates throughout time. It adapts to your body's requirements. Numerous things, such as breathing patterns, emotional states, physical posture, exercise, and sleep quality, can influence it.

5.3. Architecture of WISE System

The aforementioned sensor nodes are combined with the Arduino sensor platform, which forms the basis of the WISE development. Figure:4 presents the WISE system's implementation architecture. A number of other components are used in addition to the sensors that are integrated into WISE. First,an RFID tag needs to be attached to each unique user since a portable RFID reader that is connected to the Arduino platform makes it easier to identify various users. An additional option for the user to obtain the data is a lightweight LCD. Moreover, WISE is equipped with a WiFi module that permitsdata transfer to the cloud and subsequent access to real-time data by authorised users from anylocation at any time.

The WISE BAN data may now be processed and stored on the cloud with increased efficacy and efficiency. Data processing and storage are two of the many capabilities that are implemented via the WISE Cloud. As was discussed in previous sections, the WISE-BAN may be used to gather various sensor signals, including blood pressure, heart rate, and body temperature. Significant characteristics may be recovered to detect and identify possible cardiac illness, even if noise commonly present during data transfer, which would impair the diagnosis of the prospective disease. A system for filtering data is used to stop invalid data from being sent. Moreover, historical data is often required to identify and accurately diagnose a potential disease; for this reason, a cloud database is made to keep individual user sensor data from the WISE-BAN within the WISE-Cloud data visualisation. A web-based data visualisation strategy for illness detection and notification is implemented to make the data accessible to allowed users. Individuals who suffer from heart conditions are often quite vulnerable to sudden cardiac death. In order to protect patients from harm of this sort, WISE has to be able to monitor and understand the health of the patients. Notifications on any suspicious or odd sensor reading can also be forwarded to specified users, such as physicians and family members. The WISE-Cloud solution is built on an HTTP server and a MySQL database storage server. A web-based graphical user interface (GUI) is made; an interface depiction that displays Sensor data from the WISE-BAN is kept for each user individually within the WISE-Cloud. data visualisation. A web-based data visualisation strategy is built so that the data is accessible to permitted users only. Once the power supply is turned on, the temperature from the thermistor and the heart rate from the pulse metre sensor are recorded. The webpage displays the same data in real time after it has been posted to the WISE-Cloud database server. A similar procedure is also used to the data and blood pressure sensor. Users need this information in order to self-monitor their healthmedical professionals to identify possible illnesses. If any abnormal condition is found, an alarm will be created and sent via text message to the users' physicians or family members, as well as displayed on the LCD for the users' personal use.

6. 5G MEC-IoT-POWERED REAL-TIME REMOTE HEALTH MONITORING SYSTEM

A newer approach to providing healthcare, telemedicine can manage people's everyday health in real time at home and significantly reduce the burden associated with hospital outpatient visits. The two main demographic trends that the world is currently experiencing have made people's health issues of concern to the entire community. The first is the growing severity of the ageing population. Many elderly people will eventually have to deal with the issue of finding it difficult to get hospital medical care. The second is that the sub-health phenomena among young people is spreading, as the speed and stresses of today's society rise. The Internet of Things (IoT), 5G, artificial intelligence (AI), big data, cloud computing, and other cutting-edge technologies should be able to fully integrate the medical industry with the previously listed health problems. In particular, the telemedicine industry is continuously seeing new applications thanks to the IoT and AI made possible by 5G as shown in figure 4 (Zhang et al., 2020).

Figure 4.

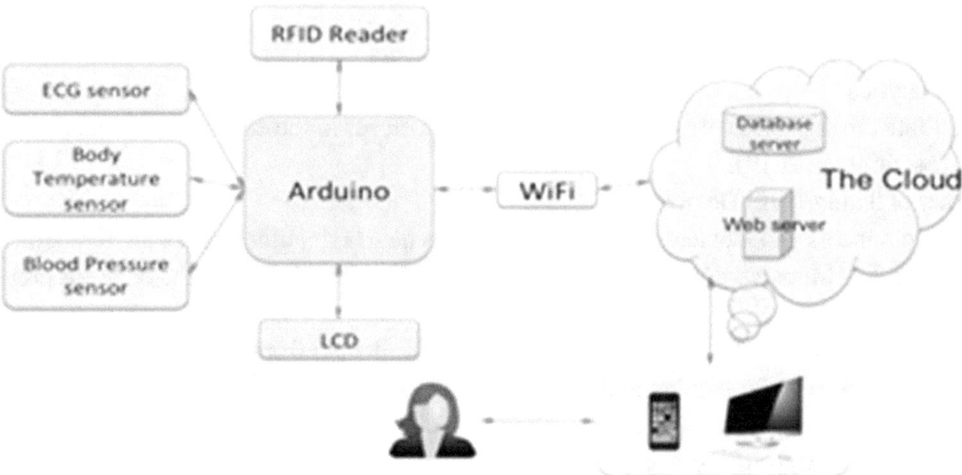

Mobile medicine, intelligent drug and device control to achieve personal medical management and health data management, remote monitoring, remote ultrasound, remote consultation, and remote surgical procedures are some of the main application scenarios of telemedicine in the medical sciences and health fields. The development of wearable biomedical devices for vital sign monitoring is now progressing rapidly. In order to create wearable biomedical devices, intelligence, compact size, low power consumption, and low cost are essential. Two of the numerous advantages of wearable health devices are the ongoing provision of medical services and the real-time perception of health data. They can monitor human characteristics and health issues in real time, helping people understand their bodily states and recognise signs early. Thanks to advancements in semiconductor technology, wearable technology has experienced considerable improvements in performance at a much lower cost and power consumption. Because of the confluence of AI and IoT, wearables are increasingly more intelligent. The development and research of wearable biomedical devices has become more important in the realm of telemedicine.

Moreover, it is critical to guarantee the rapid progress of telemedicine. Most wearable technology on the market is expected to have some sort of medical or health-related connection (Qi et al., 2017).

A wide range of vertical sectors have expressed a great deal of interest in the 5G network recently due to its many benefits, which include fast speed, large connections, and low latency. High-speed transmission and exchange of medical picture data, together with 4K/8K remote high-definition consultations, are made feasible by 5G's high-speed feature. It also improves the efficiency of diagnosis and advice, enables professionals to interact with patients at any time or place, and delivers first-rate medical resources directly to patients' homes. A plethora of medical sensor terminals, related video devices, and wearable biomedical devices can be connected thanks to 5G's large-connection capability. This will enable real-time perception and measurements, the recording and transmission of patient health information, and accurate, continuous monitoring of health information over time and space constraints.

Components:

1. 5G Network Infrastructure:
   Base Stations and Towers: Transmit and receive signals, providing high-speed connectivity.
   Core Network: Handles data routing and management for efficient communication.
2. Mobile Edge Computing (MEC):
   Edge Servers: Located close to end-users, these servers facilitate real-time data processing and analytics.
   MEC Platform: Enables software applications to run closer to the edge for low-latency processing (Nazir et al., 2019).
3. Internet of Things(IoT) Devices:
   Wearable Sensors and Devices: Collect data such as heart rate, blood pressure, temperature, etc.
   Embedded IoT Modules: Devices capable of transmitting health data to the edge for processing.
4. Cloud Infrastructure:
   Cloud Storage: Storing large volumes of health data collected from various IoT devices.
   Analytics Platforms: Processing and analyzing data for insights, trends, and alerts.
5. AI and Machine Learning Algorithms:
   Data Processing Algorithms: Analyze health data to identify patterns, anomalies, and potential risks.
   Predictive Models: Forecast potential health issues based on historical data.
6. Healthcare Applications and User Interfaces:
   Mobile Apps/Web Interfaces: Display real-time health data for users and healthcare providers.
   Alert Systems: Instant alerts for critical health changes or emergencies (Saha et al., 2020).
7. Security and Privacy Measures:
   Encryption Protocols: Ensure secure transmission of sensitive health data.
   Access Control and Authentication: Authenticate users and devices to maintain data privacy.
8. Interoperability Framework:
   Standardized Protocols: Enable seamless communication among diverse IoT devices and platforms.
   APIs and Integration Layers: Facilitate data exchange and interoperability.
9. Remote Healthcare Services:
   Telemedicine Platforms: Enable remote consultations and interventions.
   Emergency Response Systems: Immediate alerts and responses during critical health events.

A multiple-sensor network that is placed surrounding hospital beds makes up the IoT layer. Its purpose is to gather environmental and physiological data and send it to the MEC layer. There are several methods for using 4G, 5G, Wi-Fi, or Zigbee to complete the transmission duty. The system selects 5G among them in order to immediately link the Internet of Things (IoT) to the MEC layer and transfer massive amounts of high-quality, high-speed IoT sensing data every second as depicted in Figure 5. The authorised institutions, such as affiliated hospitals and the Centres for Disease Control and Prevention, can access data stored in the cloud layer as necessary. In addition, nurses may quickly respond to crises by using the monitoring terminal, which is connected to the MEC layer, to track the patients' physical conditions in real time (Duan et al., 2020).

Figure 5. The System Model's Framework

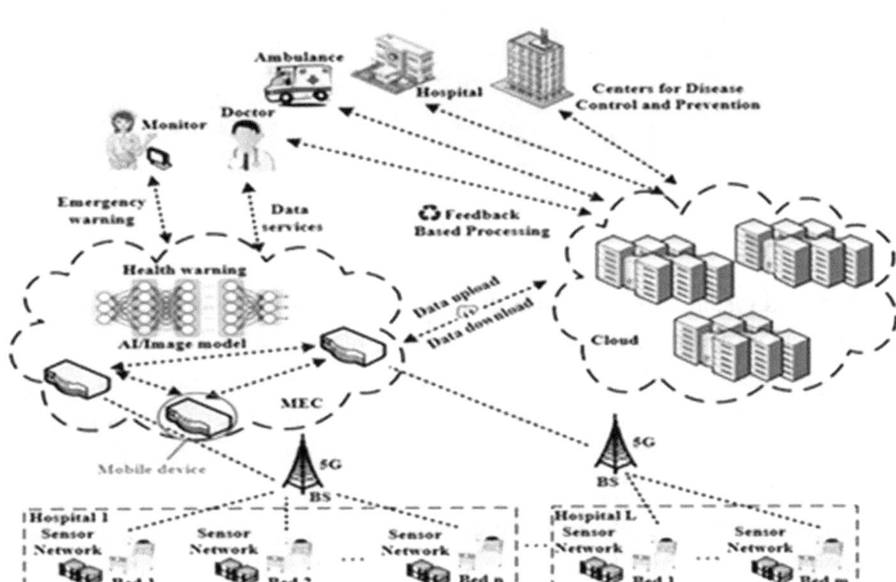

The entire process of processing and transmitting data through the MEC layer in a circumstance that is unclear. IoT-layer sensors are used by users to produce the ECG data, which is subsequently transmitted over 5G to the MEC servers for additional data processing. The data receiving, temporary data storage, artificial intelligence-powered automatic ECG diagnosis, data access, and diagnosis result generation are all handled by the MEC layer. Medical personnel rely heavily on the abundance of physiological and environmental data that hospitals collect from their patients to aid in patient diagnosis and treatment. Hospitalised patients use various types of data collected by a sensor network to accurately depict their health status. The non-hospitalized people may also make use of a similar home sensor network, or only a wearable ECG detection device that was put on upon their skin. The application situation and the user's required degree of health monitoring service will determine this.

Artificial Intelligence has recently progressed. The DL model has seen widespread use in a variety of areas, including speech and image recognition. When compared to the widely used feature extraction-based machine learning model, the performance of the DL model is significantly superior. Many professionals have provided their own categorizations of arrhythmias. Ziman et al. used spectrum transformation methods before feeding ECG data into a convolution recurrent neural network.

Figure 6. Dataflow Over the System Model

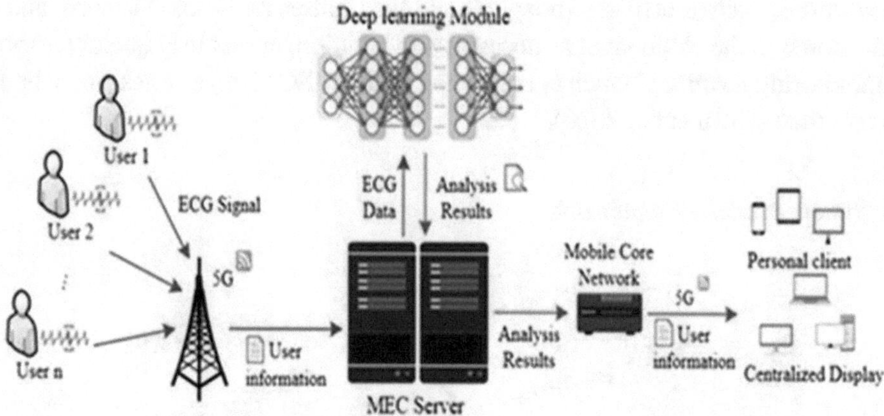

In figure:6 suggested system is made to offer large-scale users health monitoring services in a variety of situations. The cloud provides corresponding computing resources for ECG automatic diagnosis and data storage, and it permits authorized individuals or entities to perform additional disease analysis or recording through the stored data. The Internet of Things (IoT) layer is in charge of gathering the user's physiological and environmental data through a variety of sensors and uploading them to the cloud. The suggested system makes use of the MEC layer, which sits between the IoT and cloud layers, to speed up response times to emergency medical situations, decrease transmission pressure, and minimize delays in data transmission and processing. This is because the proposed service is related to medical care and is data-intensive. The data generation nodes are not accessible from the MEC layer. When utilising edge computing, data analysis operations are carried out at the network's edge as opposed to just employing cloud computing. This shortens the data transmission distance, which speeds up system operation and significantly increases the overall design of the suggested system's viability. MEC originates at the edge network. It is possible to install certain MEC hosts near to the end users. MEC hosts have enough memory and processing power. The primary benefit of the MEC layer is its ability to lower network latency thanks to the MEC host's computational and storage power. The base station serves as the actual server in this scenario. Additionally, it lessens the device's bandwidth and gets around the restrictions on the resources that are already available, including storage space and capability for processing. Prior generations of wireless networks aimed to facilitate the shift from voice-centric networks to multimedia-centric networks by offering quicker internet access. The 5G network's job is to keep content delivery, computation, control, and communication stable. It's a far more intricate and distinct work. In addition to connecting consumers, the 5G network aims to link any device or application inside the access network. Machine-to-machine communication and the Internet of Things have developed significantly as a result of the advancement of mobile technologies. Numerous telemedicine scenarios will be significantly impacted by 5G technology.

7. FUTURE DIRECTIONS WITH REGARD TO IOT ADVANCEMENTS

The emergence of IoT technology has brought great possibilities and advantages to the field of personalised healthcare. This progress is made possible in large part by the wireless body area network, which is made up of communication modules and wearable sensor equipment. Accurate detection of crises is made possible by real-time remote monitoring of patients' health situations, which guarantees prompt communication with physicians and family members. A lot of study has been done in this field, however there are still issues, which are covered in the next section. Running biomedical signal monitoring around-the-clock may be painful and invasive for people since it necessitates putting several sensors on different body areas for lengthy periods of time. Furthermore, sensors frequently have low processing and storage capacities despite producing enormous volumes of data. This not only increases processing and memory needs, but also makes data analysis more difficult. Thus, to properly extract the most relevant information, a more intelligent sensor data-filtering method must be developed. Additionally, a major problem with many sensing devices, including smartphones, is battery life, especially when using Bluetooth and WiFi connections. Therefore, a more advanced data transmission approach that maximises system performance while reducing data transmission frequency can be used as a backup. BAN has become a promising technology in the field of personalised healthcare, but it requires more attention to network security, privacy, resilience, and stability. Technically speaking, a BAN has to be more robust and tolerant to node failures brought on by damaged or low batteries. The network needs to guarantee continuous communication between nodes even in the event of outages on some of them.

The Internet of Things (IoT) has gained increasing interest in recent years because to its ability to seamlessly integrate heterogeneous intelligent devices such as smart TVs, smartphones, sensors, and many more. The wearable IoT subset of the Internet of Things is concerned with the connections and communication between wearable technology. In the meanwhile, wearable IoT has surfaced as a potential use for medical communication and data transfer, offering the required infrastructure. The healthcare industry is one such application. It is expected to transform the healthcare system and bring down healthcare expenses. There are still certain issues that need to be resolved, such developing a wearable IoT platform that is reasonably priced and ensuring its scalability, resilience, security, privacy, and other aspects (Jalali et al., 2020).

Delivering services in real time presents a variety of challenges that must be overcome. For the benefit of doctors, carers, and patients alike, user-friendly, customised, and adaptable services must be developed. For example, carers can specify the conditions and type of notification that need to be given. We should also discuss dynamic service mapping and discovery in our second section. What should be done, for example, if it turns out that a patient is having an unplanned heart attack? A medical ontology library might be established to assist in identifying the most effective and accessible materials for diagnosing certain diseases (Dhanvijay & Patil, 2019).

8. CONCLUSION

The advent of real-time IoT healthcare monitoring systems marks a watershed moment in the evolution of healthcare. This innovative ecosystem, driven by the convergence of IoT, 5G, MEC, and advanced analytics, redefines the landscape of patient care, bringing forth a paradigm shift towards personalized, proactive, and remote health management. At its core, this system revolves around the seamless integration of interconnected devices equipped with sensors and wearable capable of capturing a plethora of health metrics. These devices serve as constant health companions, monitoring vital signs, activity levels, and various biometric data points, furnishing individuals and healthcare professionals with a comprehensive real-time view of health status. The backbone of this infrastructure is the 5G network, enabling lightning-fast, low-latency communication. Complementing this, Mobile Edge Computing (MEC) strategically positions computing resources closer to the data source. This proximity facilitates swift data processing, analysis, and decision-making at the edge, ensuring near-instantaneous response times critical for healthcare interventions. However, the true power of this system lies beyond data collection; it lies in its ability to transform raw data into actionable insights. Advanced analytics and AI algorithms decode the wealth of collected data, identifying trends, anomalies, and potential health risks. Real-time alerts and notifications serve as early-warning systems, empowering healthcare providers to intervene promptly, preventing health crises and offering timely interventions tailored to individual needs (Babakerhell & Pandey, 2019).

The impact of this system extends far beyond traditional healthcare boundaries. It empowers individuals to actively engage in their health management, promoting preventive care and lifestyle changes based on real-time feedback. Moreover, it bridges geographical barriers, enabling remote patient monitoring, consultations, and access to specialized care irrespective of location, enhancing healthcare equity. Despite its promising potential, several challenges necessitate consideration. Security and privacy concerns loom large, demanding robust encryption, authentication, and stringent compliance with healthcare regulations to safeguard sensitive health data. Interoperability complexities among myriad devices and platforms require standardized protocols and cohesive integration strategies to ensure seamless data exchange and communication. The culmination of these technological advancements heralds a future where healthcare is no longer confined to clinical settings but seamlessly integrated into daily life. Remote monitoring of chronic conditions becomes the norm, significantly reducing hospital readmissions and healthcare costs. Additionally, it paves the way for more efficient clinical trials, medical research, and population health management through the aggregation and analysis of vast datasets.

In conclusion, the real-time IoT healthcare monitoring system is a transformative force poised to revolutionize healthcare delivery. It fosters a new era of patient-centric care, empowering individuals with personalized health insights while equipping healthcare providers with tools for proactive, remote, and precise interventions. As this ecosystem continues to evolve and overcome existing challenges, its potential to redefine healthcare as we know it becomes increasingly evident, promising a future where health is intelligently monitored, managed, and optimized for all.

REFERENCES

Babakerkhell & Pandey. (2019). Analysis of Different IOT Based Healthcare Monitoring Systems. *International Journal of Innovative Technology and Exploring Engineering, 8*(6S2).

Birje, M. N. (2020). Internet of things based distributed healthcare systems: A reviewJ. Data. *Information & Management*, *2*(3), 149–165.

Dhanvijay, M. M., & Patil, S. C. (2019). Internet of Things: A survey of enabling technologies in healthcare and its applications. *Computer Networks*, *153*, 113–131. doi:10.1016/j.comnet.2019.03.006

Duan, A., Guo, L., Gao, H., Wu, X., & Dong, X. (2020). Deep Focus Parallel Convolutional Neural Network for Imbalanced Classification of Machinery Fault Diagnostics. *IEEE Transactions on Instrumentation and Measurement, 69*(11), 8680–8689. doi:10.1109/TIM.2020.2998233

Jalali, A., & Lee, M. (2020). Atrial Fibrillation Prediction with Residual Network Using Sensitivity and Orthogonality Constraints. *IEEE Journal of Biomedical and Health Informatics, 24*(2), 407–413. doi:10.1109/JBHI.2019.2957809 PMID:31825883

Ke, H., Chen, D., Shi, B., Zhang, J., Liu, X., Zhang, X., & Li, X. (2020). Improving Brain E-Health Services via High-Performance EEG Classification with Grouping Bayesian Optimization. *IEEE Transactions on Services Computing, 13*(4), 696–708. doi:10.1109/TSC.2019.2962673

Lin, T., Goyal, P., Girshick, R., He, K., & Dollár, P. (2020). Focal Loss for Dense Object Detection. *IEEE Transactions on Pattern Analysis and Machine Intelligence, 42*(2), 318–327. doi:10.1109/TPAMI.2018.2858826 PMID:30040631

Lv, Q., Chen, H., Zhong, W., Wang, Y., Song, J., Guo, S., Qi, L., & Chen, C. Y. (2020). A Multi-Task Group Bi-LSTM Networks Application on Electrocardiogram Classification. *IEEE Journal of Translational Engineering in Health and Medicine, 8*, 1–11. doi:10.1109/JTEHM.2019.2952610 PMID:32082952

Nazir, Ali, Ullah, & Garcıa-Magariño. (2019). Internet of Things for Healthcare Using Effects of Mobile Computing: A Systematic Literature Review. *Hindawi Wireless Communications and Mobile Computing*.

Nie, D., Wang, L., Adeli, E., Lao, C., Lin, W., & Shen, D. (2019). 3-D Fully Convolutional Networks for Multimodal Isointense Infant Brain Image Segmentation. *IEEE Transactions on Cybernetics, 49*(3), 1123–1136. doi:10.1109/TCYB.2018.2797905 PMID:29994385

Perez, R. R., Marques, A., & Mohammadi, F. (2016). The application of supervised learning through feed-forward neural networks for ECG signal classification. *Proceedings of the 2016 IEEE Canadian Conference on Electrical and Computer Engineering (CCECE),* 1–4. 10.1109/CCECE.2016.7726762

Prodhan, U. K., Rahman, M. Z., Jahan, I., Abid, A., & Bellah, M. (2017). Development of a portable telemedicine tool for remote diagnosis of telemedicine application. *Proceedings of the 2017 International Conference on Computing, Communication and Automation (ICCCA)*, 287–292. 10.1109/CCAA.2017.8229817

Qi, J., Yang, P., Min, G., Amft, O., Dong, F., & Xu, L. (2017). Advanced internet, of things for personalized healthcare systems: A survey. *Pervasive and Mobile Computing, 41*, 132–149. doi:10.1016/j.pmcj.2017.06.018

Saha, B., Gupta, S., Phung, D., & Venkatesh, S. (2017). A Framework for Mixed-Type Multioutcome Prediction with Applications in Healthcare. *IEEE Journal of Biomedical and Health Informatics, 21*(4), 1182–1191. doi:10.1109/JBHI.2017.2681799 PMID:28328519

Saranya, E., & Maheswaran, T. (2019). IoT Based Disease Prediction and Diagnosis System for Healthcare. *International Journal of Engineering Development and Research, 7*(2), 232-237.

Shanmugasundaram & Sankarikaarguzhali. (n.d.). An investigation on IoT healthcare analytics. *International Journal of Information Engineering and Electronic*.

Wu, S., Li, G., Deng, L., Liu, L., Wu, D., Xie, Y., & Shi, L. (2019). L1-Norm Batch Normalization for Efficient Training of Deep Neural Networks. *IEEE Transactions on Neural Networks and Learning Systems*, *30*(7), 2043–2051. doi:10.1109/TNNLS.2018.2876179 PMID:30418924

Young, D. P., Keller, C. M., Bliss, D. W., & Forsythe, K. W. (2003). Ultra-wideband (UWB) transmitter location using time difference of arrival (TDOA) techniques. *The Thrity-Seventh Asilomar Conference on Signals, Systems & Computers,* 2, 1225–1229. 10.1109/ACSSC.2003.1292184

Yu, X., Yu, Z., & Ramalingam, S. (2018). Learning Strict Identity Mappings in Deep Residual Networks. *Proceedings of the 2018 IEEE/CVF Conference on Computer Vision and Pattern Recognition*, 4432–4440. 10.1109/CVPR.2018.00466

Zhang, J., Yang, L., Cao, W., & Wang, Q. (2020). Formal Analysis of 5G EAP-TLS Authentication Protocol Using Proverif. *IEEE Access : Practical Innovations, Open Solutions*, *8*, 23674–23688. doi:10.1109/ACCESS.2020.2969474

Chapter 9
Digital Health Innovations to Significantly Improve the Quality of Services in Healthcare Systems

Tarun Madan Kanade
https://orcid.org/0009-0002-0084-3107
Sandip Foundation, India

Radhakrishna Bhaskar Batule
Vishwakarma University, Pune, India

ABSTRACT

This chapter explores the synergy between digital health innovations and social networks, emphasizing their transformative impact on healthcare quality. Addressing challenges like access disparities, rising costs, and patient safety concerns, the author dissects telemedicine, EHRs, wearables, and AI, illustrating their contributions to healthcare improvement. Case studies highlight positive changes, from expanded access to informed decision-making. The role of social networks in facilitating adoption and ensuring patient engagement is crucial. The chapter introduces a framework with KPIs, underlining social networks as platforms for sharing best practices.

1. INTRODUCTION

In the rapidly evolving landscape of healthcare, digital innovations are becoming the linchpin for progress, promising to redefine the standards of service quality. This chapter seeks to unravel the intricate tapestry of current digital healthcare trends, particularly focusing on innovations that hold the potential to significantly enhance the quality of healthcare services. As we navigate the intricate amalgamation of technology and healthcare, the imperative for continuous improvement looms large. This introduction

DOI: 10.4018/979-8-3693-1934-5.ch009

sets the stage for a comprehensive exploration, illuminating the transformative power of digital health innovations and the pivotal role they play in reshaping the healthcare ecosystem.

a. Overview of Digital Health Innovations

At the heart of this chapter is a thorough examination of digital health innovations. This encompasses a spectrum of technologies, from telemedicine and wearable devices to artificial intelligence and data analytics. The overview aims to provide a panoramic view of the diverse tools and strategies under the digital health umbrella. By understanding the breadth of innovations, readers can appreciate the complexity and interconnectedness of these technologies that collectively contribute to the overarching goal of improving healthcare services (Yasmyne Ronquillo, 2023).

b. Improving Healthcare Services and Quality

The chapter accentuates the critical importance of elevating healthcare services and quality. As the healthcare landscape grapples with increasing demands, improving services becomes imperative. This section delves into the challenges faced by contemporary healthcare systems, emphasizing the need for innovations that go beyond mere convenience and actively contribute to better patient outcomes, accessibility, and overall efficiency. By elucidating the significance of this mission, the chapter positions digital health innovations as indispensable tools in the pursuit of enhanced healthcare services (Mosadeghrad, 2014).

c. Use of Social Networks for Analyzing Trends

The chapter takes an innovative approach by introducing social networks as a valuable resource for analyzing current digital healthcare trends. Social networks have evolved beyond personal connections, becoming rich repositories of health-related data. This section discusses how mining and analyzing data from these networks can unveil patterns, preferences, and behaviors relevant to healthcare. By tapping into this wealth of information, healthcare professionals can gain profound insights that shape and inform the trajectory of digital health innovations. The integration of social network analysis adds a contemporary and dynamic dimension to the exploration of digital healthcare trends in this chapter.

2. THE DIGITAL HEALTH LANDSCAPE

The digital health landscape represents a paradigm shift in the way healthcare is conceptualized, delivered, and experienced. At its essence, digital health encompasses the fusion of healthcare and technology, leveraging a myriad of digital tools and innovations to revolutionize the entire healthcare ecosystem.

a. Concept of Digital Health

Digital health is a holistic term that encapsulates the convergence of healthcare and technology to improve the efficiency, accessibility, and quality of healthcare services. At its core, digital health leverages digital tools, technologies, and platforms to enhance various aspects of healthcare delivery, from diagnosis and treatment to patient engagement and preventive care. This encompasses a wide range of technologies, including telemedicine, wearable devices, health information systems, mobile health applications, artificial intelligence, and data analytics.

Digital health aims to empower both healthcare providers and patients by facilitating seamless communication, real-time monitoring, and data-driven decision-making. It seeks to break down traditional barriers in healthcare, enabling more personalized and proactive approaches to health management. The concept extends beyond the clinical setting, embracing a comprehensive view of health that incorporates lifestyle factors, preventive measures, and patient-centered care.

b. Digital Health in Modern Healthcare Systems

The significance of digital health in modern healthcare systems is monumental, ushering in a new era of patient-centered, efficient, and accessible care. One key aspect is the democratization of healthcare information and services, allowing individuals to actively participate in their health management. Digital health facilitates remote monitoring, enabling healthcare professionals to track patient health in real-time, leading to early intervention and personalized treatment plans (Bernstein, 2022).

Moreover, it streamlines administrative processes, reducing paperwork and enhancing the overall efficiency of healthcare delivery. Telemedicine, a subset of digital health, has emerged as a critical component, providing remote consultations, especially in underserved or remote areas. This not only increases access to healthcare but also reduces the burden on physical infrastructure.

c. Role of Social Networks in Disseminating Information About Digital Health Innovations

Social networks play a pivotal role in disseminating information about digital health innovations. These platforms serve as dynamic spaces where individuals share experiences, engage in discussions, and seek information about health-related topics. Digital health information can rapidly spread through these networks, reaching diverse audiences and fostering awareness.

Social networks facilitate the viral dissemination of success stories, testimonials, and information about the latest digital health technologies. This grassroots sharing of information contributes to the adoption of innovations by building trust and credibility. Additionally, these platforms provide a space for healthcare professionals, researchers, and technology developers to engage with the public, answering queries and addressing concerns (World Health Organization, 2021).

However, the role of social networks is not without challenges, including the need for accurate information dissemination and the potential for misinformation. Understanding and navigating this dual nature of social networks is crucial for harnessing their full potential in promoting and disseminating information about digital health innovations.

3. TELEMEDICINE AND REMOTE MONITORING

Telemedicine utilizes telecommunications technology to provide healthcare services remotely, offering consultations, diagnosis, and treatment without the need for in-person visits. This approach enhances healthcare accessibility, breaking down geographical barriers and facilitating timely interventions, especially in underserved areas. It streamlines healthcare processes, reducing wait times, and encourages proactive patient engagement.

Remote monitoring complements telemedicine by continuously tracking patient health metrics through wearable devices and sensors. This real-time data allows healthcare professionals to observe vital signs and intervene promptly, contributing to a proactive and personalized approach to care. Together, telemedicine and remote monitoring empower individuals to actively participate in their health management, particularly in chronic disease scenarios, improving overall healthcare quality. These digital health solutions represent a transformative shift toward patient-centric, efficient, and accessible healthcare (Zhuravel, 2023).

a. Impact of Telemedicine on Healthcare Quality

Telemedicine, a cornerstone of digital health, has significantly transformed the landscape of healthcare delivery, profoundly impacting its quality. By leveraging telecommunications technology, telemedicine breaks down traditional barriers to healthcare access, ensuring that individuals can receive medical consultations and support remotely.

The impact on healthcare quality is multifold. Firstly, telemedicine enhances accessibility, especially for individuals in rural or underserved areas where healthcare facilities may be scarce. Patients can connect with healthcare professionals without the constraints of geographical distances, leading to timely interventions and improved health outcomes.

Secondly, telemedicine facilitates early diagnosis and intervention. Patients can seek medical advice promptly, reducing the risk of complications and enhancing the effectiveness of treatment plans. This is particularly crucial for chronic disease management, where regular monitoring and proactive interventions are key to maintaining health and preventing exacerbations (A. Shaji George, 2023).

Moreover, telemedicine contributes to patient-centered care. It empowers individuals to actively participate in their healthcare decisions, fostering a collaborative relationship with healthcare providers. This increased engagement can lead to better adherence to treatment plans, improved lifestyle choices, and overall better management of health conditions.

In summary, the impact of telemedicine on healthcare quality is substantial, addressing issues of accessibility, timeliness, and patient engagement.

b. Examples of Successful Telemedicine Programs

Numerous successful telemedicine programs showcase the tangible benefits of this innovative approach to healthcare delivery. One notable example is the Veterans Health Administration's (VA) telehealth initiatives. The VA utilizes telemedicine to provide virtual consultations, remote monitoring, and mental health services to veterans across the United States. This has not only improved access to care for veterans, especially those in rural areas, but has also demonstrated positive outcomes in terms of patient satisfaction and health outcomes (Jacqueline M Ferguson, 2021).

Another exemplary case is the Telehealth Ontario program in Canada, which provides 24/7 access to healthcare professionals via phone or online chat. This program has proven effective in reducing unnecessary emergency room visits, offering timely advice, and improving overall healthcare efficiency (Oleg Bestsennyy, 2021).

These case studies underscore the versatility and effectiveness of telemedicine in diverse healthcare settings, emphasizing its potential for scalability and positive impact on patient care.

c. Role of Social Networks in Promoting and Supporting Telemedicine Initiatives

Social networks play a crucial role in promoting and supporting telemedicine initiatives by acting as conduits for information, awareness, and community building. Platforms like Facebook, Twitter, and healthcare-specific networks serve as hubs where individuals share their telemedicine experiences, discuss the benefits, and disseminate information about available services.

Social networks contribute to the promotion of telemedicine by raising awareness about its advantages, addressing concerns, and fostering a sense of community among users. Patient testimonials and success stories shared on social media platforms act as powerful endorsements, encouraging others to explore telemedicine options.

Moreover, social networks facilitate real-time communication between healthcare providers and patients. Telemedicine providers often use social media to share updates, answer queries, and provide information about available services. This direct interaction not only enhances patient engagement but also builds trust in telemedicine as a legitimate and reliable healthcare option.

Additionally, social networks serve as platforms for healthcare professionals to collaborate, share best practices, and stay informed about the latest developments in telemedicine. This collaborative aspect contributes to the continuous improvement and refinement of telemedicine practices.

In conclusion, social networks serve as instrumental tools for promoting and supporting telemedicine initiatives, fostering a connected and informed community that actively participates in the evolution of remote healthcare delivery.

4. ELECTRONIC HEALTH RECORDS (EHRS) AND DATA ANALYTICS

Electronic Health Records (EHRs) digitize patient information, providing a centralized, accessible platform for healthcare professionals. This transition streamlines data management, fosters communication, and enhances patient care. Concurrently, Data Analytics extracts valuable insights from EHRs, allowing healthcare providers to analyze patterns and trends within patient data. This data-driven approach empowers informed decision-making, personalized treatment plans, and proactive health management.

The integration of EHRs and Data Analytics not only improves individual patient care but also contributes to broader healthcare strategies. Population health trends can be identified, facilitating resource allocation and preventive measures. Research benefits from aggregated, de-identified data, fostering medical advancements. However, ethical considerations regarding patient privacy and data security must be carefully navigated. In essence, the synergy of EHRs and Data Analytics represents a transformative leap towards efficient, informed, and patient-centered healthcare systems (Sabyasachi Dash, 2019).

a. Benefits of EHRs in Improving Patient Care and Safety

Electronic Health Records (EHRs) offer a plethora of benefits in enhancing patient care and safety. One primary advantage lies in the centralized and digital storage of patient information, allowing healthcare professionals instant access to comprehensive medical histories. This quick retrieval of data ensures that medical teams are well-informed, leading to more accurate diagnoses and tailored treatment plans.

EHRs contribute significantly to patient safety by minimizing errors. Electronic records reduce the likelihood of illegible handwriting and transcription mistakes often associated with paper-based records. Furthermore, EHRs incorporate features such as alerts for potential drug interactions or allergies, promoting medication safety.

The interoperability of EHR systems ensures seamless communication between different healthcare providers involved in a patient's care. This continuity of information prevents gaps in care, enhances care coordination, and reduces the risk of redundant or conflicting treatments.

Patient engagement is another notable benefit. EHRs often provide patients with secure access to their own health information, fostering a sense of empowerment and encouraging active participation in their healthcare journey. This transparency can lead to better-informed decision-making and improved adherence to treatment plans (Edmond Li, 2021).

In summary, EHRs significantly improve patient care and safety by ensuring timely access to accurate information, reducing errors, enhancing care coordination, and promoting patient engagement.

b. Use of Data Analytics in Healthcare Decision-Making

Data analytics has become a cornerstone in healthcare decision-making, revolutionizing how information is utilized to enhance patient outcomes and optimize healthcare processes. Through the analysis of vast datasets, data analytics provides valuable insights that guide clinical, operational, and strategic decisions.

One prominent application is predictive analytics, which involves forecasting future trends based on historical data. In healthcare, this can assist in identifying patients at risk for certain conditions, allowing for proactive interventions and personalized treatment plans. For example, predictive analytics can help prevent hospital readmissions by identifying high-risk patients and tailoring post-discharge care (Infosys BPM, 2023).

In clinical decision support, data analytics aids healthcare professionals by providing evidence-based recommendations. This ensures that diagnoses and treatment plans align with the latest medical research, ultimately improving the quality of care.

Healthcare organizations leverage data analytics for operational efficiency. It helps optimize resource allocation, streamline workflows, and identify areas for improvement. From reducing wait times to enhancing patient flow, data analytics contributes to a more efficient and cost-effective healthcare system.

In conclusion, the use of data analytics in healthcare decision-making empowers providers with actionable insights, promoting personalized care, improving clinical outcomes, and optimizing healthcare operations.

c. Social Networks can Facilitate Data Sharing and Collaboration in Healthcare

Social networks play a pivotal role in fostering data sharing and collaboration within the healthcare landscape. These platforms provide a space for healthcare professionals, researchers, and even patients to connect, share information, and collaborate on various aspects of healthcare.

One primary benefit is the rapid dissemination of medical knowledge and research findings. Healthcare professionals can share insights, discuss case studies, and stay updated on the latest advancements in their field. This real-time exchange of information accelerates the pace of medical knowledge dissemination, contributing to continuous learning and improvement in patient care.

Social networks also facilitate collaboration among healthcare professionals. Virtual communities and discussion forums allow experts from different specialties and geographic locations to collaborate on challenging cases, share best practices, and seek advice. This collaborative approach can lead to more comprehensive and effective patient care.

In the realm of patient engagement, social networks provide platforms for patients to share their experiences, connect with others facing similar health challenges, and access valuable health information. Patient communities on social networks can serve as a support system, fostering a sense of community and empowerment.

However, the use of social networks in healthcare data sharing requires careful consideration of privacy and security concerns. Striking a balance between open collaboration and safeguarding sensitive patient information is essential to ensure ethical and responsible use of these platforms.

In summary, social networks serve as dynamic tools for data sharing and collaboration in healthcare, promoting knowledge exchange, interdisciplinary collaboration, and patient engagement.

5. HEALTH INFORMATION EXCHANGE (HIE)

Health Information Exchange (HIE) is a system facilitating the secure sharing of electronic health information among healthcare providers, improving care coordination. It allows authorized professionals to access and retrieve patient data, fostering seamless communication and informed decision-making across different healthcare entities. HIE enhances patient care by providing a comprehensive view of medical histories, reducing redundancies, and ensuring timely access to critical information, ultimately contributing to improved healthcare outcomes.

a. Significance of HIE in Healthcare Interoperability

Health Information Exchange (HIE) holds paramount importance in healthcare interoperability by enabling the seamless exchange of patient data among diverse healthcare systems. It bridges gaps between different electronic health record (EHR) systems, ensuring that crucial information is accessible across various healthcare providers. This interoperability enhances care coordination, reduces duplication of tests or procedures, and contributes to a more holistic approach to patient care (What is HIE?, 2020).

b. Examples of Successful HIE Implementations

Successful implementations of HIE include the Indiana Health Information Exchange (IHIE), which connects healthcare providers statewide, improving care coordination and patient outcomes. Similarly, the Chesapeake Regional Information System for our Patients (CRISP) in Maryland has successfully facilitated data sharing among diverse healthcare entities, promoting interoperability (CHUTE, 2022).

c. Social Networks Facilitating HIE Collaboration

Social networks serve as dynamic platforms for healthcare professionals to share best practices and foster collaboration in HIE. Platforms like LinkedIn and professional forums provide spaces for discussions, enabling the exchange of insights and experiences, ultimately contributing to the advancement of HIE initiatives.

6. WEARABLE AND IOT DEVICES IN HEALTHCARE

Wearable and Internet of Things (IoT) devices have revolutionized healthcare by providing real-time health monitoring and data collection. Wearables, such as fitness trackers and smartwatches, monitor vital signs, activity levels, and sleep patterns, empowering individuals to actively manage their health. IoT devices, ranging from smart medical devices to connected implants, facilitate seamless data exchange between devices and healthcare systems. This continuous stream of data enables healthcare professionals to monitor patients remotely, personalize treatment plans, and intervene proactively. The integration of wearables and IoT devices not only enhances preventive care but also contributes to the efficient management of chronic conditions. This technological convergence marks a paradigm shift in healthcare, fostering a data-driven and patient-centric approach to well-being.

a. Impact of Wearable Devices and IoT in Healthcare

Wearable devices and the Internet of Things (IoT) have profoundly impacted healthcare by introducing real-time monitoring and personalized health insights. Wearables like fitness trackers and smartwatches enable individuals to track vital signs, exercise, and sleep patterns, promoting preventive health management. IoT extends this impact by connecting various medical devices, fostering seamless data exchange between patients, healthcare providers, and electronic health records. This interconnected ecosystem facilitates remote patient monitoring, early detection of health issues, and personalized treatment strategies, ultimately improving patient outcomes and reducing healthcare costs. The collaborative power of wearables and IoT transforms healthcare from reactive to proactive, emphasizing continuous, data-driven health management (C., 2023).

b. Real-World Applications and Benefits

Real-world applications of wearable devices and IoT in healthcare abound, showcasing their versatility. Continuous glucose monitors aid diabetic patients in managing blood sugar levels, while smart inhalers help monitor and improve asthma management. Wearable ECG monitors detect cardiac abnormalities, enabling timely interventions. In elderly care, fall detection devices enhance safety, and remote patient monitoring systems support individuals with chronic conditions. These applications not only empower patients with greater control over their health but also streamline healthcare delivery, reduce hospitalizations, and enhance overall healthcare efficiency (Li, 2019).

c. Role of Social Networks in Promoting and Reviewing Wearable and IoT Innovations in Healthcare

Social networks play a pivotal role in promoting and reviewing wearable and IoT innovations in healthcare. Platforms like Twitter, LinkedIn, and specialized forums serve as spaces where healthcare professionals, researchers, and users share information, experiences, and insights related to these technologies. This facilitates rapid dissemination of knowledge, fosters awareness, and encourages discussions around the latest advancements.

Additionally, social networks serve as channels for product reviews, allowing users to share their firsthand experiences with wearable and IoT devices. This user-generated feedback contributes to the evaluation and refinement of these technologies, guiding potential users and informing healthcare professionals about the practical implications and effectiveness of specific devices.

Moreover, social networks provide a platform for collaboration and knowledge exchange among professionals in the field. From discussing best practices to sharing research findings, these platforms foster a sense of community and facilitate continuous learning. The dialogue on social networks thus amplifies the impact of wearable and IoT innovations, promoting their adoption, and contributing to their ongoing development in the healthcare landscape.

7. ARTIFICIAL INTELLIGENCE AND MACHINE LEARNING IN HEALTHCARE

Artificial Intelligence (AI) and Machine Learning (ML) are revolutionizing healthcare by analyzing vast datasets, improving diagnostics, and personalizing treatment plans. AI algorithms interpret medical images, predict disease risks, and enhance clinical decision-making. Machine Learning models identify patterns in patient data, enabling proactive interventions and optimizing healthcare operations. This integration of AI and ML not only expedites medical research but also contributes to more precise and patient-centric healthcare. The continuous advancement of these technologies marks a transformative shift toward more efficient, data-driven, and innovative healthcare practices.

a. Use of AI and Machine Learning for Diagnostics and Treatment

The integration of Artificial Intelligence (AI) and Machine Learning (ML) in healthcare has significantly advanced diagnostics and treatment. AI algorithms process vast datasets to identify patterns and anomalies, aiding in the early detection of diseases. In diagnostics, AI enhances image analysis for radiology and pathology, improving the accuracy of medical imaging interpretations. Machine Learning models analyze patient data to predict disease risks, allowing for personalized treatment plans and interventions. Additionally, AI supports drug discovery by analyzing genetic data and identifying potential therapeutic targets. In treatment, these technologies contribute to precision medicine, tailoring approaches based on individual patient characteristics. The application of AI and ML not only expedites diagnostic processes but also fosters more effective, targeted treatments, ultimately enhancing patient outcomes (Mohd Javaid, 2022).

b. Potential for Improved Healthcare Quality Through AI-Driven Innovations

AI-driven innovations hold immense potential for improving healthcare quality across various dimensions. In diagnostics, the ability of AI to process and interpret complex medical data leads to faster and more accurate diagnoses. This, in turn, facilitates early interventions and contributes to better patient outcomes. In treatment planning, AI enables the development of personalized care strategies based on individual patient profiles, optimizing therapeutic approaches and minimizing adverse effects (Ayesha Amjad, 2023).

Moreover, AI contributes to operational efficiencies within healthcare systems. Predictive analytics can forecast patient admission rates, optimizing resource allocation and reducing hospital congestion. AI-driven technologies also enhance decision support for healthcare professionals, ensuring evidence-based practices and reducing medical errors. By automating routine tasks, AI allows healthcare providers to focus more on patient care, fostering a more patient-centric approach. Overall, AI-driven innovations have the potential to elevate healthcare quality by enhancing accuracy, efficiency, and personalized care.

c. Contribution of Social Networks to Dissemination of AI-Driven Healthcare Solutions

Social networks play a crucial role in disseminating AI-driven healthcare solutions by providing a platform for sharing insights, research findings, and practical applications. Platforms like Twitter, LinkedIn, and healthcare-focused forums create spaces for professionals to discuss the latest advancements, share success stories, and exchange knowledge.

Social networks contribute to awareness and education, ensuring that healthcare professionals and the public stay informed about the potential and challenges of AI in healthcare. These platforms also serve as channels for collaboration, fostering interdisciplinary discussions among professionals, researchers, and technology developers. The real-time nature of social networks allows for the rapid dissemination of information about newly developed AI-driven solutions, promoting their adoption and integration into healthcare practices (Abid Haleem M. J., 2022).

However, the role of social networks in disseminating AI-driven healthcare solutions requires careful navigation to address concerns related to privacy, security, and ethical considerations. Overall, social networks serve as dynamic facilitators in the dissemination and collaborative exploration of AI's transformative role in healthcare.

8. PATIENT ENGAGEMENT AND HEALTH APPS

Patient engagement is enhanced through the widespread use of health apps, fostering active participation in personal health management. These apps empower individuals to monitor fitness, track medications, and manage chronic conditions. By providing real-time health data, personalized insights, and reminders, health apps promote a proactive approach to well-being. They encourage healthier lifestyles, improve adherence to treatment plans, and facilitate communication between patients and healthcare providers. Patient engagement through health apps not only strengthens the patient-provider relationship but also contributes to a more informed and empowered healthcare community. This digital evolution marks a shift towards patient-centric care, emphasizing the importance of individuals in their healthcare journey.

a. Importance of Patient Engagement in Healthcare

Patient engagement is pivotal for improved healthcare outcomes. Actively involving patients in their care fosters a collaborative and informed approach. Engaged patients are more likely to adhere to treatment plans, make healthier lifestyle choices, and effectively manage chronic conditions. Patient engagement enhances communication between healthcare providers and individuals, ensuring a more personalized and responsive healthcare experience. Moreover, engaged patients often experience increased satisfaction with their care, leading to better overall well-being. In the era of patient-centric healthcare, fostering engagement is not only beneficial for individual health but also contributes to more efficient and effective healthcare systems (Albanians, 2023).

b. Various Health Apps and Platforms Designed to Engage Patients

A myriad of health apps and platforms are designed to engage patients in their health journey. Fitness apps track physical activity, providing personalized exercise routines. Medication management apps send reminders for prescription adherence. Chronic disease management apps offer tools for monitoring symptoms and communicating with healthcare teams. Telehealth platforms enable virtual consultations, enhancing accessibility. Personal health record apps allow individuals to manage and share their health information. These tools empower patients by providing real-time data, personalized insights, and resources, promoting active participation in their health and well-being (Krysik, 2023).

c. Role of Social Networks in Building Patient Communities and Support Networks

Social networks play a vital role in building patient communities and support networks. Platforms like Facebook, Twitter, and specialized health forums provide spaces for individuals facing similar health challenges to connect, share experiences, and offer support. Patient communities on social networks foster a sense of belonging and understanding, reducing the isolation often associated with health conditions. These networks enable the exchange of information, resources, and coping strategies, empowering individuals with knowledge. Healthcare professionals can also engage with patients, addressing concerns and providing guidance. The collaborative nature of social networks contributes to the formation of robust support systems, enhancing patient well-being and creating a dynamic environment for shared learning and advocacy.

9. QUALITY IMPROVEMENT INITIATIVES

Quality Improvement Initiatives aim to enhance healthcare delivery by systematically assessing and refining processes. These initiatives prioritize patient safety, efficiency, and positive outcomes. By employing data-driven methodologies, healthcare providers identify areas for improvement, implement changes, and continuously monitor performance. Quality Improvement Initiatives foster a culture of excellence, reducing errors, enhancing patient satisfaction, and optimizing resource utilization. This ongoing commitment to improvement ensures that healthcare organizations adapt to evolving standards, ultimately providing higher-quality care and promoting positive patient experiences.

a. Role of Digital Health in Quality Improvement Initiatives

Digital health plays a pivotal role in quality improvement initiatives by leveraging technology to enhance healthcare processes. Electronic Health Records (EHRs), telemedicine, and data analytics contribute to streamlined workflows, reduced errors, and improved patient outcomes. These digital tools enable efficient information exchange, promote evidence-based practices, and facilitate real-time monitoring. Digital health empowers healthcare providers to implement targeted interventions, personalize patient care, and optimize resource utilization, ultimately contributing to the continuous improvement of healthcare quality (Digital Transformation in Health Care: Accelerating Innovation and Efficiency, 2023).

b. Examples of Healthcare Organizations Improving Services With Digital Solutions

Numerous healthcare organizations have successfully improved services through digital solutions. Mayo Clinic's use of telemedicine expanded access to specialist consultations, enhancing patient care. Cleveland Clinic's implementation of data analytics reduced surgical complications by predicting patient risk factors. These examples showcase how digital solutions can improve efficiency, accessibility, and patient outcomes in diverse healthcare settings (Jamal H. Mahar, 2019).

c. Explain How Social Networks Can Be Utilized to Share Success Stories and Best Practices

Social networks serve as powerful platforms for healthcare organizations to share success stories and best practices. Platforms like Twitter and LinkedIn enable institutions to highlight innovative initiatives, technological implementations, and quality improvement successes. Through these networks, organizations can reach a wider audience, foster collaboration, and inspire others in the healthcare community. Social networks facilitate the dissemination of valuable insights, encouraging a culture of continuous learning and improvement in the healthcare industry. Sharing success stories on these platforms not only celebrates achievements but also contributes to the collective knowledge base, promoting a more connected and informed healthcare community (Ayodele, 2023).

10. CHALLENGES AND ETHICAL CONSIDERATIONS

Navigating challenges and ethical considerations is inherent in the evolution of healthcare technologies. Balancing innovation with patient privacy, data security, and equitable access poses complex challenges. Ensuring the responsible use of Artificial Intelligence, maintaining patient consent in data sharing, and addressing disparities in technology adoption are critical ethical considerations. Striking a harmonious balance between technological advancements and ethical principles is imperative for fostering trust, safeguarding patient rights, and promoting equitable healthcare outcomes in the ever-evolving landscape of digital health.

a. Challenges and Potential Ethical Concerns in Adopting Digital Health Innovations

The adoption of digital health innovations introduces challenges and ethical considerations. Interoperability issues, where different systems struggle to exchange information seamlessly, hinder effective healthcare coordination. Privacy concerns arise as sensitive health data becomes more susceptible to breaches. Additionally, the digital divide may exacerbate health inequalities, limiting access to those without adequate technology or digital literacy. Ethical challenges include balancing the benefits of Artificial Intelligence with the need for transparency and accountability. Ensuring patient consent, maintaining data accuracy, and addressing disparities in technology access are pivotal considerations for the responsible adoption of digital health innovations (Abid Haleem M. J., 2022).

b. Issues Related to Data Privacy, Security, and Equity

Data privacy and security are paramount concerns in the digital health landscape. Patient data, often sensitive and personal, must be safeguarded against unauthorized access and breaches. Maintaining robust security measures becomes increasingly complex with the growing volume of health data. Additionally, ensuring equity in digital health is critical to prevent the exacerbation of existing healthcare disparities. Disparities in access to technology, digital literacy, and healthcare resources can widen existing gaps, hindering the benefits of digital health from reaching all segments of the population. Striking a balance between innovation, privacy, security, and equity is essential for the ethical evolution of digital health (Metty Paul, 2023).

c. Using Social Networks to Engage in Discussions and Find Solutions

Social networks provide a dynamic platform for engaging in discussions and finding solutions to the challenges and ethical considerations in digital health. Platforms like Twitter, LinkedIn, and specialized forums facilitate collaboration among healthcare professionals, policymakers, and technology developers. These networks serve as spaces for sharing insights, best practices, and innovative approaches to address ethical concerns. Discussions on social networks contribute to a collective understanding of challenges, fostering the development of responsible guidelines and ethical frameworks. Additionally, these platforms enable the dissemination of information about successful implementations and strategies, promoting knowledge exchange and collaborative problem-solving in the evolving landscape of digital health (Jaffar Abbas, 2019).

11. FUTURE DIRECTIONS AND CONCLUSIONS

The future of healthcare lies in transformative digital advancements, with a focus on patient-centric care, Artificial Intelligence, and enhanced connectivity. As technology evolves, telemedicine and remote monitoring will become more prevalent, improving accessibility and preventive care. AI-driven diagnostics and personalized treatment plans will revolutionize healthcare outcomes. Wearable devices and IoT will continue to empower individuals in managing their health actively. Quality Improvement Initiatives will thrive through data-driven methodologies. Addressing ethical concerns and ensuring equitable access to digital health innovations will be pivotal. Social networks will play an increasingly vital role in knowledge exchange and collaboration. In conclusion, the future envisions a harmonious blend of technology and ethical considerations, fostering a dynamic and patient-centered healthcare landscape.

a. Future of Digital Health Innovations

The future of digital health innovations promises transformative changes in healthcare delivery. Continued advancements in Artificial Intelligence (AI) and Machine Learning (ML) will lead to more precise diagnostics, personalized treatment plans, and proactive health management. Telemedicine and remote monitoring will become integral components of healthcare, enhancing accessibility and preventive care. Wearable devices and the Internet of Things (IoT) will evolve to offer more sophisticated health monitoring, empowering individuals to actively participate in their well-being. Quality Improvement Initiatives will leverage data analytics for continuous enhancement of healthcare processes.

b. Key Takeaways From the Chapter

The key takeaways from this chapter include the integral role of digital health innovations in improving healthcare quality. We explored the impact of wearables, telemedicine, Electronic Health Records (EHRs), and AI-driven solutions. Quality Improvement Initiatives and the importance of patient engagement were emphasized. Challenges such as data privacy and equity were discussed. Social networks emerged as crucial platforms for collaboration and knowledge exchange.

c. Importance of Continued Analysis of Digital Healthcare Trends Using Social Networks

Continued analysis of digital healthcare trends using social networks is vital for several reasons. Social networks provide real-time insights into emerging technologies, successful implementations, and evolving challenges. The dynamic nature of healthcare requires constant adaptation, and social networks facilitate swift dissemination of knowledge. Engaging in discussions on these platforms fosters a sense of community, allowing professionals to learn from each other's experiences. Moreover, social networks amplify the collective intelligence of the healthcare community, contributing to the development of ethical guidelines and best practices. As the digital health landscape evolves, social networks serve as invaluable tools for staying informed, connected, and actively involved in shaping the future of healthcare.

12. SUGGESTED FRAMEWORK TO INDUSTRY

HealthSphere Connect is an innovative ecosystem designed to revolutionize healthcare connectivity and collaboration. It integrates cutting-edge technologies and emphasizes a patient-centric approach, fostering seamless communication and knowledge exchange among healthcare stakeholders.

MAIN COMPONENTS OF THE FRAMEWORK

1. Unified Health Platform (UHP)

The UHP integrates Electronic Health Records (EHRs), telemedicine, and Internet of Things (IoT) devices, forming a comprehensive ecosystem for patient management. AI-driven analytics enhance the platform, providing personalized diagnostics and treatment plans. This ensures seamless data exchange and a holistic approach to healthcare, optimizing patient outcomes.

2. SmartConnect Wearables

SmartConnect Wearables offer advanced devices for real-time health monitoring, empowering proactive health management. These wearables seamlessly integrate with the Unified Health Platform, enabling continuous data flow. By promoting real-time tracking and personalized health insights, they enhance patient engagement and contribute to a more connected healthcare experience.

3. Ethical AI Hub

The Ethical AI Hub implements transparent and accountable AI algorithms for diagnostics and decision support. This ensures responsible AI use, addressing ethical concerns related to patient data privacy and algorithmic transparency. The hub's focus is on maintaining patient trust and promoting ethical practices in the application of artificial intelligence within healthcare.

4. Quality Nexus

Quality Nexus is a hub for Quality Improvement Initiatives, driven by data analytics. It establishes continuous feedback loops to optimize healthcare processes. By leveraging data-driven insights, the Quality Nexus empowers healthcare providers to refine practices, enhance efficiency, and ultimately improve the quality of care delivered to patients.

Figure 1. Tarun framework for HealthSphere Connect
Image sources: (PNG wing, n.d.)

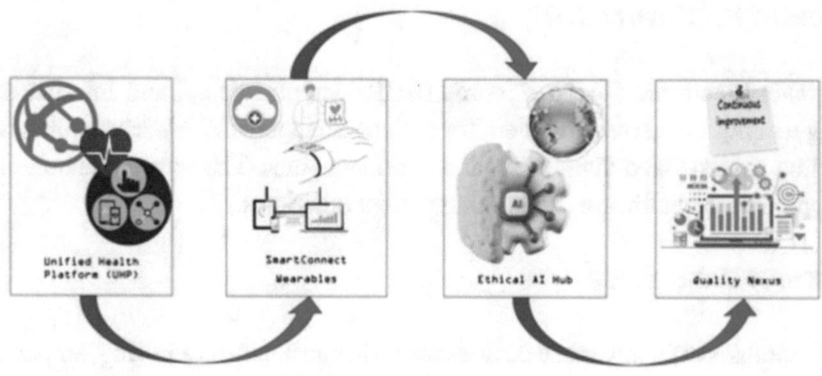

UNIQUE FEATURES OF THE FRAMEWORK

1. Patient Engagement Arcade

The Patient Engagement Arcade integrates gamification elements into healthcare to boost patient participation and adherence. It employs interactive games and incentives, creating an engaging environment that encourages healthy behaviors. The inclusion of a rewards system further motivates patients to actively manage their health, fostering a sense of achievement and sustained commitment to wellness.

2. Community Health Connect

Community Health Connect is a specialized social network within HealthSphere Connect designed for healthcare professionals. This platform facilitates the exchange of insights, best practices, and collaborative efforts on complex cases. It fosters a dynamic community where professionals can discuss challenges, share expertise, and stay updated on the latest advancements. Community Health Connect enhances interdisciplinary collaboration, contributing to a collective pool of knowledge for continuous improvement in healthcare practices.

BENEFITS OF FRAMEWORK

1. Improved Healthcare Outcomes

Proactive health management, facilitated by advanced technologies, leads to better patient outcomes. Early interventions and personalized approaches contribute to overall well-being.

2. Enhanced Communication

Improved communication, facilitated by interconnected platforms, results in better care coordination among healthcare professionals. Timely information exchange optimizes patient care and outcomes.

3. Ethical AI Practices

Implementing transparent and ethical AI practices builds patient trust by ensuring data security and responsible use of artificial intelligence in healthcare decision-making.

4. Continuous Quality Improvement

Quality improvement initiatives, powered by data analytics, ensure ongoing enhancements in healthcare processes, contributing to a dynamic and evolving healthcare system.

WHY HEALTHSPHERE CONNECT?

The name "HealthSphere Connect" encapsulates the essence of a comprehensive and interconnected healthcare ecosystem. "HealthSphere" signifies the all-encompassing scope, suggesting a holistic approach to healthcare. The term "Connect" underscores the collaborative nature of the platform, emphasizing the interconnectedness of healthcare stakeholders. This model envisions a future where healthcare transcends being merely a service, transforming into a dynamic, connected, and perpetually improving ecosystem that prioritizes collaboration, engagement, and continuous enhancement for the benefit of patients and the healthcare community.

REFERENCES

Abid Haleem, M. J. (2022). Artificial intelligence (AI) applications for marketing: A literature-based study. *International Journal of Intelligent Networks*, 119-132.

Abid Haleem, M. J. (2022). *Medical 4.0 technologies for healthcare: Features, capabilities, and applications. Internet of Things and Cyber-Physical Systems.*

Albanians, L. (2023, September 14). *The importance of patient engagement: A comprehensive overview.* Retrieved from nasscom: https://community.nasscom.in/communities/application/importance-patient-engagement-comprehensive-overview

Ayesha Amjad, P. K. (2023). A Review on Innovation in Healthcare Sector (Telehealth) through Artificial Intelligence. *Sustainability.*

Ayodele, A. (2023, June 30). *Five Social Media Platforms That Can Help Healthcare Organizations Boost Their Online Presence.* Retrieved from Linkedin: https://www.linkedin.com/pulse/five-social-media-platforms-can-help-healthcare-boost-adedotun/

Bernstein, C. (2022). *Digital health (digital healthcare).* Retrieved from TechTarget: https://www.techtarget.com/searchhealthit/definition/digital-health-digital-healthcare

C., S. (2023, June 23). *Wearable Devices and IoT in Healthcare: Revolutionizing Patient Monitoring and Transforming the Healthcare Industry.* Retrieved from Linkedin: https://www.linkedin.com/pulse/wearable-devices-iot-healthcare-revolutionizing-patient-chhabra/

Chute, D. C. (2022). *Chesapeake regional information system for our patients (CRISP).* Retrieved from Johns Hopkins Institute for Clinical & Translational Research: https://ictr.johnshopkins.edu/service/informatics/crisp/

Digital Transformation in Health Care: Accelerating Innovation and Efficiency. (2023). Retrieved from Evolved Metrics: https://evolvedmetrics.com/digital-transformation-in-health-care/

Edmond Li, J. C. (2021). Electronic Health Records, Interoperability and Patient Safety in Health Systems of High-income Countries: A Systematic Review Protocol. *BMJ Open.* PMID:34261679

Infosys, B. P. M. (2023). *The benefits of using predictive analytics in healthcare.* Retrieved from Infosys BPM: https://www.infosysbpm.com/blogs/bpm-analytics/the-benefits-of-using-predictive-analytics-in-healthcare.html#:~:text=Predictive%20analysis%20has%20proven%20effective,and%20prevent%20potentially%20negative%20outcomes

Jacqueline, M., & Ferguson, J. J. (2021). Virtual care expansion in the Veterans Health Administration during the COVID-19 pandemic: Clinical services and patient characteristics associated with utilization. *Journal of the American Medical Informatics Association : JAMIA*, 453–462. PMID:33125032

Jaffar Abbas, J. A. (2019). The Impact of Social Media on Learning Behavior for Sustainable Education: Evidence of Students from Selected Universities in Pakistan. *Sustainability.*

Jamal, H., & Mahar, M. J. (2019, March 1). *The Future of Telemedicine (and What's in the Way).* Retrieved from Consult QD: https://consultqd.clevelandclinic.org/the-future-of-telemedicine-and-whats-in-the-way/

Krysik, A. (2023, September 25). *12 Types of Healthcare Software.* Retrieved from Stratflow: https://stratoflow.com/healthcare-software-types/

Li, J. (2019, March 6). *Medical wearables offer new hope for diabetes patients.* Retrieved from TechTarget: https://www.techtarget.com/iotagenda/blog/IoT-Agenda/Medical-wearables-offer-new-hope-for-diabetes-patients

Metty Paul, L. M. (2023). Digitization of healthcare sector: A study on privacy and security concerns. *ICT Express*, 571-588.

Mohd Javaid, A. H. (2022). Significance of machine learning in healthcare: Features, pillars and applications. *International Journal of Intelligent Networks*, 58-73.

Mosadeghrad, A. M. (2014). Factors influencing healthcare service quality. *nt J. Health Policy and Management*, 77–89.

Oleg Bestsennyy, G. G. (2021, July 9). *Telehealth: A quarter-trillion-dollar post-COVID-19 reality?* Retrieved from https://www.mckinsey.com/industries/healthcare/our-insights/telehealth-a-quarter-trillion-dollar-post-covid-19-reality

Sabyasachi Dash, S. K. (2019). Big data in healthcare: Management, analysis and future prospects. *Journal of Big Data.*

Shaji George, A. H. (2023). Telemedicine: A New Way to Provide Healthcare. *Partners Universal International Innovation Journal (PUIIJ)*, 98-129.

What is HIE? (2020, July 24). Retrieved from Breadcrumb: https://www.healthit.gov/topic/health-it-and-health-information-exchange-basics/what-hie

World Health Organization. (2021). *Global strategy on digital health 2020-2025.* World Health Organization.

Yasmyne Ronquillo, A. M. (2023, May 1). *Digital Health.* Retrieved from National Library of Medicine: https://www.ncbi.nlm.nih.gov/books/NBK470260/

Zhuravel, H. (2023, August 15). *Telemedicine and Remote Patient Monitoring: Use Cases & Best Practices.* Retrieved from Binariks: https://binariks.com/blog/telemedicine-remote-patient-monitoring/

Chapter 10
Disease Monitoring and Management:
Healthcare Information Systems (HIS) in Smart Cities

R. Renugadevi
R.M.K. Engineering College, India

ABSTRACT

The world's top nations are working to find solutions to the complicated, multidimensional, and large-scale challenge of building smart cities. Control over critical aspects of the city's life cycle through computer technology and the ability to make wise operational decisions in an emergency are the two biggest benefits of a smart city. The digital transformation of healthcare, or the development of computerized clinics, communications, and intelligent systems for health monitoring and enhancing the quality of life of diverse population groups, is one of the main goals of creating a smart city. While IoT can improve human health, developing effective and safe data gathering methods for IoT healthcare monitoring systems still raises a number of restricting problems.

INTRODUCTION

The world's top nations are working to find solutions to the complicated, multidimensional, and large-scale challenge of modelling smart cities Control over critical aspects of the city's life cycle through latest technology and by making wise operational decisions during emergency are the two biggest benefits of a smart city. The digital transformation of healthcare, or the development of modern digital clinics, interactions, and intelligent systems for health monitoring and enhancing the life style of diverse population groups, is one of the main goals of creating a smart city.

This task's importance stems from many objective factors:

1) A sharp rise in the count of people living in cities while people leaving rural regions;
2) A huge intensification in the average lifespan of an individual; and

DOI: 10.4018/979-8-3693-1934-5.ch010

3) A lack of trained medical professionals due to the high expense of care needed and monitoring.

The advancement of the electronic health system is facilitated by the deployment of 5G technology and WSN. To register with the server, each user must provide a password, a smart card with a time-bounded identity, and a biometric. A reconfigurable hybrid radio communication system is developed on wireless optics and radio connectivity, addressing the idea of the hospital of the future. Utilizing optical transmission, this suggested approach reduces throughput, increases redundancy, and lessens spectrum congestion. Some writers are drawn to the topic of enemy warfare, they put in place an automated healthcare observing system to track troops' where abouts in real time.

Numerous research, for example, use a fuzzy algorithm to plan data transmission under the MAC layer to overcome the issues with energy usage in WSN. Numerous studies on energy efficiency in WSN, particularly in WBAN, have been conducted. Their goal is to enhance patient monitoring while meeting system quality requirements related to latency, energy economy, and data transfer rate (Alekya et al., 2021).

INTERNET OF THINGS-BASED HEALTHCARE SYSTEMS AND THEIR USES

People's lives are made easier by IoT-based healthcare systems and its applications in various ways, including:

1. Remote healthcare: Rather patient traveling to the hospital, wireless Internet of things solutions bring the hospital to the patient. IoT-based sensors safely collect data, are then processed by a tiny algorithm and shared with medical specialists for relevant advice.
2. Real-time monitoring: Comprehensive psychological data is gathered by IoT-powered, non-invasive monitoring devices. Data storage is managed via cloud-based analysis and gateways.
3. Preventive care: Sensor data is used by IoT healthcare systems to help identify emergencies early and notify family members. The Internet of Things allows machine learning to be used for early anomaly identification and health trend tracking (Philip et al., 2021).

Technology has evolved to a completely new level in terms of how people, technologies, and applications interact to provide healthcare solutions. IoT has tremendously improved healthcare quality by providing us with new tools and perspectives for an integrated healthcare network.

Benefits of Using IoT in Healthcare

By using IoT, healthcare activities that were laborious and prone to human error may now be automated.

Though there are countless ways the IoT might enhance healthcare, such as

- lower medical expenses.
- Errors by humans are decreased.
- The removal of distance's constraints.
- Decreased volumes of paperwork and documentation.
- Chronic illnesses are identified early on.
- enhancements to the administration of drugs.

- The urgent need for medical attention.
- Better results from the therapy.

Yang et al. (2022) conducted a comprehensive examination of intelligent Health Monitoring Systems (HMS) along with the diverse sensor components integrated into their corresponding Internet of Things (IoT) frameworks. Their analysis involved categorizing and scrutinizing relevant studies based on the incorporation of device-based and device-free techniques. The study concluded that innovative combinations of these techniques can be effectively employed to enhance existing HMS capabilities. In a study by Karatas et al. (2022), the focus shifted to exploring the application and challenges associated with big data analytics (BDA) as an exemplification of artificial intelligence (AI) techniques within the HMS domain. Their findings highlighted the pivotal role of BDA in the technological landscape of HMS. Alshamrani (2022) delved into the practicality and deployment aspects of Health Internet of Things (H-IoT) systems in smart cities. Furthermore, their investigation extended to evaluating technologies affiliated with HMS, providing insights into health monitoring through the utilization of diverse wearable sensors.

Capraro (2016) explored the integration of sensors, IoT, and AI in healthcare delivery, emphasizing the role of AI, particularly Big Data Analytics (BDA), in improving healthcare outcomes while reducing costs. The study underscored that the successful amalgamation of sensors, IoT, and AI not only lowers medical care expenses but also enhances data availability for actionable insights, thereby contributing to effective healthcare delivery. Azzawi et al. (2016) focused on IoT and AI in healthcare delivery, with a specific emphasis on security mechanisms. They proposed a novel authentication platform for IoT technologies, employing Elliptic Curve Cryptography (ECC) as a method to ensure secure healthcare applications. Sakr and Elgammal (2016) developed the SMART HEALTH framework, integrating sensors, IoT, data storage mechanisms, and AI to enhance the quality of healthcare services. Their data-driven approach aimed at facilitating health analytics for effective healthcare delivery.

Hossain and Muhammad (2016) presented an H-IoT framework that combines sensors, cloud data infrastructure, and IoT technologies for medical services. This framework primarily focuses on continuous healthcare monitoring, utilizing ECG and sensor data for seamless accessibility by healthcare practitioners. Romero et al. (2016) suggested an IoT-based approach for Parkinson's disease diagnosis and monitoring, integrating AI and sensors. They highlighted the increasing technical sophistication and acceptance of IoT and wearable sensors in healthcare, presenting opportunities for intelligent and widespread medical services. Mathew and Pillai (2016) discussed the applicability and challenges associated with AI (BDA) for deriving insights from health data, addressing the complexities and potential benefits of utilizing AI in healthcare analytics. Yeole and Kalbande (2016) explored various IoT enabling technologies and practices in healthcare delivery, with a focus on infants, adolescents, terminal diseases, acute clinic services, operating rooms, and prescription dispensers. Their study aimed at improving the efficiency of healthcare delivery systems while minimizing associated expenses.

IoT Framework

The Internet of Things (IoT) framework is broadly divided into four layers: the Sensing Layer, Communication Layer, Network Storage Layer, and Application Layer as shown in Figure 1.

Figure 1. The IoT 4-layer architecture for HMS

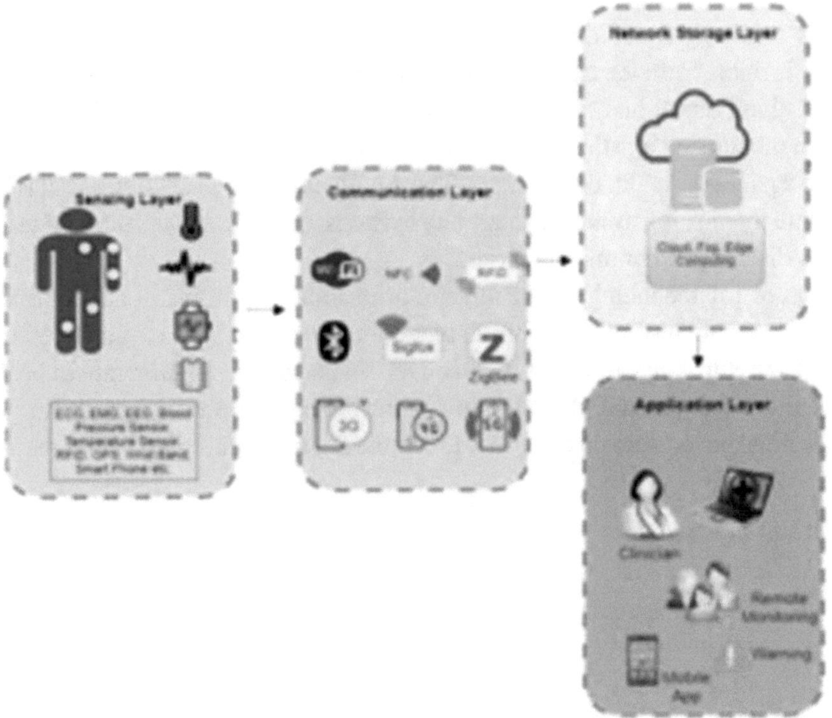

Sensing Layer

This layer, situated closest to the patient, is responsible for data collection. It consists of wearable sensors that patients carry or wear to monitor their health status. Various wearable sensors are integrated to detect physiological data such as ECG, EEG, GPS, BT, BP, and glucose measurements. Studies, for instance, by Tabassum et al. (2019) and Magaña-Espinoza et al. (2014), have successfully utilized smartphones for gathering data from the human body.

Communication Layer

In this layer, the sensor data collected in the Sensing Layer are transmitted to the Network Storage Layer using different protocols and technologies. Various protocols like ZigBee, Wi-Fi, Bluetooth, NFC, RFID, and others are employed depending on the type of sensor and data.

Network Storage Layer

Positioned as the third layer, this layer addresses the challenges posed by the increasing number of users and the corresponding growth in data size. IoT cloud-based architecture is introduced to store and manage vast amounts of data, reducing the burden on individual sensor devices.

Application Layer

The final layer is primarily focused on data visualization and employs application-based services to derive actionable insights from the extensive sensor data (health data). It facilitates easy access to data stored on the IoT cloud server and assists healthcare professionals, including doctors, nurses, and patients' families, in monitoring a patient's health status. Devices at this layer can send relevant messages to stakeholders if a patient's health deteriorates. The Application Layer encompasses various use cases, such as smart home monitoring systems, smart city systems, smart transportation systems, activity recognition systems, disease prediction, and more .

The integration of IoT technology in healthcare brings about significant advantages, ensuring that diagnostic findings are reliable and appropriate therapy can be promptly administered to patients. This technology enables doctors and caregivers to effectively manage and monitor patient health, resulting in a reduction in health response time. With IoT in healthcare, regular physical visits for patients become unnecessary, as caretakers or doctors can provide remote health tracking and diagnostics.

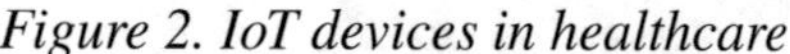

Figure 2. IoT devices in healthcare

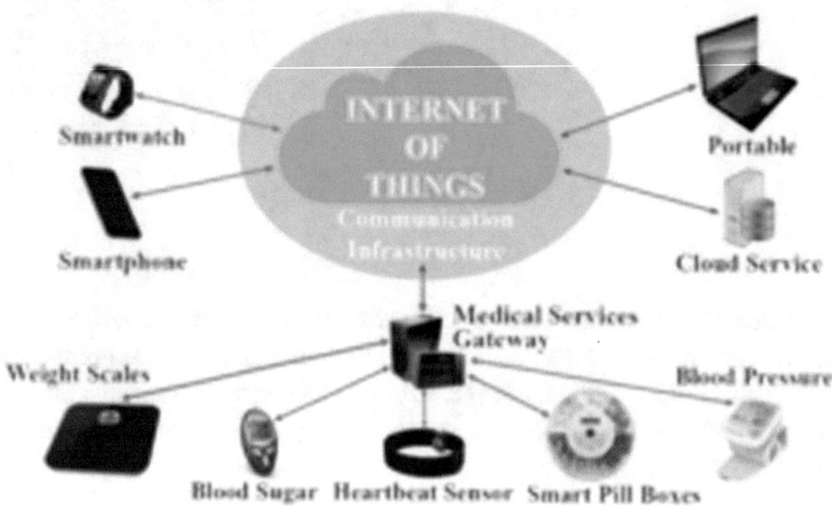

The use of Wi-Fi and sensors in hospitals allows for the identification of the relevant department when receiving detected information, streamlining communication and facilitating quicker responses (Adewole et al., 2021). In cases involving patients in intensive care, whether clinical or otherwise, IoT mechanisms enable periodic tracking. Medical sensors collect physiological data from the patient, transmit it through gateways, and store the information in the cloud. This not only enhances the quality of patient care but also contributes to a reduction in treatment costs.

A remote health monitoring system based on IoT can track a patient's health status in real-time and respond promptly to any detected health issues. As illustrated in Figure 2, a sensor device mounted on a patient can transmit vital sign data from the same location. This transmitter is connected to the hospital through a communication link or network, allowing the hospital's technology to remotely check and analyze the patient's health data (Blake, 2015). This real-time monitoring capability contributes to more proactive and personalized healthcare delivery.

There are several real-time use cases for IoT-based sensors, some of which are listed below:

1. Heart rate monitoring/cardiac monitoring devices/heart attack

IoT-based healthcare monitoring systems were the first to use health-monitoring sensors; these systems can collect and measure the required data, reliably transmit the data through various stages to the gateway and cloud server, and carry out certain edge tasks to enable low-latency prediction and decision-making for cardiac-related diseases. Certain parts use sensors to calculate heart rate. WSN technology can be used in a number of projects to continually monitor cardiac patients who require a real-time monitoring system. Numerous medical-grade sensors and equipment, including pressure, body temperature, heart rate, and pulse, are equipped with this WSN. Real-time ECG recording of a critical patient is also maintained to enable continuous monitoring of the patient.

2. Taking your body temperature

During the pandemic, COVID-19 patient sensors that measured body temperature, pulse, and SpO2 were integrated into IoT-based health monitoring systems. Through a mobile application, these devices can determine an individual's body temperature, oxygen saturation, and pulse rate.

3. Recognizing activities

Activity detection is the best way that medical wearables are now being used. The majority of fitness trackers carry out this type of identification. These days, the most widely used wearables for monitoring activity are fitness trackers. The majority of them include a very sensitive 3D accelerometer that enables the sensor to detect acceleration, even while a lot of guessing is done in the background.

4. Haemoglobin concentration and blood glucose monitoring

The Internet of Medical Things (IoMT), which is made up of equipment such as endoscopic capsules, blood-glucose monitors, heart-rate sensors, and other gadgets, is what makes up the IoMT diabetic-based WBSN monitoring system.

5. Monitoring and identification of respiration rate

There are several methods in which we can monitor the respiratory system of the human body. Some authors used advanced sensors that monitor respiration patterns. You may find a bioimpedance sensor helpful.

6. Sleep tracking

With the use of this sleep tracking software, the user may adjust their sleeping patterns and maintain a healthy life cycle. For this, a range of sensors are employed. Heart rate, pulse rate, SpO2 levels, and breathing patterns are regularly monitored by wearables; by taking these data into account, users may make well-informed decisions about the quality of their sleep.

7. Alzheimer's disease tracking and identification of anaemia

There are a number of concerns with Alzheimer's disease monitoring, which should be carefully considered. Alzheimer's cannot be diagnosed in a patient who is by themselves.

8. Clinical diagnosis and molecular diagnostics

Recent advancements in implantable devices for patient-friendly treatment and biosensors for patient-friendly diagnostics have garnered a lot of interest since they provide rapid and inexpensive healthcare applications with a lower risk of infection. Recently developed materials have been incorporated into medical equipment, enabling the quick construction of point-of-care (POC) sensor systems and implantable devices with particular functionality. The clinical diagnosis of disorders associated to albumin has been the subject of much research.

9. Detection of blood oxygen saturation

Following cardiothoracic surgery, it is critical to closely monitor patients' cardiovascular health in addition to accurately and continuously measuring intravascular oxygen levels. New data types are coming to market for wearables, such as oxygen saturation, which is the fraction of oxygen-saturated haemoglobin to total haemoglobin in the blood. This data is continually captured using oxygen-saturation (SpO2) sensors. Numerous wearables on the market already offer additional behavioural and physiological data kinds.

To efficiently manage Big Data in an IoT setting, Jennifer S. Raj (2020) presented a unique information-processing method for IoT-based healthcare-monitoring devices. Three steps make up the complete data processing process: gathering and aggregation, the process of classifying, analyzing, and making decisions based on data obtained. The trials were carried out with Python. In a simulation, this model was validated empirically by utilizing several health sensors. The characteristics were contrasted with the hierarchical Neural network models with clustering and backpropagation are used to verify performance. That model's leverage Hadoop with Apache Kafka to meet the demand for real-time data collecting as well as offline handling temporal effectiveness of the model.

A healthcare model was created by Kishor and Chakraborty (2021) utilizing seven classification algorithms. Nine distinct datasets pertaining to diseases were arranged according to categories. The effectiveness of the classifiers was assessed using four variables: AUC, accuracy, sensitivity, and specificity. This effort was divided into three stages: gathering data, pre-processing and computing, and deciding whether or not to make the results visible to doctors or other end users. The data was then stored on a cloud server. This study contrasted artificial intelligence-based health models based on previously created work. The RF classifier, in contrast to other classifiers, has the best AUC, sensitivity, specificity, and accuracy for a range of prevalent illnesses, the study's authors claim. This model may be expanded for a number of uses, including military, food availability, and weather forecasting. Kaur et al. (2019) suggested a system to evaluate the success of the proposed effort, eight datasets covering various disorders were used to collect the experimental findings. In this paper, five distinct machine learning techniques were applied. When used on the dermatological dataset, the Random Forest learning approach yielded a maximum accuracy of 97.26%, according to the scientists. Furthermore, it was said that Random Forest produced accurate and reliable findings for every dataset that was examined. The two performance measurements utilized for various machine learning approaches and datasets were accuracy and area under the curve (AUC), respectively.

An intelligent health monitoring system that uses accelerometer sensor data to identify unusual movements, such falls, was proposed by Jeong et al. (2021). The device first looks for unusual movement patterns before analyzing a person's blood pressure, heart rate, and blood type. With a smartphone, users, caretakers, and experts may verify that the patient has recorded biometric data at anytime, anyplace. An Android service environment with a Java foundation is part of this surveillance system. This monitoring system's effectiveness was assessed with the use of datasets including data from fifty distinct people. According to this concept, medical data about specific persons is protected by blockchain technology, which boosts data dependability while preserving secrecy. The collection of private medical data is tracked and saved in real-time with the use of sensor chips, a type of IoT technology. Sensitive medical data is only transmitted in real-time via a mobile device, such a smartphone. This method offers a helpful method for keeping an eye on Alzheimer's patients' day-to-day activities and giving the disease's victims high-quality treatment. This work is based on data gathered from Internet of Things (IoT) devices that measure a patient's body temperature, blood pressure, pace, and walking speed, to mention a few. The gathering of all this information and sensory data is done by the Atmega microcontroller.

Mostafa et al. (2022) suggested a platform for IoT-based health monitoring that employs a Max30100 pulse oximeter to measure BT, HR, and SpO2 levels and a NodeMCU microcontroller to acquire information from a DS18B20 temperature sensor. The readings are shown on an LCD in front of the patient as well as on the doctor's and everyone else's Blynk app-enabled phones. In order to pump disinfectant without being touched, this invention also includes an infrared (IR) sensor that recognizes items in front of it and triggers a relay. In contrast to the traditional approach, the authors claim that their project operates flawlessly and that the application just takes one minute to complete. This system is less costly than other systems on the market since it uses the NodeMCU, a less complex and expensive CPU with integrated Wi-Fi. The system is limited to cardiac patients, but it outperforms the conventional ones in terms of safety, ease of use, speed, and cost.

WIRELESS BODY AREA NETWORK

WBAN transmits data wirelessly through the body's electric field. Examples of this include connecting a music player to headphones, an electronic vehicle key from a pocket to a door unlocking system, or a control device worn around the waist to a cardiac sensor. This incredible technology is the focus of much study worldwide. IBM and MIT invented it in the US for the wearable computer viewpoint. In WBAN, sensors are used to track, gather, and send physiological data, such as temperature, electroencephalography (EEG), and electrocardiography (ECG), to a sink node. The hospital's installed LoRaWAN gateway will then transmit the collected attributes and forward to the physicians and nurses for analysis as shown in Figure 3.

WBANs are vastly different from conventional WSN in that they have network mobility that tracks an individual's motions and connection quality that adjusts based on the wearer's position. To increase the sensors' autonomy and lessen their exposure to the carriers' electromagnetic radiation, their transmission power is also maintained low. It is therefore challenging to keep a straight link between the "sink" and the other nodes in light of the body's absorption, reflection, and interference effects

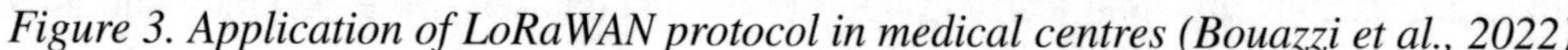

Figure 3. Application of LoRaWAN protocol in medical centres (Bouazzi et al., 2022)

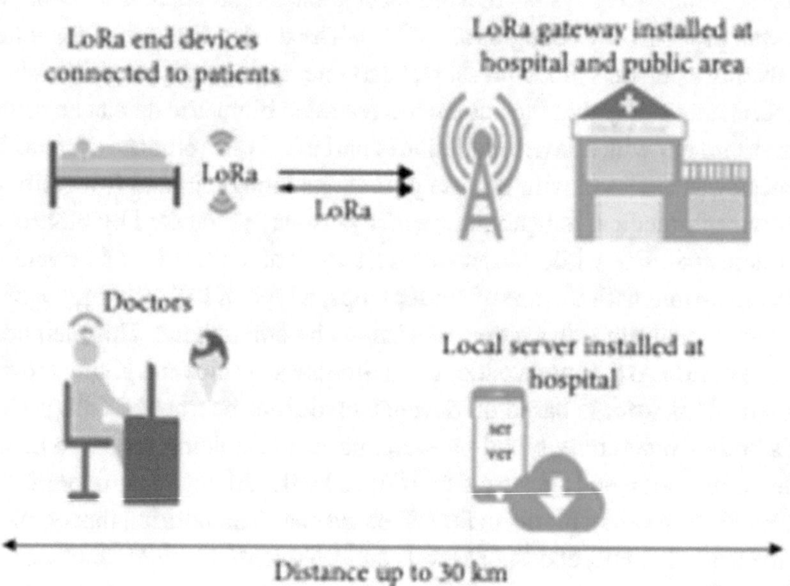

Since LoRaWAN can support wireless devices linked to the same network up to 30 km away, it can be a viable IoT solution to enhance healthcare. It can also be a useful option for changing cities into smart cities. As per the European Health Authorities guidelines, it is mandatory to adhere to temperature and CO2 levels in light of the ongoing health crisis and COVID-19 pandemic. Hospitals now have new Internet of Things sensors placed to monitor interior air quality. For instance, air quality levels exceeding 1000 parts per million are thought to be harmful to occupants' health (Bouazzi et al., 2022). These IoT solutions aim to enhance the well-being of hospital residents and nursing personnel while taking the advice of health authorities into account.

This method notifies medical staff of patients who need to be seen right away and makes it possible for them to find and identify these calls instantly. Patients can report an emergency at any moment with the use of the call button gadget. This "sensor" is small, lightweight, waterproof, and easy to clean. It has a built-in Bluetooth detector that can quickly identify and locate the device or person in question. Through an integrated speaker, it can also sense physical touch and monitor the surrounding temperature. Subsequently, vital information on patients' emergency calls and bed locations is instantly available to nurses.

Classification of Health-Monitoring Sensor

A person's health may be remotely monitored thanks to wearable technologies and data analysis. Advances in data collection methods, medical sensor technology, and wireless communications make this possible. Various devices such as smartphones, headphones, and wristwatches, wearable electronics and sensors may also be discovered in an extensive array of accessories such as clothing, hats, glasses, wristbands, socks, and shoes. Pawan Singh (2018) separated medical sensors into two categories: non-contact sensors, which comprise peripherals, and contact sensors, which include wearables and on-body devices. Therapeutic and monitoring contact sensors are two other subcategories. Again, non-contact sensors may be divided into three subcategories. The taxonomy of health-monitoring sensors is shown in Figure 4 along with instances of their uses (Singh, 2018).

This task's importance stems from many objective factors:

1) A rapid rise in the population of cities as a result of the population departure from rural regions,
2) An increase in a person's typical lifespan someone,
3) A deficiency in skilled healthcare workers and the exorbitant expense of medical oversight and therapy.

Figure 4. Classification of health monitoring system (Singh, 2018)

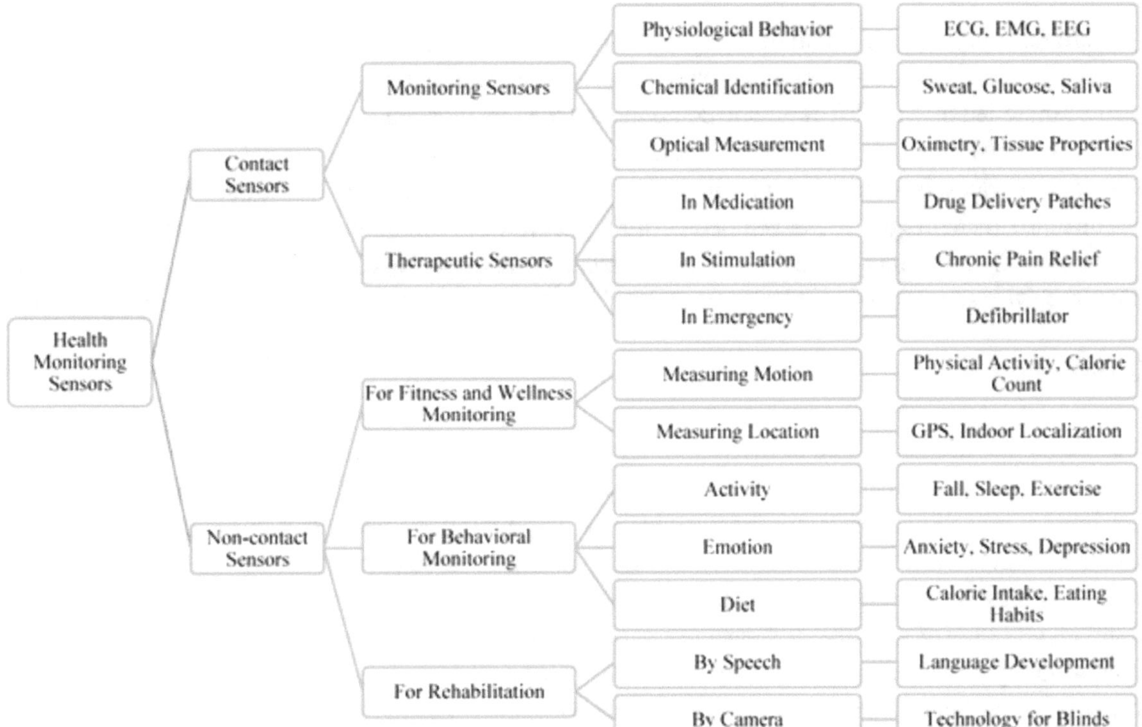

Most governments are finding it very difficult to provide these population groups with timely support since standard medical care approaches often do not match the scope or complexity of emerging health issues. To further enhance population health, the local government must also regularly support the clinics and assess their efficacy as soon as possible. Three duties are therefore pertinent.

1. An independent evaluation of the patient's state, followed by a suitable choice and communication with the clinic.
2. Verification and application of the clinic's choice (medical staff deployment and selection), as well as the compiling of data.
3. The municipal government analyses information on clinic operations and provides support as needed, such as during epidemics.

IoT Healthcare's Challenges

While IoT can improve human health, developing effective and safe data gathering methods for IoT healthcare monitoring systems still raises a number of restricting problems. These several open research challenges consist of Considerations include functionality, performance, data privacy, dependability, security, and stability. Within this segment.

Security-Based

To increase trust in using IoT in healthcare, security and privacy have to be considered throughout the design and development process. To lower security risks and safeguard privacy, security procedures must be included in every IoT layer and component. Creators must guarantee the security of IoT "things" and the systems they link to, in order for users can depend on sensors, gadgets, gateways, and Internet of Things services, ensuring their privacy, security, and confidentiality are safeguarded. Many personal and business technologies are developed without guaranteeing these elements of privacy and security. Numerous IoT-based remote health Integrated security methods have a huge effect on monitoring applications with sensors and wireless transceivers' hardware and software integrated in correspondence.

QoS-Based

QoS indicators are applicable to every sub-component of IoT architecture, ranging from individual's house to cloud-based healthcare services. It is necessary to monitor memory use to make sure that neither improper caching of data nor memory leaks are occurring. Wireless disruption causes delays and pauses in data flow, which can lead to poor signal quality, inconsistent connections, sudden disconnection, and sluggish network speeds. Energy-consumption control is another performance indicator that might result in lower stability, performance, dependability, and usefulness. For the gadgets, the process of continually gathering data is energy-intensive. After a period of drain, the battery requires time to recharge; nevertheless, the gadget cannot continually monitor during that time.

Integration-Based

Integration is the process of integrating existing tools or devices with outside technology in order to guarantee data consistency and accuracy over the duration of their lives and prepare them for future growth. Quality of life will be enhanced by extending and fusing IoT-based monitoring systems with other external devices that offer a variety of benefits. The communications, processing, and services offered by integrated information systems will all be greatly enhanced by the creation of integrated tools.

Related technologies like cloud computing and software-defined networking, are needed to expand IoT healthcare monitoring systems (Birje & Hanji, 2020).

Energy-Based

IoT devices connected to healthcare that rely on monitoring have a short battery life. Even in energy-saving mode, the gadget has some functions that must be completed, but its power supply is limited. Batteries are constantly needed for many medical devices, particularly wearables and devices for patients who require continuous status monitoring (Aghdam et al., 2021). To enable extended monitoring, the perfect system would combine power-efficient hardware architecture with low-power communications. Activity-aware energy models provide an intriguing new field of application: reduced power usage. Through the use of context-aware episodic sampling, the performance may be raised from poor to high (Birje & Hanji, 2020; Majedi et al., 2016).

Disease Prediction-Based

Thanks to its ability to accelerate early disease detection, IoT is utilised in fitness programmes, geriatric care, and the diagnosis and treatment of disorders, including chronic diseases. The future breadth of the anticipated healthcare system will progress the development of medical treatment that can predict a patient's illness early on. This will result in cheaper medical expenditures, better medical services, and better outcomes for the medical healthcare industry. Therefore, it's also necessary to create an inexpensive, independent system that monitors important metrics, sends data to the cloud or NLP, and alerts patients in a timely manner using the relevant APP for their benefit.

Conclusion

In conclusion, the future holds promising advancements for IoT healthcare monitoring systems within smart cities. The integration of IoT technology into healthcare systems has already shown tremendous potential, and ongoing innovations are poised to reshape the landscape further. Several key areas highlight the potential future advancements in this domain:

Enhanced Remote Patient Monitoring

Future IoT healthcare systems are likely to see advancements in remote patient monitoring, offering more comprehensive and real-time data. Wearable devices and sensors will become even more sophisticated, providing detailed insights into patients' health status.

Predictive Analytics and AI Integration

The integration of predictive analytics and artificial intelligence (AI) will play a crucial role in IoT healthcare monitoring. Advanced algorithms will analyze vast datasets, offering predictive insights into potential health issues, enabling proactive interventions, and personalizing healthcare plans.

Interoperability and Data Exchange

Improved interoperability among healthcare devices and systems will facilitate seamless data exchange. This will lead to a more holistic view of a patient's health by integrating data from various sources, enhancing diagnostic accuracy, and supporting more informed decision-making.

5G Connectivity and Low Latency

The deployment of 5G technology will enable faster and more reliable connectivity for IoT devices. Low latency and high bandwidth will be instrumental in transmitting real-time health data, making remote monitoring more efficient and responsive.

Blockchain for Security and Privacy

Blockchain technology is likely to be increasingly adopted to address security and privacy concerns in healthcare data. It can provide a decentralized and secure platform for managing sensitive health information, ensuring data integrity and protecting patient privacy.

Telemedicine Integration

The synergy between IoT healthcare monitoring and telemedicine will strengthen, enabling healthcare professionals to remotely assess patients and provide timely interventions. This integration will contribute to improved accessibility to healthcare services, especially in densely populated smart cities.

Community Health and Environmental Monitoring:

Future IoT healthcare systems may extend beyod individual patient monitoring to encompass broader community health and environmental monitoring. This holistic approach can help identify health trends, track the spread of diseases, and contribute to better public health management.

Smart City Infrastructure Integration

The integration of IoT healthcare systems with broader smart city infrastructure will become more seamless. Collaborations between healthcare providers, city authorities, and technology companies will lead to more efficient healthcare delivery and resource allocation.

In summary, the future of IoT healthcare monitoring within smart cities holds tremendous potential for improving healthcare outcomes, enhancing efficiency, and promoting proactive and personalized health management. As technological advancements continue, the vision of a connected and intelligent healthcare ecosystem within smart cities is likely to become a reality, benefiting both healthcare providers and the communities they serve.

REFERENCES

Adewole, K. S., Akintola, A. G., Jimoh, R. G., Mabayoje, M. A., Jimoh, M. K., Usman-Hamza, F. E., Balogun, A. O., Sangaiah, A. K., & Ameen, A. O. (2021). Intelligent IoT Systems in Personalized Health Care. Elsevier.

Aghdam, Z. N., Rahmani, A. M., & Hosseinzadeh, M. (2021). The role of the Internet of Things in healthcare: Future trends and challenges. *Computer Methods and Programs in Biomedicine*, *199*, 105903. doi:10.1016/j.cmpb.2020.105903 PMID:33348073

Alekya, R., Boddeti, N.D., Monica, K.S., Prabha, D.R., & Venkatesh, D.V. (2021). *IoT based Smart Healthcare Monitoring Systems: A Literature Review*. Academic Press.

Alshamrani, M. (2022). IoT and artificial intelligence implementations for remote healthcare monitoring systems: A survey. *Journal of King Saud University. Computer and Information Sciences*, *34*(8), 4687–4701. doi:10.1016/j.jksuci.2021.06.005

Azzawi, M. A., Hassan, R., & Bakar, K. A. A. (2016). A review on Internet of Things (IoT) in healthcare. *International Journal of Applied Engineering Research: IJAER*, *11*, 10216–10221.

Birje, M. N., & Hanji, S. S. (2020). Internet of things based distributed healthcare systems: A review. *J. Data Inf. Manag.*, *2*(3), 149–165. doi:10.1007/s42488-020-00027-x

Blake, M. B. (2015). An internet of things for healthcare. *IEEE Internet Computing*, *19*(4), 4–6. doi:10.1109/MIC.2015.89

Bouazzi, I., Zaidi, M., Usman, M., Shamim, M. Z., Gunjan, V. K., & Singh, N. (2022). Future Trends for Healthcare Monitoring System in Smart Cities Using LoRaWAN-Based WBAN. *Mobile Information Systems*, *2022*, 1–12. doi:10.1155/2022/1526021

Capraro, G. T. (2016). Artificial Intelligence (AI), Big Data, and Healthcare. *Proceedings of the International Conference on Artificial Intelligence (ICAI)*, 425.

Hossain, M. S., & Muhammad, G. (2016). Cloud-assisted industrial internet of things (iiot)–enabled framework for health monitoring. *Computer Networks*, *101*, 192–202. doi:10.1016/j.comnet.2016.01.009

Jeong, S., Shen, J.-H., & Ahn, B. (2021). A Study on Smart Healthcare Monitoring Using IoT Based on Blockchain. *Wireless Communications and Mobile Computing*, *2021*, 9932091. doi:10.1155/2021/9932091

Karatas, M., Eriskin, L., Deveci, M., Pamucar, D., & Garg, H. (2022). Big Data for Healthcare Industry 4.0: Applications, challenges and future perspectives. *Expert Systems with Applications*, *200*, 116912. doi:10.1016/j.eswa.2022.116912

Kaur, P., Kumar, R., & Kumar, M. (2019). A healthcare monitoring system using random forest and internet of things (IoT). *Multimedia Tools and Applications*, *78*(14), 19905–199. doi:10.1007/s11042-019-7327-8

Kishor, A., & Chakraborty, C. (2021). Artificial Intelligence and Internet of Things Based Healthcare 4.0 Monitoring System. *Wireless Personal Communications*, 1–17.

Magaña-Espinoza, P., Aquino-Santos, R., Cárdenas-Benítez, N., Aguilar-Velasco, J., Buenrostro-Segura, C., Edwards-Block, A., & Medina-Cass, A. (2014). WiSPH: A wireless sensor network-based home care monitoring system. *Sensors (Basel), 14*(4), 7096–7119. doi:10.3390/s140407096 PMID:24759112

Majedi, N., Naeem, M., & Anpalagan, A. (2016). Telecommunication integration in e-healthcare: Technologies, applications and challenges. *Transactions on Emerging Telecommunications Technologies, 27*(6), 775–789. doi:10.1002/ett.3025

Mathew, P. S., & Pillai, A. S. (2016). Innovations in Bio-Inspired Computing and Applications. Springer.

Mostafa, S. M. G., Zaki, M., Islam, M. M., Alam, M. S., & Ullah, M. A. (2022). Design and Implementation of an IoT-Based Healthcare Monitoring System. *Proceedings of the 2022 International Conference on Innovations in Science, Engineering and Technology (ICISET)*, 362–366. 10.1109/ICISET54810.2022.9775850

Philip, Rodrigues, Wang, Fong, & Chen. (2021). Internet of Things for in-home health monitoring systems: current advances, challenges and future directions. *IEEE Journal on Selected Areas in Communications*, *39*(2), 300-310.

Raj, J. S. (2020). A novel information processing in IoT based real time health care monitoring system. *Journal of Electronics (China)*, *2*, 188–196.

Romero, L. E., Chatterjee, P., & Armentano, R. L. (2016). An IoT approach for integration of computational intelligence and wearable sensors for Parkinson's disease diagnosis and monitoring. *Health and Technology*, *6*(3), 167–172. doi:10.1007/s12553-016-0148-0

Sakr, S., & Elgammal, A. (2016). Towards a comprehensive data analytics framework for smart healthcare services. *Big Data Res.*, *4*, 44–58. doi:10.1016/j.bdr.2016.05.002

Singh, P. (2018). Internet of things based health monitoring system: Opportunities and challenges. *Int. J. Adv. Res. Comput. Sci.*, *9*(1), 224–228. doi:10.26483/ijarcs.v9i1.5308

Tabassum, S., Zaman, M. I. U., Ullah, M. S., Rahaman, A., Nahar, S., & Islam, A. M. (2019). The cardiac disease predictor: IoT and ML driven healthcare system. *Proceedings of the 2019 4th International Conference on Electrical Information and Communication Technology (EICT),* 1–6. 10.1109/EICT48899.2019.9068821

Yang, Y., Wang, H., Jiang, R., Guo, X., Cheng, J., & Chen, Y. (2022). A Review of IoT-enabled Mobile Healthcare: Technologies, Challenges, and Future Trends. *IEEE Internet of Things Journal*, *9*(12), 9478–9502. doi:10.1109/JIOT.2022.3144400

Yeole, A. S., & Kalbande, D. R. (2016). Use of Internet of Things (IoT) in healthcare: A survey. *Proceedings of the ACM Symposium on Women in Research*, 71–76. 10.1145/2909067.2909079

Chapter 11
Intelligent System for Predicting Healthcare Readmissions

Manu Banga
GLA University, Mathura, India

ABSTRACT

Hospitalization costs accrue a huge burden on the economy; thus, we need a hospital readmission system for predicting treatment costs associated with the patient admitted at the hospital. A novel prediction model for readmissions of patients suffering from disabilities and for patients with comorbidities that pose critical health risks thereby escalating healthcare costs and posing a threat on the survival of patients is highly recommended for patients at high risk of readmission to be proactive during treatment thereby reducing readmission cost. As per data of the National Health Protection Mission hospitalized between 2016 and 2022 in India, more than 9000 patients were readmitted and took treatment after a significant lapse. This chapter proposed a machine learning framework with all key elements of patients resulting discrimination ability and predicting financial analysis to estimate targeted patients thereby identifying risk factors, and a model was tested on an Indian government repository of healthcare dataset and achieved 97.9% correct prediction readmission in hospitals.

INTRODUCTION

At this challenging moment for healthcare and the economy it is well stated that Prevention is preferable to cure but without prediction of readmission prevention is not possible. This study mainly identifies low-risk, moderate-risk and high-risk patients of readmission by computing the unstructured data research, along with its goals and objectives as human body is full of BIG DATA consists of X-Rays, diagnosis of patients for prediction of treatment needed using intelligent software systems capable of handling massive unstructured in patient readmission scenarios, the role performed by these systems is recognised in the healthcare data which has a unstructured, complex BIG DATA with characteristics are volume, variety, velocity and veracity (Abdel-Basset et al., 2021; Abdelrahman, 2020; Galetsi & Katsaliaki, 2020). The speed of healthcare data created from patient encounters and patient monitors is increasing in and out of the clinic—the second V (Velocity). More than 80 percent of medical data

DOI: 10.4018/979-8-3693-1934-5.ch011

resides in unstructured formats, such as doctors' notes, images and charts from monitoring instruments (Babu et al., 2017; Cheng et al., 2018; Forestiero & Papuzzo, 2018). The third V (Variety) and the fourth V (Veracity) deal with unsure or vague data. Most healthcare data from clinic and hospital records are afflicted with errors, as while entering data, technicians frequently attach research to the wrong person's record or copy research incorrectly. This section provides the context of the research and its aim and objectives. It then demonstrates the significance of this research. In today's digital world, life without a computer is not possible. Nearly everything around us is on an intelligent system, helping us lead life in a better way. The revolution brought by smart systems has increased global productivity and has benefited the world. Intelligent systems are useless without software. For excellence in intelligent systems, there is a strong need to develop more and more reliable software systems for healthcare.

LITERATURE REVIEW

An intelligent healthcare system discovers trends in readmission data of various departments, thereby predicting and assessing readmission rates. Organizations utilize multiple methods to examine their data to predict future events. An intelligent healthcare system is a combination of statistical analysis and various data mining techniques, such as association, classification, clustering and pattern matching. It comprises the exploration and preparation of data, defining an intelligent system, and follows its process. In the development of an intelligent healthcare system, various authors have carried out research primarily on prescriptive analytics using descriptive analytics, diagnostic analytics and predictive analytics and have proposed a framework for the healthcare industry of real-time patients using support vector machines. Good accuracy was achieved, but biased datasets resulted in false predictions (Babar et al., 2016; Bossen & Piras, 2020; Jin et al., 2016). For dealing with ambiguous, biased datasets, a framework for COVID-19 prediction was proposed using personality traits. Researchers conducted a comprehensive study of Qatar and accessed various healthcare records arising from COVID-19 (Khanra et al., 2020; Ma et al., 2018). Eminent researchers proposed a system for a hospital infrastructure management system. They surveyed designing a comprehensive system covering multispecialty domains (De Silva et al., 2015; Moutselos et al., 2018). Some researchers designed a diagnostic analytics system for heart failure readmission cases for heart patients' readmission based on pulmonary infection using naïve Bayes theorem. They achieved 71% accuracy in probability assessment (Gowsalya et al., 2014; Navaz et al., 2018; Wu et al., 2017). Researchers carried out an extrinsic survey on various healthcare data using SVM and Neural Network for predictions of heart stroke using ECG signals (Sabharwal et al., 2016; Salomi & Balamurugan, 2016). Figure 1 points to the Big Data with its dimensions for identification of patient's voluminous data.

Figure 1. Healthcare data representation

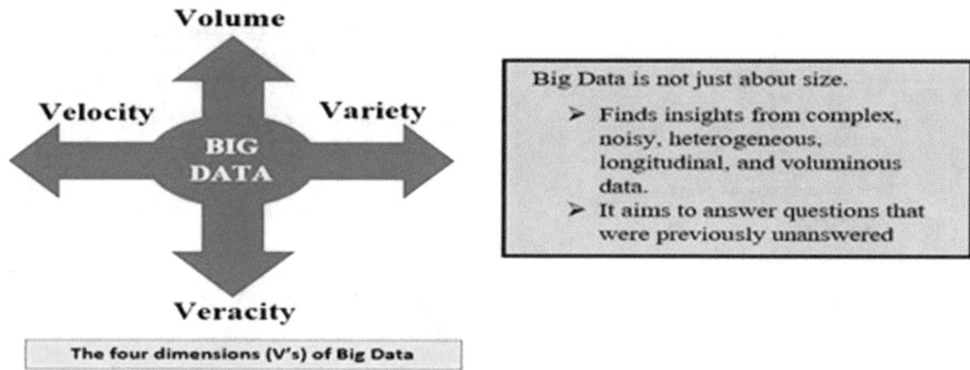

Collecting data from multiple sources from various scans, X-rays, and impressions used in daily diagnosis centers makes the body a BIG DATA generator source and this data is analyses is done with its data increasing and diminishing of patient healthcare time given at hospital using days spent by individual patients with medicines, special diet, tests based on gender, previous hospitalization history, age of the patients as patients with age above 60 years are more at risk of readmission as compared to patients of younger age similarly, research proposed prompt just-in-time model of health readmission based on attribute selection methods as feature selection pre-processing method prune the irrelevant records of the patients and based on relevant attribute of age, sorting the feature data, resolving class imbalance problem using dimension reduction thereby reducing the time-complexity of the problem (Gravili et al., 2018; Kamble et al., 2018). By adhering to the above principles not only hospitalization cost reduces but also hospital reputation also increases in the market as this model can predict the outcome before the preventive diagnosis starts. Figure 2 depicts the healthcare data collection.

Figure 2. Data collection from various test and diagnostics

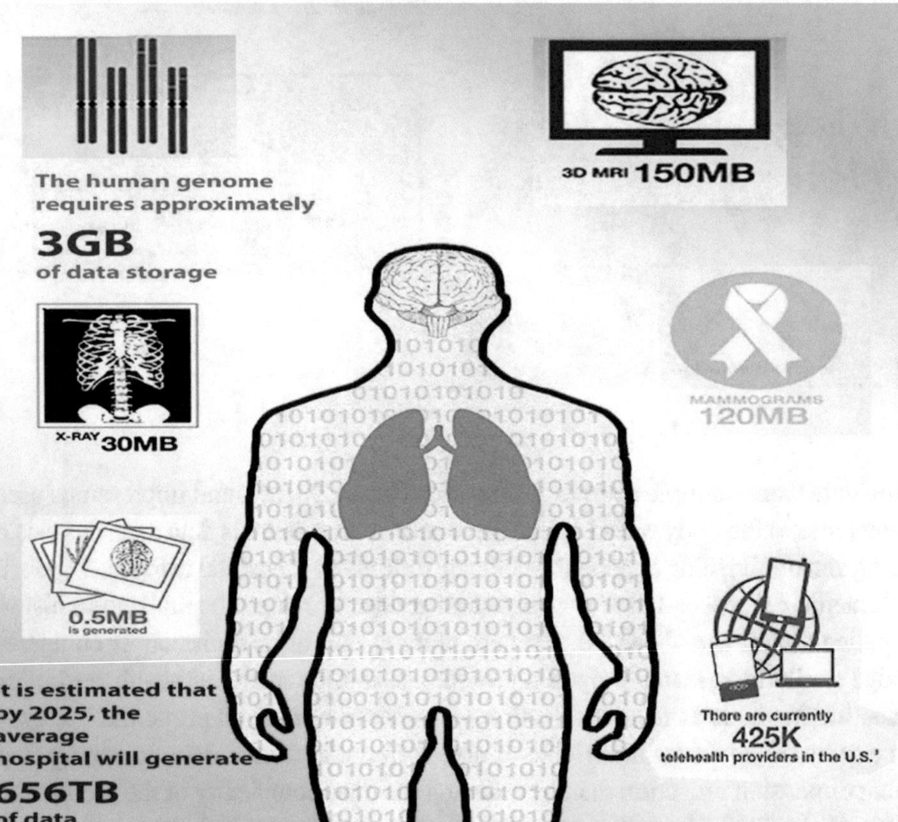

Readmission intelligent system data generated from the various sources for the identification of:

- Clinical Decision Support Systems
- Predict using preventive care model for predicting the risk of early hospitalization of patients with comorbidities
- Teleconsultation of the patients during initial phase before hospital visit through Aarogya app.
- Fraud Management for detection of billing system in Hospital raising false bills on insurance panel or other Central Government Health Scheme
- Personalized medicines of patients from Nursing Staff, attendants, daily register of the patient admitting again the hospitals.
- Preventing Healthcare methodology for the patients with disabilities giving special diet, proper medications and frequent check-ups as well as advised the doctor.

Figure 3. Data and types of origin

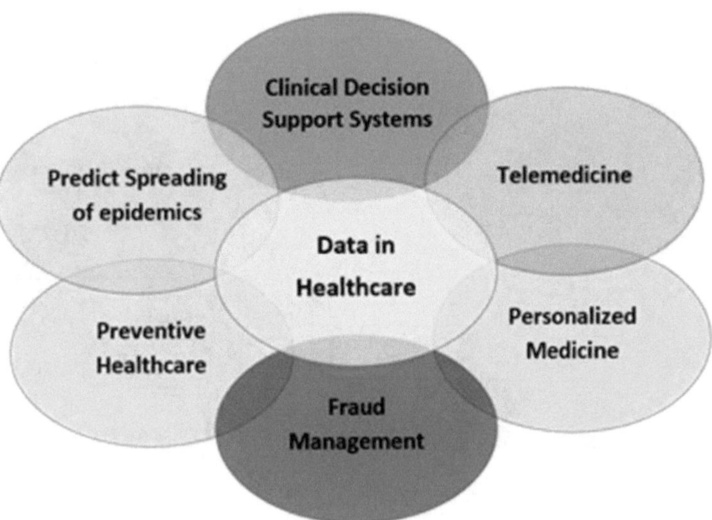

RESEARCH METHODOLOGY

By identifying patterns in readmission data from several departments, the Intelligent Healthcare System can forecast and evaluate the readmission rate. Organizations use a variety of techniques to analyses their data and forecast future events. Data mining methods including association, classification, clustering, and pattern matching are combined with statistical analysis to create the Intelligent Healthcare System. It includes data preparation and exploration, as well as defining an intelligent system and its workflow. Readmissions can be controlled by taking exploratory factor analysis of the parameter playing important role in economy and enhancing the life of the people (Kamble et al., 2018; Navaz et al., 2018), the data is well organized with parameter of preventing further deterioration of persons with disabilities as limiting our research to the persons with disabilities and the challenges taken by them in day to day activities, and coming for regular follow-up difficult for them but this model provides personalized medicines through teleconsultation thereby making system a predictive diagnostic and help in identification of fraud management thereby making decision support system and making patients clinically fit to do work as it tracks the factors responsible for the disease, looking at grass-root level thereby making searching faster retrieval and accessible by the hospitals by diagnostic analytics, and growing in this manner uses predictive analysis and make it happen for the people suffering from particular disease using Prescriptive analysis.

Figure 4. Data analytics system
Stages involved in developing intelligent system:
Stage 1: Descriptive Analytics
Stage 2: Diagnostic Analytics
Stage 3: Predictive Analysis
Stage 4: Prescriptive Analytics.

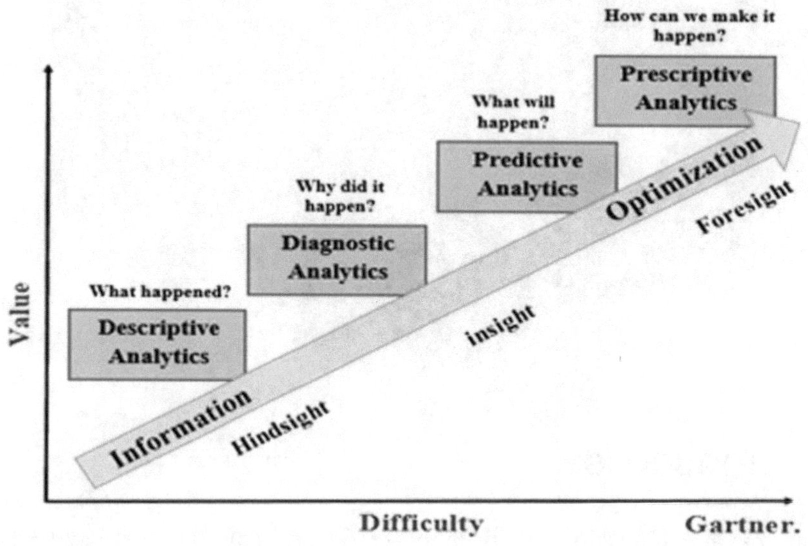

By employing above stages development of real-time healthcare readmission system can be designed but using biased datasets misclassification increases but model handled the misclassification by using boundary for separating points and attained high accuracy. Distinguished researchers proposed a system for the management of hospital infrastructure thereby building a comprehensive healthcare system that covers multiple specialization from diagnostic analytics to predictive analytics, prescriptive analytics thereby reducing deaths due to pulmonary heart diseases.

PROPOSED MODEL USING MACHINE LEARNING FOR FEATURE EXTRACTION

Feature selection is very important step in the analysis of data particularly dataset of high dimensions and attribute selection plays a significant rule in dimension reduction in selection of relevant feature parameters, using a hybrid approach for feature selection of Modified Genetic Algorithm (MGA) and Particle Swarm Optimisation (PSO) for making selection using crossover and mutation for generating new generation dataset.

Model Illustration

Based on the feature obtained classification is made as very low, low, high and very high risks of patient readmission and this categorical data is studied for the analytics of patients, first choosing a suitable population for using this model.

Proposed Algorithm for Prediction Readmission Time

Firstly the unstructured and structure dataset is loaded and features are extracted and after obtaining most relevant feature like:

1. Length of Stay of the patient: The hospital dataset loaded with the patient name with various redundancy
2. Need for Readmission based on its Severity:
3. Disabilities
4. Emergency Medical Record

Based on the above factors Patients at Risk of Readmission using patient most recent visit of four years and the likelihood of readmission using previous readmission, diagnosis and socio-demographic information of patients and on these feature for getting prediction bagging technique is used thereby underestimating patients in readmission varies from set of very low, low, moderate and high and class of patients need of no readmission thereby using algorithm optimization using Machine Learning Technique Particle Swarm Optimisation, it is improved version for selecting under estimated features and over estimated parameters and thereby played a significant role in readmission prediction. The data is loaded in a particular data structure using suitable algorithm of data mining and data feature are extracted and features are loaded with missing data using Bagging and Boosting for reducing class imbalance and misclassification as class imbalance caused wrong classification of the data, data from Set A is classified with the data of Set B but with use of F-measure Precision, Recall, Accuracy the data is classified with suitable patterns of readmission or not thereby taking attributes using Gender, Age, Patient lab tests, previous medical condition, persons with disabilities, X-Ray and the model with highest accuracy is selected and based on the feature medical history. Figure 5 explains details the entire process from feature extraction to feature selection and obtaining optimized feature subsets. This process of obtaining feature subset is repeated again till the entire dataset is extracted and loaded into model and data is divided into train dataset and test dataset, about 70 percent data is loaded into train dataset and point data is loaded into optimisation using hybrid Particle Swarm Optimisation-Modified Genetic Algorithm (MGA-PSO) as data generation made using crossover is optimised and mutation thereby getting most relevant parameters from the high multi spectral data of hospital, and again data of patients is serialized to the server using serialization and make them accessible to the use of the patients and the hospital administration thereby checking status of next follow-up advancing in this manner Big data, Cloud Computing made healthcare reach for everyone through online mode and the threat model or security of patient data is accessed by making them advance reminder for next follow though it is very difficult for the patient to reach and my this bond India has saved 15 Million Rupees otherwise it may accrue cost of treatment under National Health Mission for providing safety and treatment to all persons with disabilities as disabilities is of multiple types

- Intellectual Disability
- Locomotor Disability
- Vision Disability
- Hearing Disability
- Autism Disability

- Combination of disabilities

Figure 5 depicts the working of feature extraction for healthcare data.Due to above mentioned Disabilites persons suffering from them prevents constant follow up but with the help of cloud monitoring real time assessment of the patients diseases can cured and limitation hampering in progress of treatment can be given and feature subset is obtained.

Figure 5. Shows stages in feature extraction from healthcare

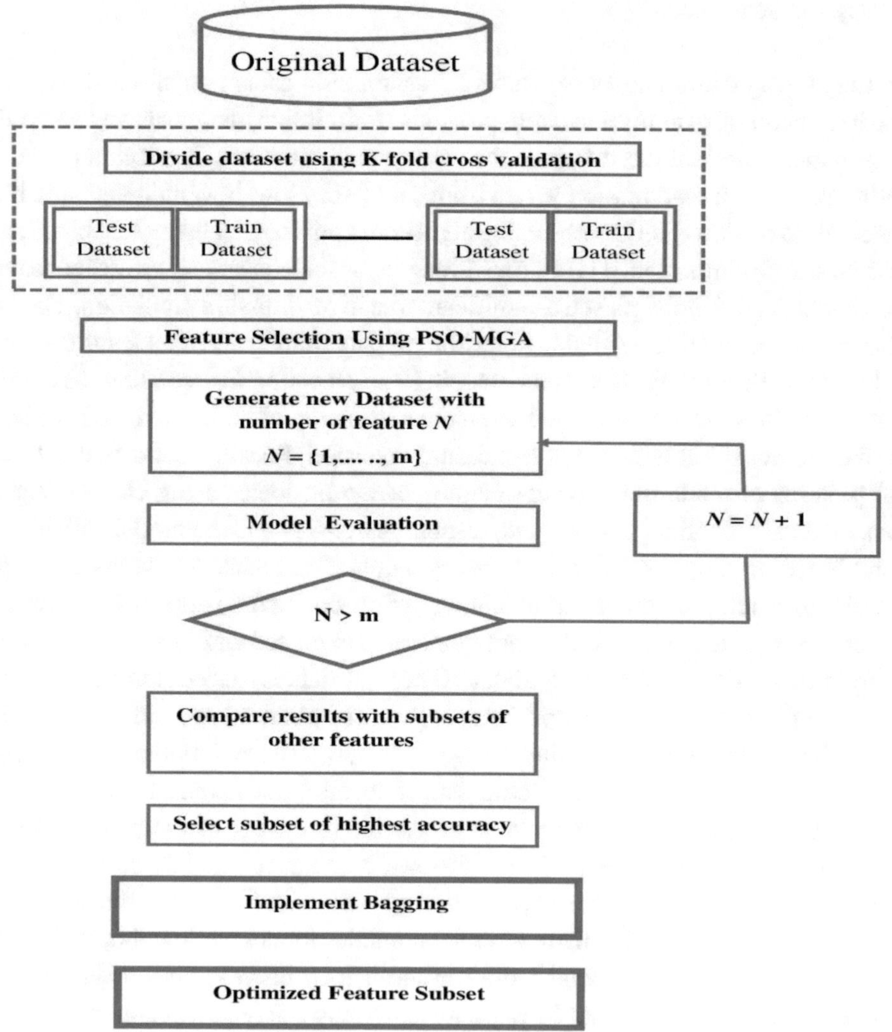

Accessing Performance of Prediction Model

Based upon the above four possible outcomes:

$$\begin{aligned}\text{TruePositiveRate}(t_p) &= \frac{\text{Positive correctly classified}}{\text{TotalNegative}} \\ &= \frac{\text{TruePositive} + \text{TrueNegative}}{\text{TruePositive} + \text{TrueNegative} + \text{FalsePostive} + \text{FalseNegative}}\end{aligned} \tag{1}$$

It species that the prediction is correctly specified and prevention is possible at the initial stage.

$$\begin{aligned}\text{TrueNegativeRate}(f_p) &= \frac{\text{Negative correctly classified}}{\text{TotalNegative}} \\ &= \frac{\text{FalsePositive} + \text{FalseNegative}}{\text{TruePositive} + \text{TrueNegative} + \text{FalsePostive} + \text{FalseNegative}}\end{aligned} \tag{2}$$

It species that the prediction is correctly specified and avoidance is possible at the initial stage for prevention.

$$\text{Sensitivity} = \text{recall} = \frac{\text{TotalPositive classified}}{\text{Total samples}} = \frac{\text{TP}}{\text{TP} + \text{FN}} \tag{3}$$

It species that the prediction is correctly specified and prevention is possible at the initial stage over all the features subset.

$$\text{Specificity} = \frac{\text{TotalNegative classified}}{\text{Total samples}} = \frac{\text{TN}}{\text{TP} + \text{FN}} \tag{4}$$

It species that the prediction is correctly specified and avoidance is possible at the initial stage for prevention over all the feature subset.

$$\text{Accuracy} = \frac{\text{TP} + \text{TN}}{\text{TP} + \text{TN} + \text{FP} + \text{FN}} \tag{5}$$

Based on the above accuracy of the model is calculated

$$\text{Precision} = \frac{\text{TP}}{\text{TP} + \text{FP}} \tag{6}$$

Based on the above precision of the model is calculated signifies correct classified to negatively classified thus misclassification can be avoided.

$$F - \text{measure} = 2.\frac{\text{Precision.Recall}}{\text{Precision} + \text{Recall}} \tag{7}$$

Based on the above precision and recall of the model is calculated signifies correct classified to negatively classified thus misclassification can be avoided and F-Score of the model is obtained

RESULTS

Using comprehensive experiment for classifying readmission as low, moderate and high as expense accrue and analyzing such huge exponential data is vey large thereby decreasing the complexity of such large database even the data is of categorial based on the fuzziness in Table 1 Readmission Prediction of patients Age, Table2: Readmission Prediction based on patient Gender, Table 3: Readmission using Admission Source Persons with Disabilities, Table 4: Readmission based on length of stay in hospital, Table 5: Readmission based on patient OPD visits, Table 6: Readmission based on Disabilities, Table 7: Readmission based on Blood Test Report, Table 8: Readmission based patient previous history, Table 9: Readmission based on patient medications and Table 10 Low, Mid, High Readmission based on laboratory tests report.

Table 1. Readmission prediction of patients age

	Total		**Readmitted in Year**		**Not Readmitted in Year**		
Age	**Occurrence**	**Occurrence Percent**	**Occurrence**	**Occurrence Percent**	**Occurrence**	**Occurrence Percent**	
Feature Age							
<= 50	3	0.3	5	0.4	27	0.3	
<=75	1310	14	164	13.5	1146	14	
<=100	780	8.3	112	9.2	668	8.2	
100+	47	0.5	5	0.4	42	0.5	

Table 2. Readmission prediction based on patient gender

	Total		**Readmitted in Year**		**Not Readmitted in Year**		
Gender	**Occurrence**	**Occurrence Percent**	**Occurrence**	**Occurrence Percent**	**Occurrence**	**Occurrence Percent**	
Feature Gender							
Male	3	0.3	5	0.4	27	0.3	
Female	1310	14	164	13.5	1146	14	

Table 3. Readmission using admission source persons with disabilities

Persons With Disabilities	Frequency	Percent	Frequency	Percent	Frequency	Percent
Feature Admission Source Panel Insurance/ TPA or Cash						
Emergency	3694	39.4	524	43.3	3170	38.8
Planned	5687	60.6	687	56.7	5000	61.2

Table 4. Readmission based on length of stay in hospital

	Total		Readmitted in Year		Not Readmitted in Year	
Age	**Occurrence**	**Occurrence Percent**	**Occurrence**	**Occurrence Percent**	**Occurrence**	**Occurrence Percent**
Based on Length of Stay in days						
1	674	7.2	86	7.1	588	7.2
2	528	5.6	75	6.2	453	5.5
3	831	8.9	72	5.9	759	9.3
4	720	7.7	68	5.6	652	8
5	373	4	41	3.4	332	4.1
6	312	3.3	64	5.3	248	3
7	209	2.2	39	3.2	170	2.1
8	143	1.5	22	1.8	121	1.5
9+	637	6.8	128	10.6	509	6.2

Table 5. Readmission based on patient OPD visits

	Total		Readmitted in Year		Not Readmitted in Year	
Age	**Occurrence**	**Occurrence Percent**	**Occurrence**	**Occurrence Percent**	**Occurrence**	**Occurrence Percent**
Based on Length of Stay in days						
No. of OPD visits						
0	6928	73.9	676	55.8	6252	76.5
1	1431	15.3	223	18.4	1208	14.8
2	492	5.2	109	9	383	4.7
3	225	2.4	82	6.8	143	1.8
4	125	1.3	37	3.1	88	1.1
5	65	0.7	22	1.8	43	0.5

Table 6. Readmission based on glucose report

	Total		Readmitted in Year		Not Readmitted in Year	
Glucose Level	**Occurrence**	**Occurrence Percent**	**Occurrence**	**Occurrence Percent**	**Occurrence**	**Occurrence Percent**
Glucose serum test result						
>200	845	9	87	7.2	758	9.3
>300	355	3.3	41	3.4	264	3.2
Normal	1927	20.5	226	18.7	1701	20.8
None	6334	67.2	857	70.8	5447	66.7

Table 7. Readmission based on blood test report

	Total		Readmitted in Year		Not Readmitted in Year	
Hb Test	**Occurrence**	**Occurrence Percent**	**Occurrence**	**Occurrence Percent**	**Occurrence**	**Occurrence Percent**
Blood Result						
>6	391	4.2	41	3.4	350	4.3
>7	1198	12.8	139	11.5	1059	13
Normal	186	2	28	2.3	158	1.9
None	7606	81.1	1003	82.8	6603	80.8

Table 8. Readmission-based patient previous history

	Total		Readmitted in Year		Not Readmitted in Year	
Number of Diagnosis	**Occurrence**	**Occurrence Percent**	**Occurrence**	**Occurrence Percent**	**Occurrence**	**Occurrence Percent**
Number of Diagnosis						
<= 1	117	1.2	12	1	105	1.3
2	599	6.4	150	12.4	449	5.5
3	1591	17	185	15.3	1406	17.2
4	1207	12.9	135	11.1	1072	13.1
5	1622	17.4	151	12.5	1479	18.1
6	1395	14.9	144	11.9	1251	15.3
7	1038	11.1	122	10.1	916	11.2
8	720	7.7	114	9.4	606	7.4
9	445	4.7	73	6	372	4.6
10	253	2.7	46	3.8	207	2.5
11	137	1.5	28	2.3	109	1.3
12	89	0.9	10	0.8	79	1
13+	160	1.7	41	3.4	119	1.5

Table 9. Readmission based on medication

	Total		Readmitted in Year		Not Readmitted in Year	
Number of Diagnosis	**Occurrence**	**Occurrence Percent**	**Occurrence**	**Occurrence Percent**	**Occurrence**	**Occurrence Percent**
Number of Medications						
151 - 175	360	3.8	56	4.6		304
176 - 200	199	2.1	29	2.4		170
201 - 225	137	1.5	19	1.6		118
226 - 250	87	0.9	12	1		75
251+	336	3.6	64	5.3		272

Table 10. Low, mid, high readmission based on laboratory tests report

	Total		Readmitted in Year		Not Readmitted in Year	
Number of Lab Test	**Occurrence**	**Occurrence Percent**	**Occurrence**	**Occurrence Percent**	**Occurrence**	**Occurrence Percent**
Number of Lab Test						
151 - 175	360	3.8	56	4.6		304
176 - 200	199	2.1	29	2.4		170
201 - 225	137	1.5	19	1.6		118
226 - 250	87	0.9	12	1		75
251+	336	3.6	64	5.3		272

CONCLUSION AND FUTURE WORK

By using above model and predicting the readmission of a patient helps in prevention by taking subtle step and reducing the extra financial burden accrue due to patient negligence and this model predicted to save Rs.150 Million Indian currency based upon current insurance, CGHS and other state level panel expenditure of government of India as per data of National Health Mission, this research can be extended using Deep Learning method for prediction of reports of persons with commodities needed readmissions or not.

REFERENCES

Abdel-Basset, M., Chang, V., & Nabeeh, N. A. (2021). An intelligent framework using disruptive technologies for COVID-19 analysis. *Technological Forecasting and Social Change*, *163*, 163–175. doi:10.1016/j.techfore.2020.120431 PMID:33162617

Abdelrahman, M. (2020). Personality traits, risk perception, and protective behaviors of Arab residents of Qatar during the COVID-19 pandemic. *International Journal of Mental Health and Addiction*, 1–12. PMID:32837433

Babar, M. I., Jehanzeb, M., Ghazali, M., Jawawi, D. N., Sher, F., & Ghayyur, S. A. K. (2016, October). Big data survey in healthcare and a proposal for intelligent data diagnosis framework. *2016 2nd IEEE International Conference on Computer and Communications (ICCC)*, 7-12. 10.1109/CompComm.2016.7924654

Babu, S. K., Vasavi, S., & Nagarjuna, K. (2017, January). Framework for Predictive Analytics as a Service using ensemble model. *2017 IEEE 7th International Advance Computing Conference (IACC)*, 121-128. 10.1109/IACC.2017.0038

Bossen, C., & Piras, E. M. (2020). Introduction to the Special Issue on Information Infrastructures in Healthcare: Governance, Quality Improvement and Service Efficiency. *Computer Supported Cooperative Work*, *29*(4), 381–386. doi:10.1007/s10606-020-09381-1

Cheng, C. H., Kuo, Y. H., & Zhou, Z. (2018). Tracking nosocomial diseases at individual level with a real-time indoor positioning system. *Journal of Medical Systems*, *42*(11), 1–21. doi:10.1007/s10916-018-1085-4 PMID:30284042

De Silva, D., Burstein, F., Jelinek, H. F., & Stranieri, A. (2015). Addressing the complexities of big data analytics in healthcare: The diabetes screening case. *AJIS. Australasian Journal of Information Systems*, *19*, 99–115. doi:10.3127/ajis.v19i0.1183

Forestiero, A., & Papuzzo, G. (2018, December). Distributed algorithm for big data analytics in healthcare. In *2018 IEEE/WIC/ACM International Conference on Web Intelligence (WI)*. IEEE Computer Society. 10.1109/WI.2018.00015

Galetsi, P., & Katsaliaki, K. (2020). A review of the literature on big data analytics in healthcare. *The Journal of the Operational Research Society*, *71*(10), 1511–1529. doi:10.1080/01605682.2019.1630328

Gowsalya, M., Krushitha, K., & Valliyammai, C. (2014, December). Predicting the risk of readmission of diabetic patients using MapReduce. In *2014 Sixth International Conference on Advanced Computing (ICoAC)*. IEEE. 10.1109/ICoAC.2014.7229729

Gravili, G., Benvenuto, M., Avram, A., & Viola, C. (2018). The influence of the Digital Divide on Big Data generation within supply chain management. *International Journal of Logistics Management*, *29*(2), 592–628. doi:10.1108/IJLM-06-2017-0175

Jin, Q., Wu, B., Nishimura, S., & Ogihara, A. (2016, August). Ubi-Liven: a human-centric safe and secure framework of ubiquitous living environments for the elderly. In *2016 International Conference on Advanced Cloud and Big Data (CBD)*. IEEE. 10.1109/CBD.2016.059

Kamble, S. S., Gunasekaran, A., Goswami, M., & Manda, J. (2018). A systematic perspective on the applications of big data analytics in healthcare management. *International Journal of Healthcare Management*, *12*(3), 226–240. doi:10.1080/20479700.2018.1531606

Khanra, S., Dhir, A., Islam, A. N., & Mäntymäki, M. (2020). Big data analytics in healthcare: A systematic literature review. *Enterprise Information Systems*, *14*(7), 878–912. doi:10.1080/17517575.2020.1812005

Ma, X., Wang, Z., Zhou, S., Wen, H., & Zhang, Y. (2018, June). Intelligent healthcare systems assisted by data analytics and mobile computing. In *In 2018 14th International Wireless Communications & Mobile Computing Conference (IWCMC)* (pp. 1317–1322). IEEE. doi:10.1109/IWCMC.2018.8450377

Moutselos, K., Kyriazis, D., Diamantopoulou, V., & Maglogiannis, I. (2018, December). Trustworthy data processing for health analytics tasks. In *2018 IEEE International Conference on Big Data (Big Data)*. IEEE. 10.1109/BigData.2018.8622449

Navaz, A. N., Serhani, M. A., Al-Qirim, N., & Gergely, M. (2018). Towards an efficient and Energy-Aware mobile big health data architecture. *Computer Methods and Programs in Biomedicine*, *166*, 137–154. doi:10.1016/j.cmpb.2018.10.008 PMID:30415713

Sabharwal, S., Gupta, S., & Thirunavukkarasu, K. (2016, April). Insight of big data analytics in healthcare industry. In *2016 International Conference on Computing, Communication and Automation (ICCCA)*. IEEE Xplore. 10.1109/CCAA.2016.7813696

Salomi, M., & Balamurugan, S. A. A. (2016). Need, application and characteristics of big data analytics in healthcare—A survey. *Indian Journal of Science and Technology*, *9*(16), 1–5. doi:10.17485/ijst/2016/v9i16/87960

Wu, J., Li, H., Liu, L., & Zheng, H. (2017). Adoption of big data and analytics in mobile healthcare market: An economic perspective. *Electronic Commerce Research and Applications*, *22*, 24–41. doi:10.1016/j.elerap.2017.02.002

KEY TERMS AND DEFINITIONS

Ayushman Bharat -National Health Protection Mission (AB-NHPM): Ayushman Bharat Yojana (ABY) is a central government-funded free healthcare coverage scheme. The scheme is focused on nearly 11 crore poor and vulnerable families in rural and urban India. It is the largest scheme of its kind in the world. ABY envisions a two-pronged, unified approach by both government and private hospitals, to provide a comprehensive healthcare on primary, secondary and tertiary levels. This is planned to be accomplished through Health and Wellness Centres (HWCs) and Pradhan Mantri Jan Arogya Yojana (PM-JAY).

Deep Learning: Deep learning is a subset of machine learning, which is essentially a neural network with three or more layers. These neural networks attempt to simulate the behavior of the human brain—albeit far from matching its ability—allowing it to "learn" from large amounts of data

Machine Learning: Machine learning is a tool used in health care to help medical professionals care for patients and manage clinical data. It is an application of artificial intelligence, which involves programming computers to mimic how people think and learn.

Model Testing: In machine learning, model testing is referred to as the process where the performance of a fully trained model is evaluated on a testing set. The testing set consisting of a set of testing samples should be separated from the both training and validation sets, but it should follow the same probability distribution as the training set. Each testing sample has a known value of the target. Based on the comparison of the model's predicted value, and the known target, for each testing sample, the performance of the trained model can be measured. There are a number of statistical metrics that can be used to assess testing results including mean squared errors and receiver operating characteristics curves. The question of which one should be used is largely dependent on the type of models and the type of application. For a regression (Regression Analysis) model, the standard error of estimate is widely used.

Model Validation: It is a phase of machine learning that quantifies the ability of an ML or statistical model to produce predictions or outputs with enough fidelity to be used reliably to achieve business objectives.

Particle Swarm Optimization (PSO): It is an artificial intelligence (AI) technique that can be used to find approximate solutions to extremely difficult or impossible numeric maximization and minimization problems.

Support Vector Machine: A support vector machine (SVM) is a type of deep learning algorithm that performs supervised learning for classification or regression of data groups. In AI and machine learning, supervised learning systems provide both input and desired output data, which are labelled for classification.

Chapter 12
Impacts of 5G Machine Learning Techniques on Telemedicine and Social Media Professional Connection in Healthcare

P. Siva Satya Sreedhar
Department of Information Technology, Seshadri Rao Gudlavalleru Engineering College, India

V. Sujay
Department of Computer Science and Engineering, Krishna University College of Engineering and Technology, India

Maderametla Roja Rani
Department of Microbiology & FST, GITAM University, India

L. Melita
https://orcid.org/0000-0001-9874-9180
Department of Computer Applications, CMR University, India

S. Reshma
Department of Artificial Intelligence and Machine Learning, Dayananda Sagar College of Engineering, India

Sampath Boopathi
Muthayammal Engineering College, India

ABSTRACT

The healthcare industry is undergoing a transformation due to the convergence of advanced technologies. This chapter explores the impact of 5G connectivity, machine learning, and social media integration in healthcare. It delves into the evolution of telemedicine, the role of social media in healthcare communication, and the emergence of 5G networks and machine learning. The chapter also discusses the foundations of 5G technology, its implications for telemedicine, and the ethical considerations of machine learning techniques in healthcare. It also highlights the potential of social media in healthcare to foster professional connections, enable collaboration, and educate patients. The chapter addresses challenges like adoption barriers, ethical dilemmas, and legal considerations, envisioning a future where these technologies integrate for efficient, ethical, and patient-centric healthcare.

DOI: 10.4018/979-8-3693-1934-5.ch012

INTRODUCTION

The healthcare industry is undergoing a transformation due to technological advancements, including 5G networks, machine learning, and social media integration. Telemedicine, once a niche concept, is now a cornerstone of modern healthcare, enabling remote access to services and bridging geographical gaps. The advent of 5G technology has amplified its potential, offering unparalleled speed, low latency, and enhanced connectivity. This technology enables real-time consultations, high-definition video conferencing, and remote monitoring of patients with unprecedented accuracy and efficiency (Schünke et al., 2022). This transformation is transforming the way healthcare is delivered and managed. The integration of machine learning algorithms and artificial intelligence (AI) in healthcare is transforming the industry towards personalized, data-driven medicine. These algorithms enable early disease detection, precise treatment planning, and the potential for foreseeing health risks before they manifest, thereby revolutionizing the way diseases are detected and managed (Salman et al., 2021).

Social media platforms significantly impact healthcare by fostering collaboration among professionals, empowering patients through education and support networks, and facilitating the dissemination of accurate medical information to a global audience. They provide a dynamic space for practitioners to share knowledge, discuss cases, and stay updated on the latest advancements in their respective fields. The integration of 5G networks, machine learning, and social media networking is transforming the healthcare industry by enhancing efficiency and fostering a more connected, informed, and collaborative ecosystem. This technological transformation is crucial for ensuring equitable access to quality healthcare, optimizing patient outcomes, and guiding the industry towards a future where technology is not just a tool but a cornerstone of compassionate and effective healthcare delivery (Zobair et al., 2021).

Telemedicine has its roots in early 20th-century experiments using radio and telephone communications for remote medical consultations. However, digital communication technologies emerged in the latter part of the century as a viable alternative to traditional in-person healthcare delivery. The primary goal was to overcome geographical barriers and bring medical expertise to underserved or remote communities (Yadav et al., 2022). Initially, telemedicine relied on basic audio and video transmission, but faced technological limitations like low-resolution images and poor audio quality. Despite these limitations, telemedicine showed immense potential in situations where immediate access to specialized care was unavailable. Remote consultations, particularly in radiology and pathology, laid the foundation for its gradual integration into mainstream healthcare (Washington et al., 2020).

The late 20th century saw the rise of the internet as a global communication medium, accelerating the evolution of telemedicine. This shift from analog to digital transmission improved audiovisual data quality, leading to more comprehensive telehealth services, including remote monitoring of vital signs, electronic health records management, and tele-surgery in specialized fields. Telemedicine has evolved significantly due to advancements in telecommunication technologies, such as broadband connections and 4G networks. These advancements enable faster and more reliable data transmission, enabling real-time interactions between patients and healthcare providers, regardless of their geographical location. This democratizes access to healthcare, offering convenience and efficiency in medical service delivery (Kumela et al., 2023).

The 5G revolution is poised to revolutionize telemedicine with its speed, low latency, and capacity to handle large data volumes. This shift will enable high-definition video consultations, remote robotic surgeries, and real-time transmission of complex medical data, surpassing previous communication technologies' limitations and paving the way for a new era in telemedicine (Afifah et al., 2021).

Social media has significantly transformed the healthcare industry by facilitating information sharing, collaboration among professionals, and patient empowerment. Platforms like Facebook, Twitter, and LinkedIn have revolutionized the way medical information is shared, discussed, and accessed by professionals and the general public, transforming the way healthcare is conducted. Healthcare practitioners are using social media to share knowledge, research findings, and best practices. Platforms like Twitter and medical forums allow professionals to exchange opinions and contribute to the collective knowledge base. This has enhanced the dissemination of medical information, broken down communication barriers, and enabled experts to collaborate on complex cases, ultimately improving patient care outcomes (Stellefson et al., 2020).

Social media platforms like Reddit and Facebook have fostered patient education and engagement through advocacy groups, forums, and health-related communities. These platforms enable individuals to share experiences, seek advice, and access information about health conditions, providing solace and support for patients as they navigate their healthcare journeys (Schillinger et al., 2020).

Social media has significantly boosted health literacy globally, empowering patients and raising awareness about preventive measures. Healthcare organizations and professionals have used platforms like Instagram and TikTok to disseminate health-related infographics, interactive campaigns, and live Q&A sessions to promote proactive health management and informed decision-making (Mheidly & Fares, 2020). However, ethical considerations and privacy concerns have emerged, with healthcare professionals balancing sharing valuable insights with protecting sensitive patient information. The integration of social media in healthcare requires careful consideration of patient confidentiality and ethical practices to ensure the best use of this platform.

5G and machine learning are transforming the way doctors interact with patients, enabling them to communicate in real-time and provide real-time assistance. 5G is faster than traditional internet, allowing doctors to communicate through video without delays and share large medical files instantly. This technology is transforming the way we live and work, allowing doctors to provide immediate care to patients from far away, enhancing the efficiency and effectiveness of healthcare (Hussain, 2020).

Machine learning, a form of artificial intelligence, allows machines to learn from vast amounts of information, similar to how we learn from books and teachers. In the medical field, this technology can help doctors detect diseases early, suggest treatments, and predict health issues before they become major problems. When combined with 5G technology, machine learning and 5G can work like a superhero team, enabling faster data sharing and analysis, enabling doctors to make quicker and more accurate decisions. This technology can also guide surgeons in real-time during surgeries (Tsao et al., 2021).

The integration of 5G and machine learning in medicine presents challenges, including ensuring patient information security and addressing the healthcare gap. However, these advancements are opening doors to faster, smarter, and better health care. With these superpowers, doctors can reach more people, detect illnesses sooner, and make treatments more effective, ultimately leading to a healthier world for everyone. Ensuring everyone can benefit from these advancements is crucial for a successful healthcare system (Devi et al., 2023).

5G TECHNOLOGY IN TELEMEDICINE

5G, the fifth generation of wireless technology, revolutionizes connectivity by offering lightning-fast speeds, low latency, and higher capacity. Operating on higher frequency bands, 5G enables faster data transmission, enabling near-instantaneous communication between devices. Its small cell technology, which deploys smaller base stations throughout an area, provides better coverage and can handle more devices simultaneously, making it ideal for densely populated urban areas. This technology enables faster data transmission and near-instantaneous communication between devices (Hameed et al., 2021).

Implications

5G technology is revolutionizing telemedicine by enabling high-definition video conferencing between doctors and patients, regardless of geographical distances. This real-time interaction allows for detailed consultations, remote diagnosis, and even surgeries conducted by remote specialists. 5G also facilitates the transfer of large medical files, ensuring accurate diagnoses and treatment plans. Remote patient monitoring using wearable devices and sensors becomes more effective. Additionally, 5G enables the integration of augmented reality and virtual reality technologies in healthcare, allowing doctors to use AR/VR for immersive training, simulations, and educational purposes (Berlet et al., 2022).

Security and Privacy

5G technology offers numerous benefits but also raises security and privacy concerns. The increased connectivity and large number of devices create a larger cyber threat surface, with potential vulnerabilities in network infrastructure. Privacy concerns arise from the vast amount of data generated and transmitted, particularly for personal health information. Robust encryption and secure transmission protocols are needed to prevent unauthorized access. As more devices become interconnected, strict regulations are needed to safeguard patient confidentiality and comply with data protection laws (Bhattacharya, 2023).

MACHINE LEARNING IN HEALTHCARE

Machine Learning in Medicine

Machine learning (ML) is a technique used in healthcare to analyze vast amounts of data and identify patterns that humans might miss. ML techniques include supervised learning, unsupervised learning, and reinforcement learning. Supervised learning uses labeled data to train algorithms for specific tasks, while unsupervised learning identifies patterns in unlabeled data, helping to find relationships between variables in patient datasets. Reinforcement learning focuses on sequential decisions, potentially aiding in treatment plans or drug dosage optimization (Lin & Hsu, 2021).

Applications

ML plays a significant role in diagnostics and treatment by analyzing medical images to detect abnormalities or diseases with high accuracy. It assists radiologists by flagging areas of concern, enabling quicker and more precise diagnoses. ML also aids in predicting diseases and assessing risks, allowing early detection for personalized treatments. In treatment, ML helps tailor therapies to individual patients through precision medicine, considering genetic, environmental, and lifestyle factors. It also assists in drug discovery by analyzing molecular structures and predicting potential drug candidates, expediting the development process (Rajula et al., 2020).

Ethical Considerations

Integrating machine learning (ML) in healthcare presents ethical challenges, including data privacy, security, and potential biases. Transparency and interpretability of ML algorithms are crucial for trust and acceptance among healthcare professionals and patients. The black-box nature of some ML models poses challenges in understanding their reasoning, especially in critical decisions. Additionally, the responsibility of errors, such as incorrect diagnoses or treatment plans, raises ethical and legal dilemmas. Therefore, robust safeguards are needed to prevent breaches and protect patient confidentiality (Muehlematter et al., 2021).

THE IMPACT OF 5G ON TELEMEDICINE

Enhancing Remote Patient Care With 5G

5G technology is revolutionizing telemedicine by enhancing the quality and effectiveness of remote patient care. Its ultra-fast speeds and minimal latency enable high-definition video conferencing between healthcare providers and patients, allowing real-time consultations with crystal-clear audiovisuals. This enhances patient-doctor interaction, bridging the gap between in-person visits and remote consultations (Boopathi, 2023b; Pramila et al., 2023; Ramudu et al., 2023; Satav, Hasan, et al., 2024). 5G's rapid data transfer capabilities facilitate the seamless transmission of large medical data files, allowing physicians to access and interpret intricate medical imaging with precision, enabling accurate diagnoses and treatment planning.

5G networks offer reliable and stable connectivity, enabling consistent patient monitoring using wearable devices and sensors. Real-time data transmission allows healthcare providers to monitor patients' vital signs, chronic conditions, and post-operative recovery, enabling timely interventions. This enhances remote patient care, ensuring seamless information flow and enhancing the quality of care, fostering a more connected and efficient healthcare ecosystem (Agrawal et al., 2024).

Real-Time Monitoring and Intervention

5G technology in healthcare revolutionizes real-time monitoring and intervention for patients, regardless of their location. Its high-speed, low-latency nature allows for seamless transmission of patient data, enabling healthcare providers to monitor vital signs and health metrics in real-time. Wearable devices equipped with sensors collect and transmit vital health data, enabling remote monitoring of patients' health status without delay (Boopathi, 2023c; Durairaj et al., 2023; Karthik et al., 2023; Reddy, Reddy, et al., 2023).

5G-enabled real-time monitoring enables immediate alerts and rapid intervention in emergencies and critical situations. It allows healthcare providers to respond promptly to patient fluctuations in vital signs, especially for chronic conditions or those requiring constant medical attention. In post-operative recovery or chronic disease management, it provides healthcare professionals with accurate patient data, enabling timely adjustments to treatment plans, medication dosages, and interventions, optimizing patient care and potentially preventing adverse health events.

5G's real-time monitoring and intervention capabilities are revolutionizing healthcare by providing reliable data streams, enabling swift responses, improving patient outcomes, and enhancing healthcare delivery efficiency.

Advancements in Surgical Procedures

The figure 1 depicts the advancements in surgical procedures and discussed below.

Step 1: Preoperative Planning and Consultation

- **Virtual Collaboration:** Surgeons can use 5G-enabled high-definition video conferencing for preoperative consultations with specialists from different locations. This allows for multidisciplinary discussions, enhancing surgical planning and decision-making.

Step 2: Augmented Reality (AR) and Virtual Reality (VR) Assisted Training

- **Training Programs:** 5G facilitates immersive AR/VR training programs for surgeons. Trainees can experience simulated surgeries and practice intricate procedures in a realistic virtual environment, enhancing their skills and preparedness.

Figure 1. Advancements in surgical procedures

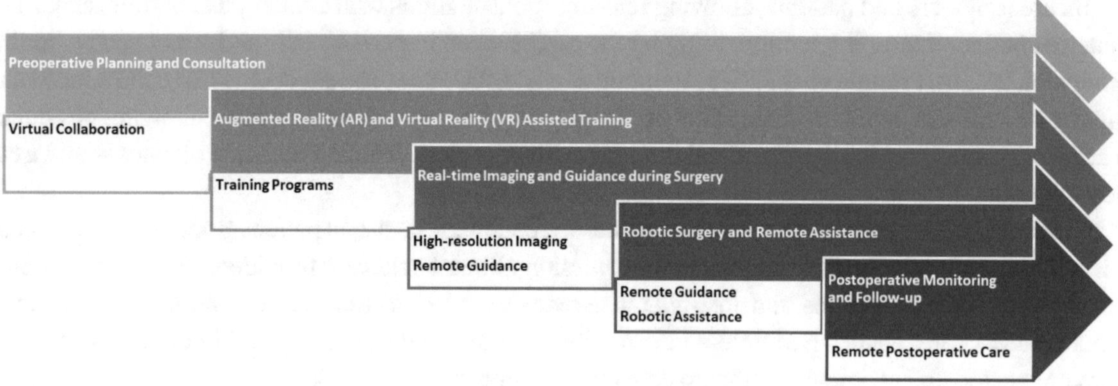

Step 3: Real-time Imaging and Guidance during Surgery

- **High-resolution Imaging:** During surgery, 5G enables real-time transmission of high-resolution imaging, such as MRI or CT scans, allowing surgeons to access detailed anatomical information instantly.
- **Remote Guidance:** Surgeons in different locations can collaborate in real-time using 5G for guidance during complex procedures. This facilitates mentoring or consultations during surgeries, potentially improving outcomes.

Step 4: Robotic Surgery and Remote Assistance

- **Robotic Assistance:** 5G enhances robotic surgical systems by reducing latency and providing real-time control and feedback. Surgeons can perform precise procedures remotely using robotic arms, aided by the high-speed and low-latency characteristics of 5G networks(Hema et al., 2023; Maheswari et al., 2023; Mohanty et al., 2023; Sundaramoorthy et al., 2023).

- **Remote Assistance:** In critical situations, expert surgeons can remotely assist or take control of robotic surgical systems via 5G networks, providing immediate support during intricate surgeries, irrespective of geographical distances(Pramila et al., 2023).

Step 5: Postoperative Monitoring and Follow-up

- **Remote Postoperative Care:** After surgery, 5G enables continuous monitoring of patients' recovery through wearable devices. Healthcare providers can remotely track vital signs, ensuring postoperative care and early detection of complications.

LEVERAGING MACHINE LEARNING IN TELEHEALTH

Machine learning (ML) is revolutionizing telehealth by processing vast patient data, providing predictive analytics and personalized insights. This enables healthcare providers to offer proactive interventions, optimize treatment plans, and tailor healthcare strategies to individual patient needs. By analyzing historical patient data and patterns, ML algorithms enable intelligent and personalized recommendations, enhancing the quality of remote healthcare services and transforming the healthcare landscape(Ingle et al., 2023; Maheswari et al., 2023; Ramudu et al., 2023; Syamala et al., 2023).

ML is crucial in bridging the gap between in-person consultations and virtual care by improving diagnostics and decision-making. Telehealth systems use ML algorithms to analyze medical images remotely, detect anomalies, and aid in rapid diagnoses. This enhances the efficiency of telehealth consultations, ensuring timely assessments regardless of patients' physical location. ML algorithms also foster proactive and preventive healthcare by continuously analyzing patient-generated data from wearables or remote monitoring devices. This early warning system allows healthcare providers to intervene preemptively, preventing adverse events and improving patient outcomes while minimizing in-person visits (Boopathi & Kanike, 2023; Maheswari et al., 2023; Zekrifa et al., 2023).

Machine learning (ML) has the potential to revolutionize telehealth, but challenges remain such as data privacy, algorithm biases, and interpretability. Ensuring ethical use is crucial to maintain patient trust and address data security concerns. The integration of ML requires ongoing validation and collaboration with healthcare professionals. Despite these challenges, ML can transform remote healthcare delivery by providing predictive insights, refining diagnostics, and enabling proactive care. However, stakeholders must navigate ethical considerations to deliver optimal virtual care experiences.

Predictive Analytics in Healthcare

Predictive analytics in healthcare uses data, statistical algorithms, and machine learning to predict future health outcomes and trends. This proactive approach helps healthcare professionals make informed decisions, identify potential health risks, and tailor personalized interventions for patients. By analyzing patient data, such as medical records, laboratory results, genetic information, and lifestyle factors, predictive models identify correlations, trends, and patterns, allowing providers to anticipate potential health issues before they manifest clinically. For example, it can predict the likelihood of a patient developing chronic conditions like diabetes or heart disease (Ramudu et al., 2023; Reddy, Reddy, et al., 2023; Ugandar et al., 2023).

Predictive analytics is a tool that helps healthcare practitioners identify health risks early, enabling early intervention and personalized interventions to prevent disease progression. It optimizes resource allocation by identifying populations at higher risk, allowing targeted interventions and improving healthcare efficiency. Predictive analytics also improves patient outcomes by enabling personalized treatment plans based on individual patient data, including genetics, demographics, and treatment response. This approach optimizes patient care, minimizes adverse effects, and enhances treatment efficacy (Boopathi, 2023b; Satav, Hasan, et al., 2024).

Predictive analytics in healthcare holds promise but faces challenges like data quality, privacy concerns, and interpretability. To effectively integrate predictive insights into clinical decision-making, ongoing education and collaboration between data scientists and healthcare providers are necessary. Despite these challenges, predictive analytics empowers providers to anticipate health risks, personalize interventions, and optimize patient outcomes. As technology advances and data utilization refines, the potential for predictive analytics to revolutionize healthcare delivery continues to grow (Kavitha et al., 2023; Pramila et al., 2023; Ugandar et al., 2023; Venkateswaran et al., 2023).

Figure 2. Personalized medicine and treatment plans

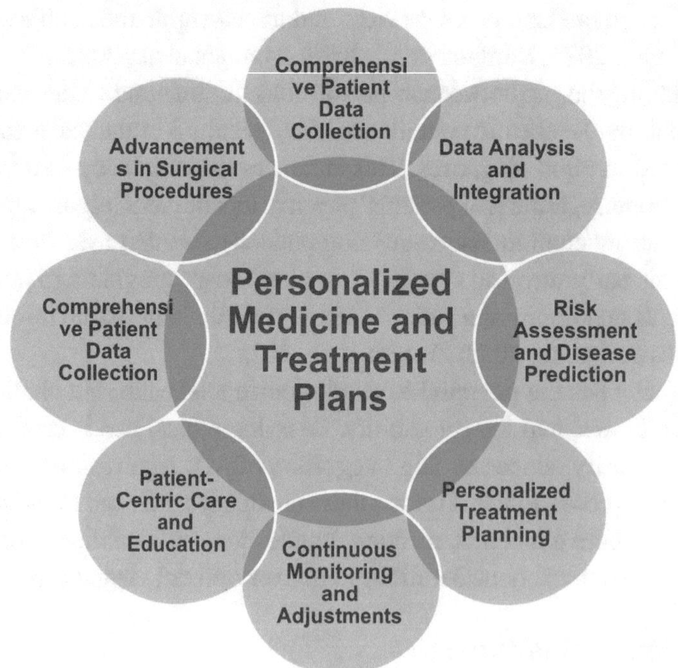

Personalized Medicine and Treatment Plans

Figure 2 illustrates personalized medicine and treatment plans and discussed below.

Step 1: Comprehensive Patient Data Collection

- **Gathering Medical History:** Healthcare providers collect detailed patient medical histories, including genetic information, past illnesses, family medical history, lifestyle factors, and treatment responses(Boopathi, 2023b, 2023c; Karthik et al., 2023).
- **Utilizing Advanced Diagnostics:** Employing advanced diagnostic tools such as genetic testing, biomarker analysis, and imaging techniques to gather comprehensive patient-specific data.

Step 2: Data Analysis and Integration

- **Machine Learning Algorithms:** Leveraging machine learning and predictive analytics to analyze vast datasets and identify patterns and correlations within the collected patient data.
- **Integration of Multi-Omics Data:** Integrating multi-omics data (genomics, proteomics, metabolomics) to gain a holistic understanding of the patient's biological makeup.

Step 3: Risk Assessment and Disease Prediction

- **Risk Stratification:** Using predictive models to assess individual patient risk factors for certain diseases or adverse health outcomes based on the analyzed data.
- **Early Disease Prediction:** Predicting the likelihood of developing specific diseases or conditions based on the patient's genetic predisposition and lifestyle factors.

Step 4: Personalized Treatment Planning

- **Tailoring Treatment Strategies:** Designing treatment plans that are unique to each patient, considering their genetic makeup, disease risks, and individual responses to therapies.
- **Precision Drug Selection:** Selecting medications based on genetic markers, predicting treatment response, and minimizing adverse effects.
- **Lifestyle Recommendations:** Providing personalized lifestyle modifications, including diet and exercise plans, to complement medical interventions.

Step 5: Continuous Monitoring and Adjustments

- **Remote Monitoring Technologies:** Utilizing wearable devices and remote monitoring tools to continuously track patient health metrics and treatment responses.
- **Feedback Loop:** Implementing a continuous feedback loop where treatment efficacy and patient response are assessed, allowing for adjustments to the treatment plan as necessary.

Step 6: Patient-Centric Care and Education

- **Patient Engagement:** Engaging patients in their care by educating them about their personalized treatment plans and involving them in decision-making processes.
- **Empowering Self-Management:** Providing resources and support for patients to actively participate in managing their health through personalized strategies.

AI-ASSISTED DECISION MAKING IN CLINICAL SETTINGS

Enhancing Clinical Decision Making With AI

The Figure 3 highlights the potential of AI in improving clinical decision making.

- **Data Analysis and Pattern Recognition:** AI algorithms process vast amounts of patient data, including medical records, diagnostic images, laboratory results, and real-time monitoring data. These algorithms excel in recognizing patterns and correlations within this data, aiding in more accurate diagnoses and treatment planning(Boopathi & Kanike, 2023; Dhanya et al., 2023; Ravisankar et al., 2023; Ugandar et al., 2023).

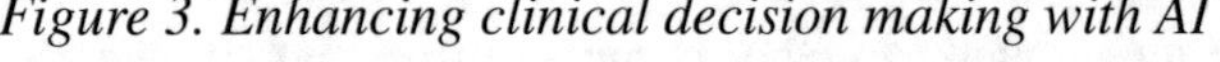

Figure 3. Enhancing clinical decision making with AI

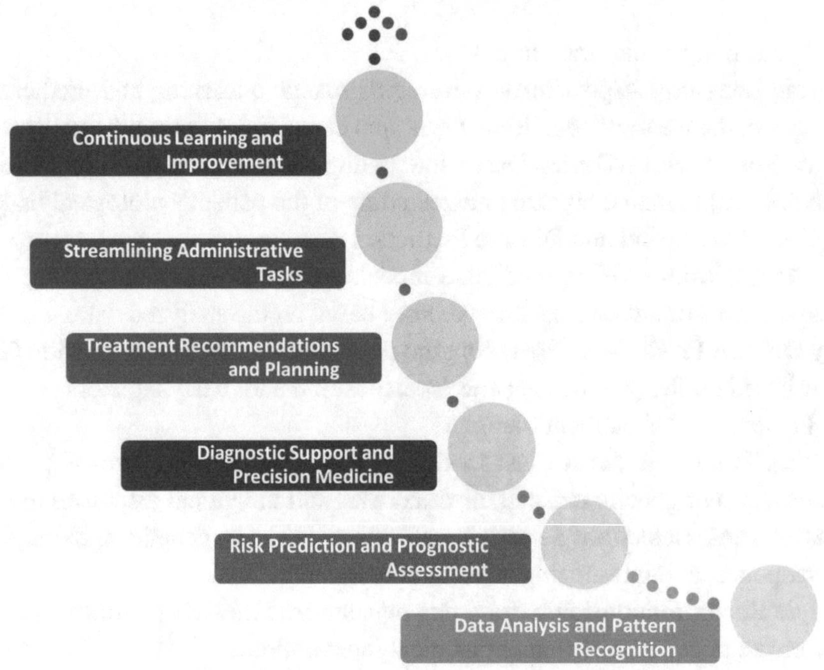

- **Diagnostic Support and Precision Medicine:** In diagnostic settings, AI algorithms assist clinicians by analyzing medical images (such as X-rays, MRIs, CT scans) to detect abnormalities or subtle patterns that might escape human observation. Moreover, AI enables precision medicine by analyzing genetic and molecular data to tailor treatments based on individual patient characteristics.
- **Risk Prediction and Prognostic Assessment:** AI models predict patient outcomes and assess risks by analyzing historical data and patient-specific variables. These models assist in predicting disease progression, identifying individuals at higher risk for certain conditions, and recommending personalized interventions for better health management(Boopathi, Khare, et al., 2023; Reddy, Gaurav, et al., 2023; Sengeni et al., 2023).
- **Treatment Recommendations and Planning:** AI-powered decision support systems provide treatment recommendations by synthesizing patient data and medical knowledge. These systems offer insights into optimal treatment options, dosage adjustments, and potential adverse effects, aiding clinicians in selecting the most effective and personalized treatment plans.
- **Streamlining Administrative Tasks:** AI streamlines administrative tasks by automating documentation, scheduling, and coding processes. Natural language processing (NLP) algorithms help convert voice or text inputs into structured data, reducing the administrative burden on healthcare professionals.

- **Continuous Learning and Improvement:** One of AI's strengths is its ability to continuously learn from new data inputs and adjust its algorithms. This iterative learning process enables AI systems to evolve and improve their accuracy over time, staying updated with the latest medical knowledge and best practices.

Despite its potential benefits, AI-assisted decision-making raises ethical considerations such as transparency, accountability, and biases within algorithms. Human oversight remains crucial to ensure that AI recommendations align with patient needs, clinical judgment, and ethical guidelines, fostering a collaborative approach between AI systems and healthcare professionals.

SOCIAL MEDIA'S ROLE IN PROFESSIONAL HEALTHCARE NETWORKING

Professional Networking and Collaboration

- **Knowledge Sharing and Information Dissemination:** Social media platforms serve as dynamic spaces where healthcare professionals share insights, research findings, and best practices within their specialized fields. Discussions on platforms like Twitter, LinkedIn groups, or specialized forums facilitate the exchange of information, keeping professionals updated with the latest advancements in healthcare(Schillinger et al., 2020; Stellefson et al., 2020).
- **Collaboration and Networking Opportunities:** Healthcare professionals use social media to connect with colleagues, experts, and peers globally, transcending geographical boundaries. This interconnectedness fosters collaboration on research projects, facilitates mentorship, and creates avenues for seeking advice or second opinions on challenging cases.
- **Professional Development and Continuous Learning:** Social media platforms host diverse content formats, including webinars, podcasts, and educational resources, enabling healthcare professionals to access continuing medical education (CME) opportunities conveniently. These platforms offer a wealth of information and facilitate discussions on emerging trends, enhancing ongoing professional development.
- **Patient Education and Engagement:** Healthcare professionals utilize social media to educate patients, debunk myths, and provide accurate medical information. By engaging with patients through credible sources, professionals empower individuals to make informed healthcare decisions and foster better doctor-patient relationships(Boopathi, 2023a; Durairaj et al., 2023; Sharma et al., 2024).
- **Advocacy and Influencing Policy:** Social media allows healthcare professionals to advocate for public health issues, raise awareness about healthcare disparities, and influence policy discussions. Amplifying their voices on these platforms, professionals contribute to shaping healthcare policies and addressing societal health challenges.

Utilizing Social Platforms for Medical Collaboration

The figure 4 illustrates the use of social platforms for medical collaboration and explained here.

- **Virtual Communities and Professional Groups:** Social platforms like LinkedIn, professional forums, and specialty-specific groups on platforms such as Facebook or Reddit provide spaces for healthcare professionals to join communities focused on their specialties. These communities enable discussions, sharing of insights, and seeking advice on complex cases, fostering collaboration among peers (Hussain, 2020; Tsao et al., 2021).
- **Global Networking and Expertise Sharing:** Healthcare professionals use social platforms to connect with colleagues worldwide, transcending geographical barriers. This global networking opens avenues for sharing expertise, seeking second opinions, and collaborating on research projects or international initiatives.
- **Real-Time Communication and Collaboration:** Social platforms offer instant messaging, video conferencing, and collaborative tools that facilitate real-time communication. Healthcare teams can engage in discussions, exchange information, and work collaboratively on patient cases, enhancing interdisciplinary collaboration (Boopathi, 2023b; Kavitha et al., 2023; Maguluri et al., 2023; Sankar et al., 2023).
- **Crowd-Sourcing and Problem Solving:** Platforms like Twitter or specialized medical forums allow professionals to crowd-source information and seek input from a wide range of experts. This collaborative problem-solving approach helps in finding innovative solutions to complex medical challenges.
- **Continuing Medical Education (CME) and Knowledge Dissemination:** Healthcare professionals utilize social platforms to access educational resources, webinars, and research updates. These platforms offer a space for sharing new discoveries, guidelines, and advancements in various medical fields, contributing to continuous learning and professional development.
- **Facilitating Research and Clinical Trials:** Social platforms serve as conduits for recruiting participants, sharing study findings, and promoting awareness about ongoing clinical trials or research projects. Collaborative efforts through these platforms accelerate the pace of research and dissemination of findings.

Figure 4. Utilizing social platforms for medical collaboration

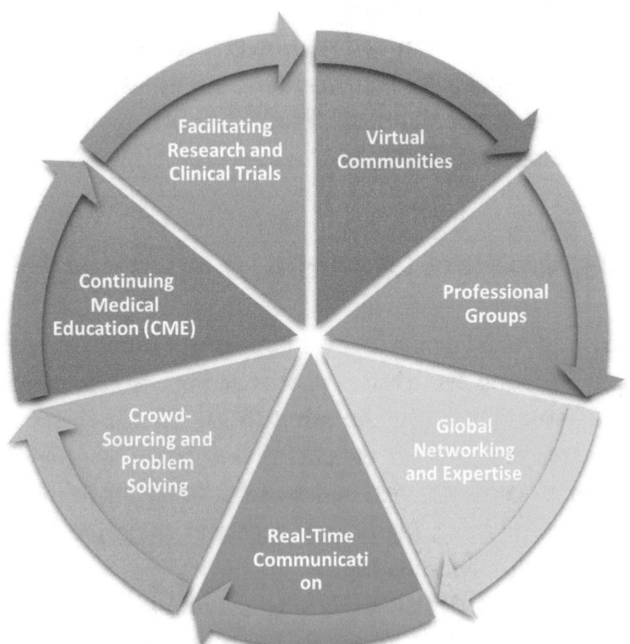

Patient Education and Engagement

- **Sharing Reliable Medical Information:** Healthcare professionals utilize social platforms to share accurate and verified medical information in accessible formats. This includes infographics, articles, or videos explaining medical conditions, treatment options, and preventive measures. By disseminating reliable information, professionals empower patients to make informed decisions about their health(Stellefson et al., 2020).
- **Fostering Health Literacy:** Social platforms serve as educational hubs where healthcare professionals promote health literacy by explaining complex medical concepts in easy-to-understand language. Professionals clarify misconceptions, answer common questions, and engage in Q&A sessions, enabling patients to better understand their health concerns(Mheidly & Fares, 2020).
- **Advocating Preventive Care and Wellness:** Through social platforms, healthcare professionals advocate for preventive care strategies and wellness initiatives. They offer guidance on healthy lifestyles, diet, exercise, and mental health, encouraging patients to adopt proactive measures for overall well-being.
- **Engaging in Patient-Centric Discussions:** Professionals facilitate patient-centric discussions on social platforms, encouraging patients to actively participate in healthcare decisions. These discussions involve patient testimonials, sharing experiences, and addressing concerns, fostering a supportive community environment.
- **Empowering Self-Management and Support:** Healthcare professionals use social platforms to provide resources, tools, and self-management tips for patients managing chronic conditions.

They create support networks where patients can share experiences, seek advice, and offer mutual support, promoting self-care and resilience.

- **Enhancing Doctor-Patient Communication:** Social platforms can improve doctor-patient communication by serving as channels for patients to ask questions, clarify doubts, or seek additional information outside scheduled appointments. Professionals respond to patient queries, fostering a more connected and informed relationship.

INTEGRATION OF 5G, MACHINE LEARNING, AND SOCIAL MEDIA

The integration of 5G, ML, and social media is revolutionizing various industries like healthcare, communication, and technology, offering significant benefits and needs(Hameed et al., 2021).

Enhanced Connectivity and Data Transmission (5G): 5G's high-speed, low-latency networks provide faster and reliable data transmission, enhancing healthcare by providing quick access to large medical files, real-time remote consultations, and seamless diagnostic data sharing. This improved connectivity facilitates machine learning algorithms' access to extensive datasets, enhances predictive analytics, and enables real-time decision-making.

Advanced Data Processing and Decision-Making (Machine Learning): The integration of 5G technology in machine learning algorithms allows for quick access to large datasets, enhancing the accuracy and efficiency of these models. This real-time data from 5G networks enables swift analysis and processing, thereby enabling predictive analytics in healthcare, aiding in diagnostics, treatment planning, and personalized medicine (MacEachern & Forkert, 2021; Varoquaux & Cheplygina, 2022).

Amplified Reach and Communication (social media): Social media platforms are vital for information dissemination, reaching a wide audience. Integrating them with 5G and ML creates a collaborative ecosystem for knowledge sharing. This benefits healthcare professionals by facilitating real-time discussions, expert collaborations, and sharing medical information with patients seeking reliable healthcare (Agrawal et al., 2024; Rahamathunnisa et al., 2023; Satav, Lamani, et al., 2024).

Personalized and Responsive Healthcare Solutions: The integration of 5G-powered machine learning algorithms and social media can provide personalized healthcare solutions, enabling patients to receive real-time medical advice and tailored treatments. This integration empowers individuals to make informed health choices, enhancing patient engagement and education.

Synergy between Telemedicine and AI/ML

- **Intersection:** Telemedicine integrated with AI/ML algorithms enables remote diagnostics, personalized treatment plans, and predictive healthcare analytics.
- **Impact:** This intersection allows for real-time consultations, accurate diagnostics through image analysis, and personalized care recommendations, improving access to healthcare and optimizing treatment outcomes.

Integration of Wearable Tech and Data Analytics

- **Intersection:** Wearable devices connected to data analytics platforms collect continuous health data.
- **Impact:** The integration allows for remote patient monitoring, early detection of health issues, and proactive interventions, enhancing preventive care and chronic disease management.

Convergence of 5G, IoT, and Remote Surgery

- **Intersection:** 5G's high-speed connectivity enables IoT devices to facilitate remote surgeries with minimal latency.
- **Impact:** Surgeons can perform intricate procedures remotely using robotic tools, guided by real-time imaging and haptic feedback, expanding access to specialized care worldwide.

Social Media Engagement and Patient Education

- **Intersection:** Social media platforms serve as avenues for patient education and engagement.
- **Impact:** Healthcare professionals leverage social media for patient education, creating interactive content, fostering support communities, and disseminating credible health information, promoting health literacy and patient empowerment.

Blockchain in Health Data Security and Interoperability

- **Intersection:** Blockchain technology ensures secure and interoperable health data exchange.
- **Impact:** It enhances data security, enables secure sharing of patient records across healthcare systems, and facilitates accurate, real-time access to patient information, fostering continuity of care(P. R. Kumar et al., 2023; Sundaramoorthy et al., 2023).

AI in Drug Discovery and Precision Medicine

- **Intersection:** AI accelerates drug discovery processes and facilitates personalized medicine.
- **Impact:** AI-driven drug development streamlines research, identifies potential drug candidates, and tailors treatments based on individual patient characteristics, leading to more effective and targeted therapies(Rebecca et al., 2023).

Virtual Reality (VR) and Mental Health Interventions

- **Intersection:** VR technology offers immersive experiences for mental health interventions and therapy.

- **Impact:** VR-based therapy aids in managing anxiety disorders, phobias, and PTSD, providing immersive exposure therapy and improving mental health treatment outcomes.

FUTURE TRENDS AND POSSIBILITIES

Artificial Intelligence (AI) and Machine Learning (ML) Integration

- **Predictive Analytics:** AI-driven predictive analytics will continue to evolve, enabling early disease detection, personalized treatment plans, and precision medicine.
- **Clinical Decision Support:** AI-powered decision support systems will assist healthcare professionals in making more informed and accurate clinical decisions, improving patient outcomes.

Telemedicine and Remote Healthcare

- **Expanded Reach:** Telemedicine will become more ubiquitous, extending access to healthcare in remote areas and improving patient-provider connectivity.
- **Remote Monitoring:** Wearable devices and IoT will enable seamless remote patient monitoring, facilitating proactive healthcare management (Kumar B et al., 2024).

Personalized Medicine and Genomics

- **Genomic Medicine:** Advances in genomics and precision medicine will drive tailored treatments based on an individual's genetic makeup and molecular characteristics.
- **Targeted Therapies:** Targeted therapies and gene editing technologies will revolutionize treatment approaches, providing more effective and personalized interventions.

5G-Powered Healthcare Solutions

- **Enhanced Connectivity:** Widespread adoption of 5G will enable faster data transfer, supporting real-time diagnostics, remote surgeries, and IoT applications in healthcare.
- **Edge Computing:** Edge computing facilitated by 5G will optimize data processing and analysis, enhancing the efficiency of healthcare systems.

Virtual and Augmented Reality in Healthcare

- **VR/AR-based Therapies:** VR/AR applications will expand in healthcare, aiding in patient rehabilitation, medical education, and mental health treatments.

- **Surgical Training and Simulation:** VR/AR technologies will provide immersive training for surgeons, allowing simulated practice for complex procedures (Boopathi, Pandey, et al., 2023; Nishanth et al., 2023; Rahamathunnisa et al., 2023; Sampath et al., 2022).

Patient-Centric Technologies and Engagement

- **Health Apps and Wearables:** Patient-focused mobile health apps and wearable devices will empower individuals to take proactive roles in managing their health.
- **Remote Consultations:** Virtual care platforms will offer seamless remote consultations, improving patient engagement and healthcare accessibility.

***Blockchain for Data Security and Interoperability*:** Blockchain technology will facilitate secure and interoperable health data sharing across healthcare systems, ensuring privacy and data integrity.

CHALLENGES AND FUTURE DIRECTIONS

Addressing Adoption Barriers

- **Interoperability Issues:** Integration and compatibility between different healthcare systems pose challenges in sharing and accessing patient data seamlessly.
- **Resistance to Change:** Healthcare professionals may face resistance in adopting new technologies due to workflow disruptions and learning curves.
- **Financial Constraints:** Cost implications and investment requirements for implementing new technologies hinder widespread adoption, particularly in resource-limited settings.

Ethical and Legal Concerns

- **Data Privacy and Security:** Safeguarding patient data from breaches and ensuring data privacy remain critical concerns in healthcare technology adoption.
- **Algorithm Bias and Transparency:** Ethical considerations surround algorithmic biases and the transparency of AI/ML decision-making in healthcare.
- **Regulatory Compliance:** Navigating complex regulatory frameworks and ensuring compliance with evolving healthcare laws and standards poses challenges.

Predictions for the Future of Healthcare Technology

- **AI-Powered Personalization:** AI-driven healthcare solutions will become increasingly personalized, tailoring treatments and interventions to individual patient characteristics.

- **Rise of Remote Healthcare:** Telemedicine and remote monitoring will become integral components of healthcare delivery, enhancing access and continuity of care.
- **Advancements in Genomic Medicine:** Genomics will play a more prominent role in healthcare, guiding precision medicine and targeted therapies.
- **Expanding Role of Wearable Devices:** Wearable technology will continue to evolve, enabling continuous health monitoring and proactive health management.
- **Blockchain for Data Security:** Blockchain technology will gain traction for secure health data exchange, enhancing interoperability and data integrity.
- **Integration of Virtual/Augmented Reality:** VR/AR applications will further integrate into healthcare, transforming medical education, therapy, and surgical simulations.

Future Directions

- **Enhancing Interoperability:** Addressing interoperability challenges through standardized protocols to enable seamless data exchange between healthcare systems.
- **Ethics-Centric AI:** Developing ethical frameworks and governance models to ensure responsible AI use and transparency in decision-making processes.
- **Affordable Access:** Innovations focusing on cost-effective solutions to make advanced healthcare technologies more accessible and affordable.
- **Collaboration and Education:** Encouraging collaboration between tech developers, healthcare providers, and regulators while prioritizing ongoing education and training for healthcare professionals.

IMPLEMENTATION STRATEGIES

Figure 5 illustrates the strategies for implementing social media through 5G/ML and elaborated below.

Telemedicine and 5G Integration

- **Real-time Consultations:** Healthcare providers leverage 5G's high-speed connectivity for seamless, high-definition video consultations. For instance, remote diagnosis and monitoring of chronic conditions like diabetes or heart disease are conducted in real time, improving patient care(Devi et al., 2023; Lin & Hsu, 2021).
- **Remote Surgical Assistance:** Surgeons perform or guide surgeries in remote locations using robotic systems powered by 5G's low latency. Experts from distant locations provide real-time guidance, enhancing surgical precision and expanding access to specialized care.

Figure 5. 5G/ML/social media implementation strategies

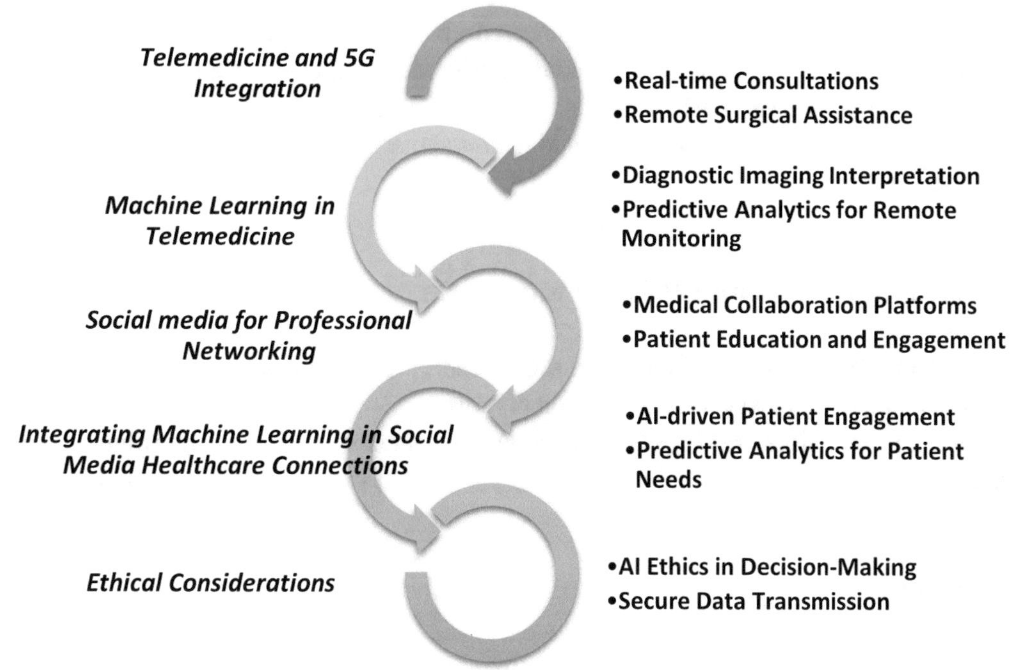

Machine Learning in Telemedicine

- **Diagnostic Imaging Interpretation:** ML algorithms analyze medical images like X-rays or MRIs, aiding in swift and accurate diagnostics. For instance, detecting anomalies or early signs of diseases using AI-based image recognition enhances diagnostic accuracy(Salman et al., 2021; Varoquaux & Cheplygina, 2022).
- **Predictive Analytics for Remote Monitoring:** ML algorithms predict health trends using patient data from wearables. This allows for proactive interventions in chronic disease management, reducing hospital admissions.

Social media for Professional Networking

- **Medical Collaboration Platforms:** Healthcare professionals engage in discussions, share expertise, and seek advice on platforms like Twitter, LinkedIn groups, or specialized forums. This enables global networking, interdisciplinary collaboration, and knowledge sharing (Schillinger et al., 2020; Stellefson et al., 2020).
- **Patient Education and Engagement:** Professionals utilize social media to disseminate medical information, conduct health-related discussions, and build communities. For instance, hosting live sessions on Facebook or Instagram educates patients on managing specific health conditions.

Integrating Machine Learning in Social Media Healthcare Connections

- **AI-Driven Patient Engagement:** ML-powered chatbots on social platforms provide accurate health information, offer basic medical advice, or guide patients to appropriate resources.
- **Predictive Analytics for Patient Needs:** Analyzing social media data using ML helps identify healthcare trends, allowing professionals to address emerging health concerns or disseminate targeted health campaigns.

Ethical Considerations and Privacy Measures

- **Secure Data Transmission:** Implementation of encryption protocols ensures secure transmission of patient data over 5G networks and social platforms.
- **AI Ethics in Decision-Making:** Healthcare professionals validate ML algorithms to ensure unbiased, ethical decision-making in diagnostics and patient interactions on social media platforms.

CONCLUSION

The vision of a new healthcare era is a transformative shift driven by technological innovation, patient-centricity, and commitment to advancing medical care, with key themes shaping its trajectory.

- The fusion of 5G, artificial intelligence, machine learning, and other cutting-edge technologies lays the foundation for a healthcare revolution. These innovations enable real-time data analysis, personalized treatments, and remote healthcare access, redefining the possibilities for patient care.
- Central to this transformation is the elevation of patient empowerment. Accessible health information, remote consultations, and wearable tech empower individuals to take an active role in their health management, fostering a proactive approach to wellness.
- As technology accelerates healthcare progress, ethical considerations and regulatory frameworks become paramount. Ensuring patient privacy, addressing algorithm biases, and establishing robust ethical guidelines are crucial for responsible technology adoption.
- The future of healthcare hinges on collaboration—between tech developers, healthcare providers, policymakers, and patients. Continuous education and training equip healthcare professionals to navigate evolving technologies effectively.
- Advancements in healthcare technology must prioritize inclusivity, ensuring that innovations are accessible to diverse populations and across various socio-economic landscapes.

The future of healthcare is one where it goes beyond boundaries, providing personalized, accessible, and ethical care to all. This is a world where technology enhances human capabilities, patient empowerment is prioritized, and collaborative innovation fosters a healthier, more connected world. A commitment to ethics, education, and inclusivity will drive this transformation towards a fundamental right for all.

REFERENCES

Afifah, K., Yulita, I. N., & Sarathan, I. (2021). Sentiment Analysis on Telemedicine App Reviews using XGBoost Classifier. *2021 International Conference on Artificial Intelligence and Big Data Analytics*, 22–27.

Agrawal, A. V., Shashibhushan, G., Pradeep, S., Padhi, S. N., Sugumar, D., & Boopathi, S. (2024). Synergizing Artificial Intelligence, 5G, and Cloud Computing for Efficient Energy Conversion Using Agricultural Waste. In B. K. Mishra (Ed.), Practice, Progress, and Proficiency in Sustainability. IGI Global. doi:10.4018/979-8-3693-1186-8.ch026

Berlet, M., Vogel, T., Gharba, M., Eichinger, J., Schulz, E., Friess, H., Wilhelm, D., Ostler, D., & Kranzfelder, M. (2022). Emergency telemedicine mobile ultrasounds using a 5G-enabled application: Development and usability study. *JMIR Formative Research*, *6*(5), e36824. doi:10.2196/36824 PMID:35617009

Bhattacharya, S. (2023). The impact of 5g technologies on healthcare. *Indian Journal of Surgery*, *85*(3), 531–535. doi:10.1007/s12262-022-03514-0

Boopathi, S. (2023a). Deep Learning Techniques Applied for Automatic Sentence Generation. In K. Becerra-Murillo & J. F. Gámez (Eds.), Advances in Educational Technologies and Instructional Design. IGI Global. doi:10.4018/978-1-6684-3632-5.ch016

Boopathi, S. (2023b). Internet of Things-Integrated Remote Patient Monitoring System: Healthcare Application. In A. Suresh Kumar, U. Kose, S. Sharma, & S. Jerald Nirmal Kumar (Eds.), Advances in Healthcare Information Systems and Administration. IGI Global. doi:10.4018/978-1-6684-6894-4.ch008

Boopathi, S. (2023c). Securing Healthcare Systems Integrated With IoT: Fundamentals, Applications, and Future Trends. In A. Suresh Kumar, U. Kose, S. Sharma, & S. Jerald Nirmal Kumar (Eds.), Advances in Healthcare Information Systems and Administration. IGI Global. doi:10.4018/978-1-6684-6894-4.ch010

Boopathi, S., & Kanike, U. K. (2023). Applications of Artificial Intelligent and Machine Learning Techniques in Image Processing. In B. K. Pandey, D. Pandey, R. Anand, D. S. Mane, & V. K. Nassa (Eds.), Advances in Computational Intelligence and Robotics. IGI Global. doi:10.4018/978-1-6684-8618-4.ch010

Boopathi, S., Khare, R., Jaya Christiyan, K. G., Muni, T. V., & Khare, S. (2023). Additive Manufacturing Developments in the Medical Engineering Field. In R. Keshavamurthy, V. Tambrallimath, & J. P. Davim (Eds.), Advances in Chemical and Materials Engineering. IGI Global. doi:10.4018/978-1-6684-6009-2.ch006

Boopathi, S., Pandey, B. K., & Pandey, D. (2023). Advances in Artificial Intelligence for Image Processing: Techniques, Applications, and Optimization. In B. K. Pandey, D. Pandey, R. Anand, D. S. Mane, & V. K. Nassa (Eds.), Advances in Computational Intelligence and Robotics. IGI Global. doi:10.4018/978-1-6684-8618-4.ch006

Devi, D. H., Duraisamy, K., Armghan, A., Alsharari, M., Aliqab, K., Sorathiya, V., Das, S., & Rashid, N. (2023). 5g technology in healthcare and wearable devices: A review. *Sensors (Basel)*, *23*(5), 2519. doi:10.3390/s23052519 PMID:36904721

Dhanya, D., Kumar, S. S., Thilagavathy, A., Prasad, D. V. S. S. S. V., & Boopathi, S. (2023). Data Analytics and Artificial Intelligence in the Circular Economy: Case Studies. In B. K. Mishra (Ed.), Advances in Civil and Industrial Engineering. IGI Global. doi:10.4018/979-8-3693-0044-2.ch003

Durairaj, M., Jayakumar, S. M., Karpagavalli, V. S., Maheswari, B. U., & Boopathi, S. (2023). Utilization of Digital Tools in the Indian Higher Education System During Health Crises. In C. S. V. Negrão, I. G. P. Maia, & J. A. F. Brito (Eds.), Advances in Logistics, Operations, and Management Science (pp. 1–21). IGI Global. doi:10.4018/978-1-7998-9213-7.ch001

Hameed, K., Bajwa, I. S., Sarwar, N., Anwar, W., Mushtaq, Z., & Rashid, T. (2021). Integration of 5G and block-chain technologies in smart telemedicine using IoT. *Journal of Healthcare Engineering*, *2021*, 1–18. doi:10.1155/2021/8814364 PMID:33824715

Hema, N., Krishnamoorthy, N., Chavan, S. M., Kumar, N. M. G., Sabarimuthu, M., & Boopathi, S. (2023). A Study on an Internet of Things (IoT)-Enabled Smart Solar Grid System. In P. Swarnalatha & S. Prabu (Eds.), Advances in Computational Intelligence and Robotics. IGI Global. doi:10.4018/978-1-6684-8098-4.ch017

Hussain, W. (2020). Role of social media in COVID-19 pandemic. *The International Journal of Frontier Sciences*, *4*(2), 59–60. doi:10.37978/tijfs.v4i2.144

Ingle, R. B., Swathi, S., Mahendran, G., Senthil, T. S., Muralidharan, N., & Boopathi, S. (2023). Sustainability and Optimization of Green and Lean Manufacturing Processes Using Machine Learning Techniques. In N. Cobîrzan, R. Muntean, & R.-A. Felseghi (Eds.), Advances in Finance, Accounting, and Economics. IGI Global. doi:10.4018/978-1-6684-8238-4.ch012

Karthik, S. A., Hemalatha, R., Aruna, R., Deivakani, M., Reddy, R. V. K., & Boopathi, S. (2023). Study on Healthcare Security System-Integrated Internet of Things (IoT). In M. K. Habib (Ed.), Advances in Systems Analysis, Software Engineering, and High Performance Computing. IGI Global. doi:10.4018/978-1-6684-7684-0.ch013

Kavitha, C. R., Varalatchoumy, M., Mithuna, H. R., Bharathi, K., Geethalakshmi, N. M., & Boopathi, S. (2023). Energy Monitoring and Control in the Smart Grid: Integrated Intelligent IoT and ANFIS. In M. Arshad (Ed.), Advances in Bioinformatics and Biomedical Engineering. IGI Global. doi:10.4018/978-1-6684-6577-6.ch014

Kumar, B. M., Kumar, K. K., Sasikala, P., Sampath, B., Gopi, B., & Sundaram, S. (2024). Sustainable Green Energy Generation From Waste Water: IoT and ML Integration. In B. K. Mishra (Ed.), Practice, Progress, and Proficiency in Sustainability. IGI Global. doi:10.4018/979-8-3693-1186-8.ch024

Kumar, P. R., Meenakshi, S., Shalini, S., Devi, S. R., & Boopathi, S. (2023). Soil Quality Prediction in Context Learning Approaches Using Deep Learning and Blockchain for Smart Agriculture. In R. Kumar, A. B. Abdul Hamid, & N. I. Binti Ya'akub (Eds.), Advances in Computational Intelligence and Robotics. IGI Global. doi:10.4018/978-1-6684-9151-5.ch001

Kumela, A. G., Gemta, A. B., Hordofa, A. K., Dagnaw, H., Sheferedin, U., & Tadesse, M. (2023). Quantum machine learning assisted lung cancer telemedicine. *AIP Advances*, *13*(7), 075301. doi:10.1063/5.0153566

Lin, T.-W., & Hsu, C.-L. (2021). FAIDM for medical privacy protection in 5G telemedicine systems. *Applied Sciences (Basel, Switzerland)*, *11*(3), 1155. doi:10.3390/app11031155

MacEachern, S. J., & Forkert, N. D. (2021). Machine learning for precision medicine. *Genome*, *64*(4), 416–425. doi:10.1139/gen-2020-0131 PMID:33091314

Maguluri, L. P., Ananth, J., Hariram, S., Geetha, C., Bhaskar, A., & Boopathi, S. (2023). Smart Vehicle-Emissions Monitoring System Using Internet of Things (IoT). In P. Srivastava, D. Ramteke, A. K. Bedyal, M. Gupta, & J. K. Sandhu (Eds.), Practice, Progress, and Proficiency in Sustainability. IGI Global. doi:10.4018/978-1-6684-8117-2.ch014

Maheswari, B. U., Imambi, S. S., Hasan, D., Meenakshi, S., Pratheep, V. G., & Boopathi, S. (2023). Internet of Things and Machine Learning-Integrated Smart Robotics. In M. K. Habib (Ed.), Advances in Computational Intelligence and Robotics. IGI Global. doi:10.4018/978-1-6684-7791-5.ch010

Mheidly, N., & Fares, J. (2020). Leveraging media and health communication strategies to overcome the COVID-19 infodemic. *Journal of Public Health Policy*, *41*(4), 410–420. doi:10.1057/s41271-020-00247-w PMID:32826935

Mohanty, A., Jothi, B., Jeyasudha, J., Ranjit, P. S., Isaac, J. S., & Boopathi, S. (2023). Additive Manufacturing Using Robotic Programming. In S. Kautish, N. K. Chaubey, S. B. Goyal, & P. Whig (Eds.), Advances in Computational Intelligence and Robotics. IGI Global. doi:10.4018/978-1-6684-8171-4.ch010

Muehlematter, U. J., Daniore, P., & Vokinger, K. N. (2021). Approval of artificial intelligence and machine learning-based medical devices in the USA and Europe (2015–20): A comparative analysis. *The Lancet. Digital Health*, *3*(3), e195–e203. doi:10.1016/S2589-7500(20)30292-2 PMID:33478929

Nishanth, J. R., Deshmukh, M. A., Kushwah, R., Kushwaha, K. K., Balaji, S., & Sampath, B. (2023). Particle Swarm Optimization of Hybrid Renewable Energy Systems. In B. K. Mishra (Ed.), Advances in Civil and Industrial Engineering. IGI Global. doi:10.4018/979-8-3693-0044-2.ch016

Pramila, P. V., Amudha, S., Saravanan, T. R., Sankar, S. R., Poongothai, E., & Boopathi, S. (2023). Design and Development of Robots for Medical Assistance: An Architectural Approach. In G. S. Karthick & S. Karupusamy (Eds.), Advances in Healthcare Information Systems and Administration. IGI Global. doi:10.4018/978-1-6684-8913-0.ch011

Rahamathunnisa, U., Sudhakar, K., Murugan, T. K., Thivaharan, S., Rajkumar, M., & Boopathi, S. (2023). Cloud Computing Principles for Optimizing Robot Task Offloading Processes. In S. Kautish, N. K. Chaubey, S. B. Goyal, & P. Whig (Eds.), Advances in Computational Intelligence and Robotics. IGI Global. doi:10.4018/978-1-6684-8171-4.ch007

Rajula, H. S. R., Verlato, G., Manchia, M., Antonucci, N., & Fanos, V. (2020). Comparison of conventional statistical methods with machine learning in medicine: Diagnosis, drug development, and treatment. *Medicina*, *56*(9), 455. doi:10.3390/medicina56090455 PMID:32911665

Ramudu, K., Mohan, V. M., Jyothirmai, D., Prasad, D. V. S. S. S. V., Agrawal, R., & Boopathi, S. (2023). Machine Learning and Artificial Intelligence in Disease Prediction: Applications, Challenges, Limitations, Case Studies, and Future Directions. In G. S. Karthick & S. Karupusamy (Eds.), Advances in Healthcare Information Systems and Administration. IGI Global. doi:10.4018/978-1-6684-8913-0.ch013

Ravisankar, A., Sampath, B., & Asif, M. M. (2023). Economic Studies on Automobile Management: Working Capital and Investment Analysis. In C. S. V. Negrão, I. G. P. Maia, & J. A. F. Brito (Eds.), Advances in Logistics, Operations, and Management Science. IGI Global. doi:10.4018/978-1-7998-9213-7.ch009

Rebecca, B., Kumar, K. P. M., Padmini, S., Srivastava, B. K., Halder, S., & Boopathi, S. (2023). Convergence of Data Science-AI-Green Chemistry-Affordable Medicine: Transforming Drug Discovery. In B. B. Gupta & F. Colace (Eds.), Advances in Computational Intelligence and Robotics. IGI Global. doi:10.4018/978-1-6684-9999-3.ch014

Reddy, M. A., Gaurav, A., Ushasukhanya, S., Rao, V. C. S., Bhattacharya, S., & Boopathi, S. (2023). Bio-Medical Wastes Handling Strategies During the COVID-19 Pandemic. In C. S. V. Negrão, I. G. P. Maia, & J. A. F. Brito (Eds.), Advances in Logistics, Operations, and Management Science. IGI Global. doi:10.4018/978-1-7998-9213-7.ch006

Reddy, M. A., Reddy, B. M., Mukund, C. S., Venneti, K., Preethi, D. M. D., & Boopathi, S. (2023). Social Health Protection During the COVID-Pandemic Using IoT. In F. P. C. Endong (Ed.), Advances in Electronic Government, Digital Divide, and Regional Development. IGI Global. doi:10.4018/978-1-7998-8394-4.ch009

Salman, O. H., Taha, Z., Alsabah, M. Q., Hussein, Y. S., Mohammed, A. S., & Aal-Nouman, M. (2021). A review on utilizing machine learning technology in the fields of electronic emergency triage and patient priority systems in telemedicine: Coherent taxonomy, motivations, open research challenges and recommendations for intelligent future work. *Computer Methods and Programs in Biomedicine*, *209*, 106357. doi:10.1016/j.cmpb.2021.106357 PMID:34438223

Sampath, B. C. S., & Myilsamy, S. (2022). Application of TOPSIS Optimization Technique in the Micro-Machining Process. In M. A. Mellal (Ed.), Advances in Mechatronics and Mechanical Engineering. IGI Global. doi:10.4018/978-1-6684-5887-7.ch009

Sankar, K. M., Booba, B., & Boopathi, S. (2023). Smart Agriculture Irrigation Monitoring System Using Internet of Things. In G. S. Karthick (Ed.), Advances in Environmental Engineering and Green Technologies. IGI Global. doi:10.4018/978-1-6684-7879-0.ch006

Satav, S. D., Hasan, D. S., Pitchai, R., Mohanaprakash, T. A., Sultanuddin, S. J., & Boopathi, S. (2024). Next Generation of Internet of Things (NGIoT) in Healthcare Systems. In B. K. Mishra (Ed.), Practice, Progress, and Proficiency in Sustainability. IGI Global. doi:10.4018/979-8-3693-1186-8.ch017

Satav, S. D., Lamani, D. K. G., H., Kumar, N. M. G., Manikandan, S., & Sampath, B. (2024). Energy and Battery Management in the Era of Cloud Computing: Sustainable Wireless Systems and Networks. In B. K. Mishra (Ed.), Practice, Progress, and Proficiency in Sustainability (pp. 141–166). IGI Global. doi:10.4018/979-8-3693-1186-8.ch009

Schillinger, D., Chittamuru, D., & Ramírez, A. S. (2020). From "infodemics" to health promotion: A novel framework for the role of social media in public health. *American Journal of Public Health*, *110*(9), 1393–1396. doi:10.2105/AJPH.2020.305746 PMID:32552021

Schünke, L. C., Mello, B., da Costa, C. A., Antunes, R. S., Rigo, S. J., de Oliveira Ramos, G., da Rosa Righi, R., Scherer, J. N., & Donida, B. (2022). A rapid review of machine learning approaches for telemedicine in the scope of COVID-19. *Artificial Intelligence in Medicine*, *129*, 102312. doi:10.1016/j.artmed.2022.102312 PMID:35659388

Sengeni, D., Padmapriya, G., Imambi, S. S., Suganthi, D., Suri, A., & Boopathi, S. (2023). Biomedical Waste Handling Method Using Artificial Intelligence Techniques. In P. Srivastava, D. Ramteke, A. K. Bedyal, M. Gupta, & J. K. Sandhu (Eds.), Practice, Progress, and Proficiency in Sustainability. IGI Global. doi:10.4018/978-1-6684-8117-2.ch022

Sharma, D. M., Venkata Ramana, K., Jothilakshmi, R., Verma, R., Uma Maheswari, B., & Boopathi, S. (2024). Integrating Generative AI Into K-12 Curriculums and Pedagogies in India: Opportunities and Challenges. In P. Yu, J. Mulli, Z. A. S. Syed, & L. Umme (Eds.), Advances in Higher Education and Professional Development. IGI Global. doi:10.4018/979-8-3693-0487-7.ch006

Stellefson, M., Paige, S. R., Chaney, B. H., & Chaney, J. D. (2020). Evolving role of social media in health promotion: Updated responsibilities for health education specialists. *International Journal of Environmental Research and Public Health*, *17*(4), 1153. doi:10.3390/ijerph17041153 PMID:32059561

Sundaramoorthy, K., Singh, A., Sumathy, G., Maheshwari, A., Arunarani, A. R., & Boopathi, S. (2023). A Study on AI and Blockchain-Powered Smart Parking Models for Urban Mobility. In B. B. Gupta & F. Colace (Eds.), Advances in Computational Intelligence and Robotics. IGI Global. doi:10.4018/978-1-6684-9999-3.ch010

Syamala, M. C. R., K., Pramila, P. V., Dash, S., Meenakshi, S., & Boopathi, S. (2023). Machine Learning-Integrated IoT-Based Smart Home Energy Management System. In P. Swarnalatha & S. Prabu (Eds.), Advances in Computational Intelligence and Robotics (pp. 219–235). IGI Global. doi:10.4018/978-1-6684-8098-4.ch013

Tsao, S.-F., Chen, H., Tisseverasinghe, T., Yang, Y., Li, L., & Butt, Z. A. (2021). What social media told us in the time of COVID-19: A scoping review. *The Lancet. Digital Health*, *3*(3), e175–e194. doi:10.1016/S2589-7500(20)30315-0 PMID:33518503

Ugandar, R. E., Rahamathunnisa, U., Sajithra, S., Christiana, M. B. V., Palai, B. K., & Boopathi, S. (2023). Hospital Waste Management Using Internet of Things and Deep Learning: Enhanced Efficiency and Sustainability. In M. Arshad (Ed.), Advances in Bioinformatics and Biomedical Engineering. IGI Global. doi:10.4018/978-1-6684-6577-6.ch015

Varoquaux, G., & Cheplygina, V. (2022). Machine learning for medical imaging: Methodological failures and recommendations for the future. *NPJ Digital Medicine*, *5*(1), 48. doi:10.1038/s41746-022-00592-y PMID:35413988

Venkateswaran, N., Kumar, S. S., Diwakar, G., Gnanasangeetha, D., & Boopathi, S. (2023). Synthetic Biology for Waste Water to Energy Conversion: IoT and AI Approaches. In M. Arshad (Ed.), Advances in Bioinformatics and Biomedical Engineering. IGI Global. doi:10.4018/978-1-6684-6577-6.ch017

Washington, P., Leblanc, E., Dunlap, K., Penev, Y., Kline, A., Paskov, K., Sun, M. W., Chrisman, B., Stockham, N., Varma, M., Voss, C., Haber, N., & Wall, D. P. (2020). Precision telemedicine through crowdsourced machine learning: Testing variability of crowd workers for video-based autism feature recognition. *Journal of Personalized Medicine*, *10*(3), 86. doi:10.3390/jpm10030086 PMID:32823538

Yadav, S., Bhole, G. P., & Sharma, A. (2022). Telemedicine using Machine Learning: A Boon. *Emerging Computational Approaches in Telehealth and Telemedicine: A Look at The Post COVID-19 Landscape*, 70.

Zekrifa, D. M. S., Kulkarni, M., Bhagyalakshmi, A., Devireddy, N., Gupta, S., & Boopathi, S. (2023). Integrating Machine Learning and AI for Improved Hydrological Modeling and Water Resource Management. In V. Shikuku (Ed.), Advances in Environmental Engineering and Green Technologies. IGI Global. doi:10.4018/978-1-6684-6791-6.ch003

Zobair, K. M., Sanzogni, L., Houghton, L., & Islam, M. Z. (2021). Forecasting care seekers satisfaction with telemedicine using machine learning and structural equation modeling. *PLoS One*, *16*(9), e0257300. doi:10.1371/journal.pone.0257300 PMID:34559840

Chapter 13
Understanding Digital Health Innovations to Improve the Quality of Services in Healthcare Systems:
A Progressive Outlook

Vijit Chaturvedi
Amity Business School, Amity University, Noida, India

ABSTRACT

The chapter highlights developments in the healthcare industry, opportunities and challenges behind the role of various stakeholders in establishing a well pronged healthcare infrastructure, role of technology in shaping digital healthcare systems, and the shift in digital healthcare innovation from a clinician-centric to a patient-centric approach. The chapter also emphasized measures and strategies to avoid digital inequality, which may happen due to varied external and internal geographic, political, socio economic, technological, and regulatory reasons. Another important aspect that needs attention whenever innovations in digital healthcare is discussed is advancement in digital research. How digitalization in healthcare is transforming prevention to management of health conditions is shown, and the role of digital therapeutics (DTx) is also discussed.

1. INTRODUCTION TO HEALTH CARE INDUSTRY: DEVELOPMENTS AND TRANSITIONS

1.1 Healthcare Industry: Developments

In the present time across the world healthcare system is emphasizing on how to ensure progressive and comprehensive development in healthcare industry. Innovation and development in healthcare has been witnessing leaps and bounds in growth. It is seen right from healthcare financing, role of pharmaceuticals,

DOI: 10.4018/979-8-3693-1934-5.ch013

healthcare institutions, different communities and public, digital healthcare and upskilling of nursing workforce along with development in workforce diversity. Kleinman and Dougherty, 2013.

Unequal development across borders is also largely contributed to health facility, infrastructure, accessibility, affordability, and sustainability of a health ecosystem thus demanding cooperation from all stakeholders, scalability, and sense of accountability on the part of all stakeholders.

It is evident from the history that right from 1854 to 1908 there have been remarkable advancement in the growth of healthcare industry wherein quality improvement initiatives of Nightingale to Barton's contribution of Sanitary commissions to growth in Sterilization way back in 1879 to technological interventions in 1895.This was further accelerated by growth of pharmaceuticals in 1881-1995 and development of healthcare financing till 1945 and quick progression of healthcare financing and role of industry in production of related sources from 1908.

Heath care is amongst the fastest growing sector with vast pace specially after pandemic understanding the relevance and the need of both present and futuristic development. It is seen in number of aspects right from medical institutions, medical tourism, equipment manufacturing, different kinds of services and networks for both internal and external customers. There is a direct and strong relationship between healthcare system and economic growth as 10% increase in life expectancy thus contributing to economic growth. Whether talked at family, state, country, or Universal level holistic health this is one aspect which is fundamental for peace and security for all geographies World health organization defines Innovation in health care as a new and better solution with a transformative ability to augment a better developing oriented health to people. It includes inclusion of effective health care policy, practices, systems, product, process, and program along with technologies to ensure right development. Thus, it is a combination of diffusion, adoption, and invention in healthcare.

It is evident from healthcare information and Management system Society that more than 80 percent of countries have augmented investment in Health care infrastructure, digitally innovative ecosystem by adopting digital healthcare tools in next five years. In Indian Context too the investment in healthcare with digital adoption is $372 Billion and public health spending to increase by 2.5% of country's GDP by 2025.

The history and development in Healthcare has been seen transformative changes since ages, starting from Home remedies wherein home related remedies like different kind of spices vegetables and common items were used to cure entreat different diseases this was a reactionary approach in which people based upon their understanding of medicinal properties of plants just by hit and trial method tried to provide treatment based upon herbalism which is long and will trusted remedy for different ailments. Followed by this was ancient pharmacology which also gained lot of attention based upon different practices which is as old as Mesopotamia who used to call it right kind of medical diagnosis.

During 19th century there had been several technological chemical and processor spaced on biological advances which provided a new route to the physician and development of different process and methodology for treating elements. History speaks about during the beginning of 20th century the foundation of modern healthcare began to evolve wherein anaesthetics use of different kinds of interceptor sceptics in the growth of vaccination to avoid different kind of ailments also picked.

In the history of healthcare evolution there has been a remarkable development which is also known as therapeutic revolution which during 20th century helped in indicating specific diseases the effectiveness of medicine das grew attention during development of vaccinations related to diseases like leprosy tuberculosis plague and malaria which were the most life taking and challenging problems affecting different geographies and gradually these developments gave rise to a complete globalization of medicines.

1.2 Challenges and Intervention During Healthcare Evolution

Across the globe the development of healthcare industry has been different, if been talked about developments in West right from colonial times in 1700's there were few upper-class physicians that emigrated in colonies and played a significant role in development.

Those times the biggest challenges were mortality amongst children and infants as discussed earlier some common problems like malaria, TB, diphtheria, yellow fever was highly fatal. Somewhere during 1735 medical society started getting formed and 1765 was the medical college at Philadelphia been built, the medical department of King's college during 1770 awarded American M.D degree. There have been several challenges right from lack of resources, trained professionals to unknown reasons, poor diagnosis, and lack of medical intervention that during Civil war more than war disease took toll of lives of soldiers. Whether it was measles, mumps, chicken pox, typhoid or other problems, Union army hospitals being the only rescue with available knowledge.

During Industrial revolution, unions and organized healthcare picked attention as the Country leaders also believed that no country could prosper wherein countrymen are sick and poor. With more manufacturing jobs picking up there was also need of ensuring allowance sand social security of different kinds to ensure wellbeing and thus insurance also and ensuring life and dependents of family of workmen was also thought important.

During the great depression moment different health related bills were approved and old age benefits were approved. After IInd World War health insurance debate picked attention and employer sponsored insurance which will stabilize well-being of people was thought important. During 1950's medical advancements and costs moved with high velocity wherein effects of Penicillin acted as an eye opener for people, slowly polio vaccine ushered in and successfully helped society to be protected against this dreadful ailment.

During 1960s National health expenditure was calculated, and GDP was found to be strongly affected by them also different studies have indicated how National health cost directly affects Economy of country (Raghupathi V, Raghupathi W,2020).

Gradually in 1970 National Health Insurance picked attention followed by several health insurance and social insurance policies at country across, post 1980's with advent of technology there have been remarkable changes in automated Healthcare system. The above discussion sheds light on how healthcare has evolved overtime. with gradual advent of technology there have been vast developments wherein electronic health records transformed the ways of development. The electronic recording of patients has made system more efficient with better implementation efforts.

During 1980's computers evolved and GUI with network technologies completely revamped the way system worked, administrative information among healthcare-oriented computer system and diagnosis related groups. Cost related factors were the most dominant factors. Development of standards that govern the structure of medical terminology with appropriate records are necessary.

Throughout 20th century there have been revolutionary developments in technology development. In 1993 DICOM which was a benchmark for digital imaging and communication in medicine came to practice which provides a diverse scope for patients, procedures, equipment's, and images.

From 2000-2010 Medical support system developed largely with development also in Nursing care and other clinical data availability. Today as per one of the reports of WHO more than 66%of countries have defined strategy and plans for digital healthcare and electronic health records with prescription of paperless and verifiable quality is available. These technologies which evolved as a mere data management aspect to moving from a local to a global architecture so that communication between the hospitals, research centres and moving to a shift from hospital centric to customer centric approach is picking. The transition from technical information utilization to strategic decision making is possible only by this technological intent.

1.3 Transition With Technology: Shift From a Clinician- to Patient-Driven Approach With Artificial Intelligence and Robotics in Healthcare

Artificial intelligence has revamped the way in which different stakeholders have been benefitted, with algorithms of different kinds it assists doctors and medical professionals in geocoding, health data, epidemic and syndromic surveillance as well.AI techniques helps to design and develop different kinds of drugs and helps in giving a personalized patient care, predictive models based on same can helps to develop decision making.AI is found to benefit diagnosis of patients like 3D mapping solutions of patients body, robotics in healthcare has picked lot of attention for rehabilitation robots that helps in providing physical support and automate procedure also.

Thus, the role of AI in automating health areas includes-Predictive medicine, patient data diagnostics, better clinical decision making, quality management, technology awareness and awareness along with training of professionals, intelligent machines play a pivitol role in setting transparency, setting responsibility, generating two-way communication and development of AI application. With large availability of data business models based on insights can be designed and developed based on predictive analytics based on AI decisions high quality treatment, patient diagnostic, analysing past data, present data and making future prediction is possible (Secinaro, S., Calandra, D., Secinaro, A. et al. (2021).

In healthcare there has been wide application of Precision medicine-predicting what protocol to be used for patient attributes and treatment context. Machine learning and precision medicine requires a defined and applied database for effective treatment. Thus, supervised learning helps in identifying right outcome.

There has been wide usage of Neural network also which since 1960, involving deep learning also called as neural network which helps in predicting outcomes. Usage of deep learning in radiomics used in detection of radiomics and imaging for clinical trial with image analysis also helps in early detection in cancerous cases. Deep learning is also used in form of Natura language processing with speech recognition, text analysis, translation, and different approach to it namely statistical and semantic.

Statistical is based on machine learning, speech recognition, and in healthcare its application lies in analysing unstructured notes and transcribe patient interaction with the help of Conversational AI. Similarly Expert system that require human experts and based on knowledge domain, they are based on data and machine learning algorithms that are unbiased by traditional rules.

Application of robots similarly has revolutionized the way in which healthcare has been quite different, with AI capabilities the embedded brains help in augmenting intelligence. Surgical robots provide power to surgeons for improving their ability and creating precise and minimal invasive actions. Robotic surgery is widely used in head, neck, gynaecologic, prostrate and in different other critical organs. Similarly, Robot Process automation is not dependent on robots, it is a well cushioned program for combination of workflow, business rules and different presentation layer with semi-intelligent users and using technologies like image recognition.

Recent advancement includes IBM's Watson which has considerably helped in diagnosing different ailments like cancer and its treatment it uses a combination of machine learning and an LLP capability it is a combination of process system with technology which are based upon cognitive services and uses speech language vision and different programmed procedures, it is highly applicable in case of cancer treatment which is arity area across the geographies.

Another application of technology for healthcare includes Google's collaboration with health delivery network for effective development of different prediction models which helps clinicians to handle severe and critical situations like sepsis and cardiac issues, based upon AI image interpretation algorithm it helps in making predictive decision and thus offers a good example of clinical success machines which also is supported by right treatment protocols. These combinations help in not only writing diagnosis but also effective patient treatment.

There is also a defined role of genetic profiles which are taken care by right specialized medical practitioners which helps in identifying different genetic variants and develop either new drugs for combination or focus upon improvement of the concurrent medicine. AI and predictive models also help in solving issues like these which help human clinicians to get support with business insight.

Along with the technical aspect another important issue which is moving from technical centric to customer centric or patient centric approach AI has been helpful in keeping the patient and related members highly engaged has been a common challenge for more than 300 clinical leaders and different healthcare professionals to take care of patient engagement and the majority suffering from high level of disengagement provided different choices available. The application of search engine-based optimization targeted content use of messages helps in effectively contextualizing AI capabilities also for patient engagement.

It is also helpful to predict different behaviors of patients with the help of electronic sensors biosensors smartphones, conversational interfaces which help in highly customizing the whole pathway of treatment.

Not only for technical or invasive and noninvasive medical treatment AI also helps in saving time and bringing efficiency when it comes to administrative applications in healthcare wherein it finds substantial scope and what's the efficiency exercise. There are several documentations to be maintained at healthcare institutions starting from claims, routine documentation of patients, follow up for revenue and medical records maintained electronically, different institutions also deploy use of chat bots for patient interaction and follow up for their wellness and providing services like telehealth. These are NLP based applications which help in bringing efficiency for all the stakeholders of healthcare structure.

Another important area wherein AI is highly helpful in making healthcare highly accelerated is a concern which is a bigger concern for all health institutions across with technological interventions and role of AI in generating an A well automated healthcare administration in all the pillars, it also has equal challenge of displacement of the existing workforce. According to one of the studies which Deloitte conducted along with Oxford Martin institute it was found that a substantial percentage of jobs at different levels may be replaced by adoption of technology. Let us equal cost of automation technologies but this all additively has impact on labor market the growth and future of these health institutions which is also affected by social regulatory political technological and other aspects as well.

Digital health care refers to use of information and communication technologies to understand health issues and challenges and thus prescribing it effectually in more customized and precise way. Digital health has led to complete transformation in medical and health practices progress. It has revolutionized completely the ways in which right from diagnosis, treatment, care, and prevention of health conditions are confronted and resolved.

The wide spectrum of digital healthcare innovations is not limited to technologies and information tools alone but is significantly oriented to the requirements and responsibilities of the stakeholders. With advanced developments in the field of Artificial intelligence, IoT, Neural mapping, Deep learning, telemedicine, Robotics in diagnosis and surgical intervention to predictive based counselling the procedural or operational aspect is highly strengthened, however there is another side which first needs attention.

These includes understanding the stakeholders in ensuring excellence in digital healthcare innovation to be sustained not only for short term but with a futuristic perspective. This field of innovations in digital healthcare involves clinicians, researchers, public health, technologies for managing data, intelligence in technologies, appropriate diagnosis, drug development, health solutions for various ages and types, ensuring development of mobile apps with a supportive function and virtual connectivity to all beneficiaries along with right progression of Health care Policy at Government level along with effective assessment and Governance.

It is important that technological adoption to ensure workflow management is important but equally important is upskilling and looking for scope for improvement as with technology the future of patient lies in which cannot be detailed whether it is with digital information or application in any other direct or indirect service. But there should be planned interventions especially in context to some specific branches like radiology with AI intervention in radiology including deep learning models which are based upon imagine exercise skilling is important which will act as a facilitator for correct diagnosis and treatment and give right feedback and preparation of patient with trust and appropriate medical intervention (Davenport T, Kalakota R.,2021).

Thus, with advent in knowledge-based system can help in solving specific issues like fuzzy logic that helps in solving prediction of disease like cholera, Machine learning helping in analysis using algorithm, Image and signal processing helps in in generating interpretation form large data. Thus, AI can be of great help especially in areas wherein human resources are less, designing treatment plans, appropriate medication, drug creation, solving public health problems. (Columbia.edu,2023)

2. STRATEGIES TO AVOID DIGITAL INEQUALITIES IN HEALTHCARE

2.1 Understanding Digital Healthcare

Digital healthcare helps in employing required information with the help of communication technologies so that a well questioned health and lifestyle can be maintained for a wider population. Thus, with the help of technological competencies and more patient centric approach based on data which is widely available of customer base digital health data has picked a lot of attention in recent past. Today with changes and disruption in every field healthcare sector is not untouched. The current shift with more of patient centricity and values-based health care directly gets benefitted when digital health data with the help of recent and most contemporary medical practices helps in creating a real world which is free from any kind of inequalities.

With the help of telehealth and telemedicine mobile based services and rise in data science with the help of suitable analytical techniques digital health helps in connecting the 3 important stakeholders patients' physicians and procedure in an effective way thus helping both preventive and predictive digital health becoming possible saving lives of millions. (Mumtaz H, et.al,2023)

Digital health has immense potential and transformational capacity to make healthcare a new form which is not limited by resources and increase access, quality, ethical aspects, and efficiency in healthcare delivery.

There are several challenges when it comes to equity in digital healthcare solutions amongst which lack of evidence high concern for privacy at governance level how the data will be kept secure and different ethical issues are major ones. It is important to be sensitive for health data especially when it is about privacy of people when digital tools are a support. Both at government as well as at private level this is a challenge.

There are also challenges when it comes to health outcome because involved the efficiency of solution. Another challenge when it comes to health equity is of socio-economic status demographic role of separate groups like minorities elder people low-income groups to whom making realised the benefit of digital health solution because of literacy issues becomes difficult.

It is true that with respect to technological progress we are moving towards 5G and development of most modern communication infrastructure and health infrastructure but still digitising medical records comprehensive information high quality healthcare with the help of advent tools like smartphones different algorithm for diagnosis platforms for taking feedback from customer and business insightful healthcare models based on artificial intelligence which are promoting patient centricity and high patient engagement also leading to health empowerment. This has helped in health companies and a better ecosystem of health created.

2.2 Digital Health Equity and Inclusion: Status and Challenges

Digital health equity not only are dependent upon country level policy but have their own challenges including how to engage and assure trust when it comes to digital health, resource constraints understanding the wider and dense population, varied expectation of customers budget issues, stakeholders involvement insufficiency, standardization of process and procedures, availability of evaluation framework, training and development of healthcare staff and lack of coordination at different levels both strategic and operational.

Another important challenge is healthcare disparity with respect to health data available of separate groups in populations communities' demographics medical conditions, quality of data available and maintaining its reliability is also a challenge. How to maintain the electronic health records to understand the risk at which the majority population is, and the expected outcomes also sometimes depreciate the rising trend of utilising digital healthcare administration.

Another important challenge is in terms of productivity in equity which is because of differences in technological availability and computing capabilities across the healthcare industry. Lack of infrastructure proper software and technological adoption along with fear and trust factors with some social issues also becomes barrier to health equity. In recent past improvement in data security with rising big data management in healthcare records also needs appropriate protection understanding in recent past lot of data hacking cases and ransom attack on different clinical computer networks requires technological and IT interventions to keep it protected.

Another important trend which is picking attention is Ambi balance when it comes to digital health. It requires a relational and multifaceted understanding that complete implications of digital health BP accompanied with different dimensions which may vary as per practices resulting into both positive and negative outcomes. It is important to ensure the technological support whether it is wearable or an algorithm that dependability and appropriate ability of the digital device is suitable accessible and matching.

Another key factors which affect the right implications of digital health is the requirement and understanding of patients which in most of the cases due to trust data security and correct congruence between patient needs and values becomes challenged. It is important that right engagement and participation of healthcare professional with the patient to communicate correctly and ensure right adoption of digital health is initiated along with an assurance of its adherence in long run.

Communication and trust building is also amongst crucial factors that affect digital environment when it comes to health management along with infrastructure and policy or governance issues. There is a need to standardise data sharing and ethical transaction standards between health institutions and the public, sometimes the challenges also include over gathering of data and improper integration into decision making, sometimes lack of research basis and uninformed consent for data collection and its method of usage also limits and weekends the trust with the digital health system. Crucial factors which affect the future of digital health with equity is availability of trained and professionals in the health care well conversant with both technology and technical procedure, lack of clarity on policies structure and the defined standing operating procedures along with both financial and non-potential resources affect the strengthening of digital health interventions.

There is also a strong rule of culture and work environment which helps different health institutions as well as the social gambit to adapt to these technologies with trust and fairness. With momentum from clinic centric to patient centric approaches there is a need to have a specific digital health technology employment in a specific as well as generic manner.

2.3 Universal Digital Health: An Equitable Perspective

Digital transformation in health rising enormously there is a strong need to have an integrated way of questioning individuals' communities and country to ensure the universal health equity and availability along with accessibility for all in a sustainable manner is important. Achieve this universal health mission, the role of digital health facilitated through technology is of prime importance it is not only applicable in one geography but makes sense globally. The role of different stakeholders ranging from policy makers to healthcare providers to public different community's social media business environmental factors geographic factors and the futuristic expectations are equally important.

With increasing importance of digital health application there are equal challenges when it comes to comparing digital skills globally cording to research almost 37% of the world population has not used Internet in 2020 will the majority being represented by developing countries thus this reflects cognitive disability because of educational socio economic and socio demographic factors along with living conditions which make things more chronic and hindering way of using digital healthcare. Thus, to delimit this factor providing appropriate adjustment and adapting to digital technologies and thus strengthening the most vulnerable group will directly and both indirectly empower and make potentially capable resources and remove the segregation amongst the population.

There have been numerous global initiatives and programmes at national sectoral and local level to ensure digital wellbeing becomes a right for all. According to World Health Organization the global digital health strategy 2020-25 there have been different initiatives from World Economic Forum this has led to a great advancement when it comes to digitally advanced society both in Europe and North America.

Since global health access is important across the geographies there is a need to urgently look for what are the digital solutions available when it comes to access based upon developed and developing economies. It is important that for making digital health accessible for everyone there should be a mutual knowledge exchange at different levels across the countries to ensure that whether it is through research scientific discoveries technological development and data analysis matched with correct algorithms the implications based upon country specific sector specific group specific and elemental specific are available for the required population.

There can be certain initiatives and strategies by way of which this gap can be bridged namely-

1. There is a need to collaborate academic knowledge with the expertise available which will help in engaging different stakeholders will help in creating digital health networks help and involving different nongovernmental organization and governmental initiatives for different kind of groups.
2. There is a need to educate the health professionals and different communities about universal health equity for everyone through different mediums as well as by conducting mass awareness programs ranging from conferences to symposium.
3. It important to conduct research in a participatory approach known as community based participatory research so that different geographies can be benefited by way of this.
4. Identifying and understanding correct parameters that affect socio economic differences and access off digital health irrespective of inequalities of opportunity should be conducted. This is possible when from the beginning stage an environment off inclusivity is strengthened in the initial stages of both research as well as exchange creation of different collaborative centres will also significantly affect the accessibility and coverage of digital health.
5. There should be upscaling upskilling inconsistent ways of healthcare professionals viren the concept of digital health for all can be emphasised at both primary secondary and higher level for ensuring successful implementation of digital health literacy.

Thus, there is a key role of different stakeholders reject from citizens to academicians to policymakers to it experts to healthcare professionals' society and different communities to deploy the capability of digital health in a bad manner and thus help in producing the health differences across the geography. This will have a larger impact for the wellbeing of economy at large.

2.4 Digital Exclusion and Intervention

It is a bigger challenge when it comes to economic development because it is not limited to simply access of services, but it also is inclusive of access to skill set devices right attitude and a required personality along with social and motivational based barriers that affect an individual societal and country level development.

It is not possible to create cushioned and one size fitting all approach for everyone accessing digital health thus the need of diverse groups individual characteristics requirement is important to be classified so that to stablish trust and sustainable relationship, becomes easier this will help in ensuring correct digital engagement.

Another important group which might be having digital skills and might be easily available on social media would not be feeling engaged with the healthcare online this is a very challenging situation where it is difficult to engage people with health care digitally here in the role of social media to educate them about different benefits associated with digital engagement is important.

An important help to circumvent the invoice issue can be by developing trust as it is a known fact that to make digital banking related transaction people use technology but when it comes to health pay hesitant thus to victor over their confidence also using technology for health also will improve largely.

It is important that right information should also be accessed so that the incorrect information or misleading information should not lead to losses and evading trust amongst the people and thus leading to them feeling disengaged for an extended period. It is important to have a human touch irrespective of digital healthcare uptake which will help in putting human touch along with technical intervention as and when required contact with the trusted healthcare professionals and related associates is primarily important whether it is related to physical or mental illness. Thus, there is a big challenge off digital by default which contributes to digital division and leading to disadvantage is it needs to be managed sensitively wherein a combination of need to access face to face and digitally available should be balanced.

Thus, it can be understood that in order to achieve digital access for better health correct gap measurement and documentation of digitally engaged and unengaged must be improvised followed by training and right skill development of the health care professionals correct intervention of government policy through both online and offline channels should be promoted, data related to reasons of health inequalities at different geographies should be measured and with Co-opted approach based upon the analysis health interventions should be implemented.

3. DIGITAL INNOVATIONS IN HEALTHCARE

3.1 Need of Digital Innovation in Healthcare

Digital transformation has been progressing since advent of digital technology which will benefit society largely and help in development of healthcare industry. Healthcare solutions based on technology helps in making system efficient, seamless, affordable, improvement in healthcare solutions and improvising level of medical care.

There is a direct relation between development in digital healthcare and its application in various therapies and procedures. This will help in also utilizing massive data which is available to be utilized through new therapies and best practices to improve wellbeing, reduce cost, and help provide new opportunities.

This will also give rise to effective development in medical education and create opportunities in healthcare sector. The role of IoT, Artificial intelligence, cloud computing and social media is important in this along with rising opportunities of telecommunications and financial services. Whether it is usage of patient's internet or by usage of digital health applications via phone it is important to take a right decision about their health. With rising role of patient in healthcare in today's scenario it is more of consumer health services with more characteristic like ease, efficiency, speed, immediacy, quality, and cost. It is important to find out what strategic challenges are involved when it comes to implementation of these healthcare technologies (Stoumpos AI, Kitsios F, Talias MA, 2023).

3.2 Advancements in Digital Innovation

A significant report of Digital authority tools found there is a drastic change in digital tools in healthcare which includes rise of on demand healthcare because today's consumers of healthcare have also changed understanding their busy schedules demand and prefer quick, affordable, and quality services. Compared to past decade more mobile based services are preferred.

With more than 4 billion people today on internet it is quite evitable that when used with effectiveness of available customers in form of users the possibility of digital transformation in different offers and services in healthcare can be expanded. Consumers prefer to go online to find details of medical information because with growth of Gig Economy the availability of service providers are readily available. The role of medical practitioners also becomes highly engaging and accessible when on demand healthcare providers also help in meeting the requirement.

Another important factor is right utilization of Big Data managed by digital authoring tools which helps in increasing quality and reduction in *errors of medication, facilitates preventive care,* big data analysis helps in identifying creative ad preventive plans for holding the frequent flyer tendency to stable customers as well as helps in ensuring more accurate staffing based on estimated future admission, allocating resources and right way of dealing with patients.

Also, use of virtual reality in procedures, facilitating virtual reality simulations to both residents and doctors to perform more effective with the help of wearables, headsets and in helping patients with various disabilities to perform effectively. Digital marketing tools are expected to grow as a market to $5.1million by 2025 with increased usage, it also helps in curing patients with different kind of anxiety, stroke, stress disorders.

A bigger benefit of digital technology is supported by wearables technology, this is becoming increasingly popular because patients are more expecting and like prevention and maintenance and thus demanding information about health. This helps in monitoring health effectively including different devices like heart rate sensors, various kinds of exercise trackers, sweat meters and various kinds of oximeters. The major benefits why these devices make sense is it helps in personalizing health experience, helps in providing better insurance incentives and better gamification opportunities.

It also has opened new avenues in "Redditive" healthcare and better insight-based models can be build based on different AI tools as well that can help in different ways like using maximums searched words by different seekers for health or different medical conditions, it will help business to identify how much human resource planning is needed as well. Virtual reality helps in providing right training to doctors, wearable devices helping inn improving preventive medicine, artificial intelligence helps in personalizing the treatment.

3.3 Artificial Intelligence Tools for Healthcare Transformation

There are various apps and tools(Robotic) like Moxi, a hospital designed assisting nurses for stocking and fetching supplies .Based on AI technology there are chatbots and virtual health assistants which helps in providing assistance, global healthcare chatbots are projected to reach $3143.3 million by 2025. It also contributes in specific areas like precision medicine, medical imaging, genomics and also in drug discovery correctly. Machine learning helps in quick development of drug based on learned algorithms. Thus, it can help in reducing costs and help health organizations. Similarly, Blockchain technology has completely revamped the healthcare sector, it helps in preventing data breaches, helps in maintaining effective and accurate medical records and cut costs.

Similarly advanced growth in 5G also mobile which helps in providing medical training, practicing at own with the help of headsets, 5G drones can help in delivering to toughest geographic areas, like deliver defibrillators to help cardiac arrest patients. (Digital Authority partners. (digitalauthority.me,2023)

According to a study by Deloitte centre for Health solutions in context to digital healthcare solutions there are certain factors important, health system considers digital capabilities as a basic path to transform relationship with consumers. It is important to assess the digital state to optimize opportunities for digital transformation. It is important to set KPI to challenge and overcome the addition to budgetary constraints. For organization there are several factors like communication, ownership, transparency, culture which support development of digital culture in organization.

3.4 Benefits of Digital Adoption

High patient satisfaction and engagement, Improved quality of care and patient outcomes, revenue growth, better customer satisfaction, better data sharing and collaboration, reduced regulatory and compliance risk.

Along with this developing a design thinking approach is important. The report emphasized that journey of patient is not only limited to while it is in hospital but before and after as well, which can be leveraged by adoption of digital tools. The use of Business Intelligence tools and BI capabilities matter lot when it comes to customer satisfaction. Based on different health interviews it was found that ROI based on initiatives taken is equally important as it helps in deciding based on BI models and capabilities which tools and interventions are making sense. Thus data, talent and budget are amongst the top factors that affected successful implementation as well can become challenges when talked about effective digital transformation. With the above factors the reports talk that role of defining C level support is equally important as partners with team and other teams for effectively.

Leadership and managing change within are found to be crucial factors when it comes to adoption of tools. It is important to create digital leadership and governance structure with business Strategy, build a culture for digital leadership, focus on how next generation talent can be developed, high level of flexibility and scalability of implementation to manage and evolve technologies, develop KPI which are highly scalable, measurable and accountable to connect service provider with the targeted customer when it comes to effectual health service (Chuke A, Hendricks J, Wurz J, Shudes C, 2021).

There are various tools that are finding space for transforming tomorrow.

Ultronics is a digital tool that with the aid of artificial intelligence has potential to diagnose heart disease and save millions of lives and thus save millions by proactive diagnosis. There are number of self-service tools as well that helps in streamlining scheduling, electronic payment auto renewal of prescriptions, to manage health without any hassles. There are number of wellness tools as well which helps in monitoring fitness by coaching, real time consultation, wearable technology, clinical decision making is also equally important.

Financial Transparency tools are also gaining attention in today's time as the tools will give access to financial aspects of health care abd help customers in comparing the prices as well as benefits related to better development

3.5 Digital Therapeutics: A New Supplement for Innovation in Healthcare

With advancement in technological innovation, it is now quite sure to say that technology enabled medical interventions with planned tools and software's identifying, diagnosis, prevention and treatment of different ailments have become possible. These are evidence-based therapeutics which help in ensuring effective intervention.

Dr Joseph Kvedat from Boston USA initiated the development of a program in which application of technology which is free from the limitations of space time and personal limitations can be developed.

The term e-patient was first coined by Dr Tom Ferguson in 1999 refers to patients who are equipped, enabled and empowered with respect to their healthcare decision.

DTX are founded on basis of software programs which can be understood as a type of software medical device without requiring a hardware. Since it uses consumer mobile smartphones, tablets to connect else DTX does not requires any FDA regulated hardware.

It is a new category wherein evidence-based solution which are proven and adhere to certain regulation are directly delivered to patients with software and helps in combating different ailment like diabetes, certain kind of pain and others. As part of m -Care intelligence digital therapeutics helps in strengthening clinical evidence and helping large scale usage.

There are three essential elements in this including –

- Product with which disease can be treated
- Managing the present condition of patient
- Improve the health function.

The basic principles of Digital Therapeutics alliance are to-

- Help and prevent medial disorder or disease
- Help in including design, manufacture, and quality of best practices
- Incorporate and maintain product development and process of usage
- Engage end users in development and appropriate use of product
- Ensure safety and privacy of patient
- Effective product development, deployment and sustaining good practices.
- Publish outcome of different trials conducted and getting it published in right journals
- Appropriate clinical validation and regulatory status
- Ensure regular studies for product performance.

Based on different studies conducted it was found that whether it is the ace of diabetes or pain or even a specific mental behaviour therapeutics has without an error helped in providing quality solutions. In another solution there is also availability of cognitive behavioural therapy that focuses on improving outcome of Type 2 diabetic people, similarly how by conducting awareness programs, glucose monitoring devices, virtual physicians, peer support and with the help of health coaches helps in improving health metrics. (Omada, Better Therapeutics). Another organization like Akili interactive also helps in providing a prescription video game-based treatment which aims at improvising ability of young children with hyperactivity disorder, attention deficit etc.

To ensure the healthy and effective implementation of health it is important to recommend certain specific criteria for efficacy of digital therapeutics and to also be supported by randomized clinical trials (Vaidya, A (2023).

DTx are direct to customer apps and are helpful for different problems chronic insomnia, panic and also in substance disorders etc. They are strong basis for providing health equity since can be sued independently or adjunct to medication as well.

3.6 Digital Therapeutics Market: A Vivid landscape

There are various DTX products in the market that are available like Sleepio which is for sleeping disorders, Livongo and Omada for diabetes prevention, though they are not cleared by Food and Drug administration (FDA) still they are commercially available through employee health insurance. Different countries are also working actively on regulating these products and introducing specific controlled policy understanding health and safety.

DT x has immense potential when it comes to preventing and managing chronic issues like diabetes, this segment is seen to grow at a vast speed and potential almost 3X of pharma companies and in India the workforce deployed is 429.8 million which is expected to grow larger.

DTx is seen as a fast-growing alternative to fight against chronic issues. It uses wearables, health monitoring devices and self-reporting tools. For providing value-based care in cost effective manner investing in development of wearables and devices is important to prepare people for health equity. Digital medicine consists of software and hardware supported by evidence to measure or intervene in the service of human health. Example of digital health entities and health system includes health information clinical care administration tools.

Digital diagnostics, digital biomarkers and patient monitoring and different devices are example of digital medicine and for remote patient monitoring devices. Like digital sensors, wearable design and Virtual reality and artificial intelligence. DT x relies on algorithm for action and information management which is easy to generate, collate and analyse the health data.

One of the organisations developed AI based Robot which nudges people to take medicine timely to avoid non adherence of medication, the robot matches with usage of psychology modelling to tailor their interaction and ensure dosing. Another initiative is developing of a pill with ingestible sensor small and coated with copper and magnesium, it generates signal post the dose is consumed at skin of patient wherein it is controlled by sensor.

The sensor can also record activity, heart rate, sleep quality, temperature etc. Similar these are seen to be helpful for oncology patients, Hepatitis and Diabetes 2 patients to be extended to use for HIV patients and even for patients with bipolar II disorders and schizophrenia.

Thus, it can be concluded that DTx helps in providing personalized and evidence-based care which helps in self-agency control and specifically in patient solutions, some common ones being Labbe and Aaron.

Similarly, AI tailored medication also helps in offering customized solutions and a better trial and error for seeking appropriate therapy. This helps in also identifying specific biology-based requirement which helps doctors in diagnosing in more customized way.

AI language models have also been a great support system to improve medication dictation tools that helps to save professional to save time for data entry kind of job.

Health aligned Wearables have been revolutionary that have brought the closest possibility, right from Fitbit to Apple watch there has been lot of exponential growth which promotes consistent monitoring on health from routine to long term.

Role of Connected Devices whether it is robotics to telemedicine there are different mobile apps that have helped patients and caregivers to connect and make health services more efficient.

Augmented and Virtual Reality support from training to surgery have also augmented usage of technology in supporting healthcare.

Genetic Testing is also another advancement that helps in serving multipurpose right from tracing the ancestors to analysing the genes for predicting medical issues and provide customized solution. Today with development of AI even problems like Dememtia can be treated, human speech can be detected easily and cured. From telemedicine to remote procedures health innovation has transformed todays equity-based health inclusion.

The above discussion thus delved in how digital healthcare helps not only in moving towards building a strong empowered development of Nations, which contribute towards physical, mental, psychological well being of individuals and systems.

Thus, with progressively growing business models and insight generation capability through data usage facilitated by technologies and digital research the growth and future of innovation in digital combination of health care excellence will be achieved successfully. This will help in fulfilling the goal of equitable, affordable, quality healthcare services to all right from rural to urban to all communities to vulnerable through digital support and right investment.

4. CONCLUSION

The Chapter aimed at determining different factors and sources along with environmental factors that led to vast and quick development with a rich history of development in healthcare. Across the geographies the major strength preventive mechanism to keep a country growing and sustainable is Good Health at less cost and better services. It is pertinent to note that today's competitive and disruptive world demands a quick, efficient, and agile system which can serve heterogeneity. With rising demands, environmental constraints, competitiveness, government regulation, technological advancement sand biological changes and challenges due to global factors maintaining the complete health is a dauntful task.

It is also important to take care of big data generated through different activities that healthcare institutions generate like Biomedical research, patients' records, other hospital routine reports, this requires right infrastructure, management, organizing and generation of data with strong integration of technology. This way medical therapies and biomedical research will help in generating personal medicine outcome (Dash, S., Shakya war, S.K., Sharma, M. et al. (2019).

The stakeholders when it comes to healthcare management and administration is no longer limited to Clinical practitioners alone but inclusive of all primary and secondary customers, a complete quality perspective when it comes to quality, trust, engagement and sustained efficient services. With a complete shift from clinician centric to patient centric support the role of technology is primary. It is equally important to adhere to ethical values and system to ensure fairness and equity with inclusiveness in healthcare.

Thus, for a sustained healthcare system it is important to ensure right skeuomorphism with developments on consistent level, affordability, enhanced bionic humans upskilling and reducing errors at all levels (Thimbleby H. (2013).

It is important that healthcare organization needs to lessen down bureaucratic aspects to be more agile and adopt future. It is important to be innovative and reduce the conservative approach.

New approaches are consistently adopting new measures to integrate cloud with existing technologies, deeper AI infusion for deployment of chatbots for appointment to intelligent vice integration and telemedicine, Infrastructure development and deployment of mobile portal.

There are smarter therapies like insulin pens, auto injectors, smart packaging will help in clinical and business operation. Today's healthcare has completely revitalized with personalized approach wherein genomic profile to back-end healthcare technology society determines health much faster than any human physician.

Thus, digital health which is now an emerging and growing field helps in healthcare innovation and healthcare technology to support healthcare organization. With technology a whole better advancement in Genomic Era is expected, thus relating the future of genetics in medicine will help future health organization to grow fast. Thus, lot of challenges associated with next generation sequencing, application of technology in genomic information of patients and customizing treatment based on it, understanding genetic variations, any chromosomal abnormality and ethical implications associated with genomic data is important to be understood to sustain a healthy humankind.

Amongst the 16 UN SDG the third goal is of good health and Wellbeing, hi line with the goal it is important thar whether it is fighting against the HIV, Child immunisation or dreadful diseases like TB or malaria it is important that access to healthcare at affordable cost is to be adhered.

The aim of Sustainable goals is to make a commitment towards ending these and a bigger purpose being to provide universal health to all. Thus, increased investment in healthcare and support system to confront the challenges of social to resource inadequacies sometimes is important for achieving bigger target of "Health for all".

REFERENCES

Chuke, A., Hendricks, J., Wurz, J., & Shudes, C. (2021) Digital transformation, From a buzzword to an imperative for health systems. *Deloitte Insights*. https://www2.deloitte.com/us/en/insights/industry/health-care/digital-transformation-in-healthcare.html

Dash, S., Shakyawar, S. K., Sharma, M., & Kaushik, S. (2019). big data in healthcare: Management, analysis and future prospects. *Journal of Big Data*, *6*(1), 54. doi:10.1186/s40537-019-0217-0

Davenport, T., & Kalakota, R. (2019). The potential for artificial intelligence in healthcare. *Future Health J.*, *6*(2), 94-98. https://csd.columbia.edu/sites/default/files/content/docs/ICT%20India/Papers/ICT_India_Working_Paper_43.p doi:10.7861/futurehosp.6-2-94

Kleinman & Dougherty. (2013). Assessing quality improvement in health care: Theory for practice. *Pediatrics*, *131*(1), S110–S119. PMID:23457146

Mumtaz, H., Riaz, M. H., Wajid, H., Saqib, M., Zeeshan, M. H., Khan, S. E., Chauhan, Y. R., Sohail, H., & Vohra, L. I. (2023, September 28). Current challenges and potential solutions to the use of digital health technologies in evidence generation: A narrative review. *Frontiers in Digital Health*, *5*, 1203945. doi:10.3389/fdgth.2023.1203945 PMID:37840685

Raghupathi, V., & Raghupathi, W. (2020, May 13). Healthcare Expenditure and Economic Performance: Insights from the United States Data. *Frontiers in Public Health*, *8*, 156. doi:10.3389/fpubh.2020.00156 PMID:32478027

Secinaro, S., Calandra, D., Secinaro, A., Muthurangu, V., & Biancone, P. (2021). The role of artificial intelligence in healthcare: A structured literature review. *BMC Medical Informatics and Decision Making*, *21*(1), 125. doi:10.1186/s12911-021-01488-9 PMID:33836752

Stoumpos, A. I., Kitsios, F., & Talias, M. A. (2023, February 15). Digital Transformation in Healthcare: Technology Acceptance and Its Applications. *International Journal of Environmental Research and Public Health*, *20*(4), 3407. = doi:10.3390/ijerph20043407 PMID:36834105

Sustainable Development Goals, Good Health and Wellbeing. (n.d.). https://www.un.org/sustainabledevelopment/health

Thimbleby H. (2013). Technology and the future of healthcare. *J Public Health Res.*, *2*(3), e28. Doi: doi:10.4081/jphr.2013

Vaidya, A. (2023). *What Are Digital Therapeutics and Their Use Cases.* https://mhealthintelligence.com/features/what-are-digital-therapeutics-and-their-use-cases

Chapter 14
The Benefits of Social Media Platforms for Medical Practitioners:
Building a Global Medical Network

Arpita Nayak
https://orcid.org/0000-0003-2911-0492
KIIT School of Management, KIIT University, India

Atmika Patnaik
University of Cambridge, UK

Ipseeta Satpathy
KIIT School of Management, KIIT University, India

Sukanta Kumar Baral
https://orcid.org/0000-0003-2061-714X
Indira Gandhi National Tribal University, India

B. C. M. Patnaik
KIIT School of Management, KIIT University, India

ABSTRACT

Social media has significantly impacted the way medical professionals interact, collaborate, and share their perspectives. It has enhanced healthcare and medical education by facilitating knowledge exchange and fostering global networking. Social media platforms also serve as a virtual center for professionals to search for global work opportunities. They are powerful promotional tools for medical meetings and conferences, attracting attendees worldwide and encouraging collaboration. They provide access to diverse viewpoints, encouraging alternative approaches to healthcare challenges. This digital connection can lead to collaborative research partnerships, joint initiatives, and the exchange of best practices, creating a global network of subject matter experts. This chapter provides an overview of the benefits of social media platforms for medical practitioners in building a network.

DOI: 10.4018/979-8-3693-1934-5.ch014

INTRODUCTION

Social media tools, such as Twitter, have transformed how medical practitioners disseminate information and interact with the public. Twitter has swiftly grown in popularity among vascular surgeons as a means of sharing research findings and exchanging information. As to one study, social media comments on vascular surgical articles are linked to a spike in the total amount of literature citations, signifying greater scientific influence. Twitter, in particular, is being used as an instructional instrument for ongoing medical education and research methods. In 2013, the European Journal of Vascular and Endovascular Surgery (EJVES) recognized the importance of social media presence and established a Twitter account. It has developed since then to highlight key publications, guidelines, and free/open-access studies (Chaudhuri & Prendice,2023). Social media has the potential to tremendously help medical practitioners by providing them with timely access to cutting-edge knowledge and research, allowing them to keep up to speed on the most recent breakthroughs in their area. It provides a forum for medical professionals to enhance their reputation by demonstrating their knowledge and sharing vital thoughts with a larger audience. Social media makes networking easier, allowing medical professionals to interact with colleagues, specialists, and possible partners all around the world. It can garner financial opportunities for medical research and initiatives by reaching out to a worldwide audience. Medical professionals may use social media to market events and employment opportunities to a global audience for free (Bhasin,2017). Medical practitioners may use social media channels to enhance their views and engage in advocacy activities. These venues, whether supporting public health programs, increasing awareness of rare illnesses, or campaigning for healthcare policy reforms, give a large audience and tools for mobilizing support. Social media knowledge may be utilized in patient care as well. Healthcare practitioners may utilise these platforms to convey vital health information to patients, increase patient involvement, and promote preventative activities. This patient education allows people to make educated health decisions and encourages collaborative doctor-patient partnerships (Giroux & Moureau,2020). Social media for healthcare has revolutionized lives in the modern digital era, altering how we interact, communicate, and obtain information. Healthcare professionals (HCPs) have access to a variety of social media technologies for increasing professional training and learning, ranging from wikis to VR games. For example, they may use these technologies to increase organizational visibility, improve patient care quality, and give training to improve quality. Social media networks, in various forms, offer significant benefits that unite physicians all over the world. These platforms provide chances for professional growth, ongoing education, and worldwide professional involvement. They enable medical professionals to look for employment openings, promote meetings, engage in case discussions, and network with other medical community members. Social media also allows healthcare practitioners to construct social and professional networks and swiftly and broadly disseminate information. It offers a platform for gaining access to health information, specialized clinical expertise, and engaging in research efforts. Furthermore, social media facilitates peer-to-peer and clinician-to-patient communication for consultations, while also enhancing institutional branding and speeding up interactions between healthcare professionals (Alasnag et al.,2021; Ventola,2014). People believe social media more than any other conventional advertising channel, which influences their choice of healthcare providers. According to one survey, 8 out of 10 Online users in the US seek health information online, with 74% using social media. Furthermore, 41% of patients believe that social media influences their choice of physician or facility for care. As shown in "Figure 1", respondents in the survey responded to the question on the importance of social media as a helpful tool (Popa,2022).

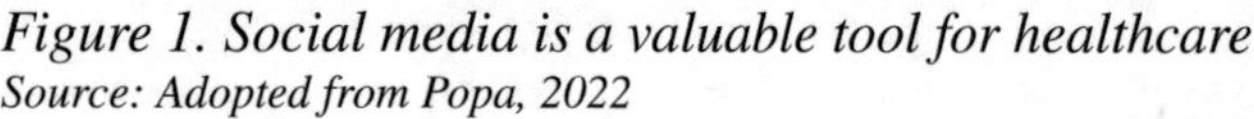

Figure 1. Social media is a valuable tool for healthcare
Source: Adopted from Popa, 2022

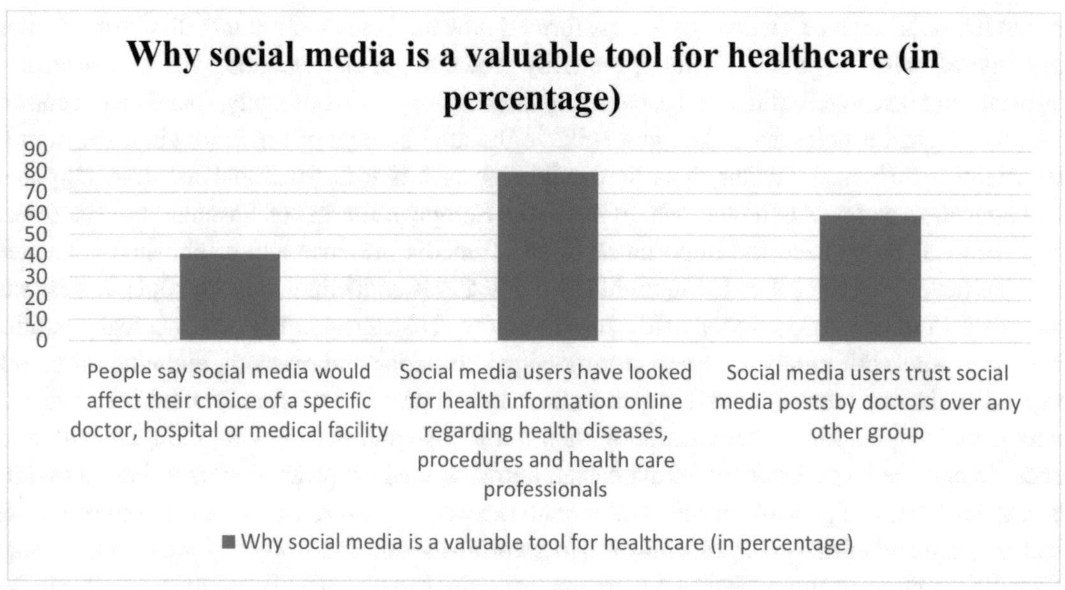

Social media platforms have evolved into vital instruments in the fields of research, education, and clinical practice, providing a plethora of advantages. They not only increase the exposure of research products, but they also encourage scholarly networking, allowing experts to interact and engage on a worldwide scale. Social media profiles that are ethically controlled have emerged as viable tools for post-publication discussion in the context of medical publications. They act as meeting places for important authors to debate and elaborate on their works, thus broadening the societal consequences of their work. This dynamic engagement enriches academic discourse and invites a larger audience to explore these intellectual contributions. Furthermore, social media aggregators play an important role in tracking and producing alternative analytics. These indicators provide academics with useful insights about current subjects and significant publications in their respective domains, offering a new perspective on the effect of research articles. Traditional citations, while important, are no longer the only way to assess the influence of a research work. To promote their accomplishments, publishers are increasingly displaying both traditional citations and new metrics. This all-encompassing method provides a more complete picture of a journal's influence and importance in the academic world. The Scopus database, which counts not just standard citations but also other metrics, is a notable example of this comprehensive approach. This dual monitoring ensures a more comprehensive assessment of the influence of an indexed item, adding to a more thorough understanding of its relevance (Zimba & Gasparyan, 2021). Social media is the digital age's connecting tissue, bridging gaps, and bringing people together. It's a place where geographical borders dissolve, allowing us to reach out to friends, relatives, and acquaintances no matter how far away they are. We not only share our opinions and experiences on these platforms, but we also meet like-minded people, broadening our social circles and forming new ties. It serves as a clearinghouse for the exchange of information, ideas, and expertise, keeping us up to date on current events and trends. Furthermore, it serves as a platform for self-expression and creativity, allowing us to demonstrate our skills and feel a sense of belonging. Aside from personal relationships, social media serves as a portal to companies, organizations, and brands, allowing for direct contact and involvement. In a nutshell, it is the digital glue that holds our world together (Quesenberry,2020). During the last decade, the increased use of social media (SM) and medical apps (applications) has enhanced healthcare delivery and continued medical training in a variety of ways, including interaction between physicians and patients and scientific online conversations. Prior to the COVID-19 pandemic, Saudi Arabia pioneered the use of telemedicine. The Saudi Ministry of Health (MOH) has created a number of apps to aid in healthcare delivery. One example of transforming healthcare delivery is the "Mawid" App, which allows clients to arrange appointments for health services. "Mawid" was founded in 2017, and the number of users exceeded 2.5 million in 2018 (Kheir et al.,2022). The internet now provides access to an array of health information, including factsheets on how to quiet a colicky infant and videos on how to do a heart transplant. In 2014, 87% of US adults reported accessing the Internet, with 72% looking for health information. Additionally, a large number of respondents who viewed health information online reported that the data they saw will "likely" or "very likely" influence their future choices regarding health care (Campbell et al.,2016). Social media platforms have brought in a new age for the medical community, providing a myriad of outlets for linking practitioners worldwide. These digital platforms serve as virtual gathering places for healthcare professionals to congregate, share information, and interact on a never-before-seen scale. Medical practitioners may utilise social media to interact with colleagues, mentors, and experts from all around the world, allowing them to communicate beyond geographical boundaries. This worldwide network not only allows for the exchange of information and best practices, but it also allows for real-time conversations on cutting-edge research, novel therapies, and new healthcare trends (Chiang,2021). Platforms for medical journals that are ethically regulated improve intellectual dialogue and increase the social effect of research publications. The importance of social media in sharing information, participating in meaningful debates, and catalyzing joint efforts is highlighted by its function in cementing relationships within the medical fraternity. As we go through the digital era, it becomes clear that social media has become a vital instrument in establishing a tight-knit global medical network, enhancing the profession with the collective expertise of practitioners worldwide. Social media platforms have evolved into useful tools for medical practitioners, promoting cooperation, aiding information transmission, and keeping experts up to date on the most recent research trends. In our increasingly linked world, embracing these platforms can increase the reach and impact of medical research (Lopez et al.,2019). The Importance of building networks is vital as it helps medical professionals to remain up to speed on the latest breakthroughs and best practices in their area. Networking allows for cooperation and knowledge exchange with colleagues, which leads to professional growth and development. Medical practitioners can have access to multiple viewpoints and ideas from experts with varying backgrounds and experiences through networks, which improves their understanding of healthcare practices. Networking may lead to employment possibilities such as job referrals, mentorship, and research project partnerships. Building a strong network may give emotional support and a feeling of community, particularly during difficult times. Networks can make it easier to share resources, information, and knowledge, resulting in better patient care and outcomes (Ahmed,2017). Social Media serve as a virtual connection allowing mentors and students to communicate in real time across geographic borders. Social media offers medical trainees unparalleled opportunities to provide guidance, transmit expertise, and exchange medical information and thoughts. Experienced doctors may readily share their clinical experience with trainees, guiding them through challenging scenarios, clinical decision-making, and evidence-based practices. By offering continuing medical innovation, research breakthroughs, and developing therapies, access to social media enables continuous learning, a cornerstone of medical education. Furthermore, these seminars support collaborative research efforts by allowing physicians and trainees to engage in multidisciplinary dialogue and contribute to the advancement of ongoing medical knowledge. Social media platforms, in particular, provide a dynamic, knowledge-rich environment that supports networking, mentorship, and continual professional development for physicians and other healthcare professionals.

PROJECT COLLABORATION: SOCIAL MEDIA BRIDGING THE GAP BETWEEN MEDICAL PRACTITIONERS

In the medical profession, collaborative initiatives entail working with diverse teams to reach research goals and address challenging scientific and biological concerns. These studies highlight the value of collaboration and teamwork in clinical and laboratory research. Building a team with a unified research aim and ensuring psychological safety for all members is required for successful collaboration (Patel et al.,2021). Collaborative initiatives bring together specialists from many professions, such as physicians, researchers, and scientists, to address complicated medical problems. Collaboration gives for a more thorough approach to issue resolution and a broader viewpoint. Researchers may more effectively tackle difficult medical issues by pooling resources and expertise medical research collaboration can lead to the discovery of novel medicines and interventions, eventually improving patient outcomes. Researchers can create more effective and personalized ways of patient care by merging various viewpoints and skills. Collaborative initiatives encourage the exchange of resources, data, and expertise, resulting in enhanced research efficiency. Researchers can prevent duplication of effort and make faster progress by collaborating (Nyström et al.,2018). Collaborative initiatives need clear communication as well as the formulation of ground rules and principles. This helps to reduce possible disputes and ensures that everyone in the team is working towards the same objective. Collaboration projects in medical research are important for medical practitioners because they allow for the exchange of interdisciplinary experience and information, allowing for a more holistic approach to patient treatment. Collaboration initiatives can help medical practitioners by providing access to a varied variety of knowledge, including researchers, scientists, and clinicians, which can improve problem-solving abilities and lead to novel treatments and interventions. Collaboration initiatives can increase research efficiency, allowing medical practitioners to avoid duplicating efforts and move forward more swiftly. They can develop more effective and personalized methods of patient treatment by working together, thereby improving patient outcomes. Furthermore, collaborative projects aid in conflict resolution by providing clear communication channels and norms that ensure all team members are working towards the same goal. This encourages medical practitioners to operate in a supportive and collaborative setting (Zalatoris et al.,2017). The phrase "social media" has a broad and shifting definition. In broad terms, the phrase refers to technologies powered by the internet that enable individuals and groups to congregate and interact; exchange information, ideas, personal messages, photographs, and other content; and, in some circumstances, interact contemporaneously with other users of the site. Social media is sometimes known as "Web 2.0" or "social networking." Healthcare professionals from all around the world may utilize social media platforms to share their knowledge, skills, and research findings with peers from all over the world. This enables cooperation as well as the exchange of thoughts and knowledge. Medical practitioners may use social media to interact and network with one another regardless of distance or nation. This allows people to network professionally, seek guidance, and cooperate on initiatives (Stukus et al.,2019). Medical information, research articles, and instructional materials may all be found on social media sites. Medical professionals may use these tools to expand their expertise, remain up to speed on new advances, and cooperate on projects. Healthcare personnel may use social media technologies to collaborate on projects in real time, regardless of their physical location. This encourages collaboration and enables the sharing of ideas and skills. Social media platforms connect healthcare professionals with specialists from across the world, permitting them to seek advice, share expertise, and collaborate on projects from a range of perspectives. The European Society of Intensive Care Medicine (ESICM) has announced that its LIVES conference will be online in 2021. This allowed everyone who was interested to join, regardless of geography. Facebook, Twitter, and online forums create a virtual social environment in which healthcare practitioners may exchange expertise and cooperate. Healthcare practitioners may rapidly adapt to computer-mediated collaborative endeavours and other kinds of social media, permitting them to communicate and participate in real-time with coworkers. Contributing to healthcare knowledge-sharing groups on social media channels provides practitioners with knowledge that improves their capacity to contribute to project cooperation (Alali,2018). Project teams may connect to a larger network of specialists and stakeholders by utilizing social media, allowing them to gain varied viewpoints and ideas. Social media may also aid in the development and maintenance of professional ties, which are essential for effective project cooperation. The foundation of connectedness is given by social media platforms, which serve as a portal for people to interact and share. Enhancing medical collaboration has been identified as an important strategy for reforming the healthcare system. Collaboration in health care has been found to enhance patient outcomes by reducing unnecessary adverse pharmaceutical responses, morbidity and mortality rates, and prescription dosage management (Bosch & Mansell, 2015). Patients and physicians can engage and participate on social media platforms for clinical care, research, and patient support, regardless of geography. This is especially beneficial for patients and experts who are geographically dispersed, such as those working in the field of unique and orphan diseases. Medical practitioners can utilise social media to get current health information, professional clinical expertise, and to participate in the most recent research endeavours. This enables the flow of ideas, experience, and resources regardless of geographic location. Social media platform technological advancements will enable ever-better venues for patients and professionals to connect and participate, eventually improving the quality of life. (Stephens,2014). Throughout the COVID-19 pandemic, scientists and medical experts from all around the world worked together to study the virus. Social media has been used to exchange data, discuss discoveries, and coordinate research activities in real time, allowing for the development of therapies and vaccinations to be accelerated. Social Media acted as a savior in the mode of connectivity. Healthcare knowledge is always developing as new clinical evidence becomes accessible. It has been claimed that clinical practice recommendations are typically out of date within 6 years after release. Individual practitioners can benefit from alerts of freshly released research and pipeline data via social media networks. Many journals have turned to social media to provide end consumers with updates and healthcare information (Son,2017). Doctors can utilise e-health networks, which are supported by social media devices, to access forums, seek or share medical knowledge online, and find literature, permitting them to interact and conveniently connect. Practitioners in e-health organizations may contact each other at any time and from any place in the world, resulting in improved connectivity and information transfer. In e-health communities, the density of the physicians' information dissemination network is generally high, indicating that doctors are closely connected and information is quickly transmitted. Doctors with higher professional titles have geographic features, familiarity, trust, and high degrees of reciprocity in e-health communities, making them more likely to influence the behavior of other doctors and receive duplicate information in the network (Abbasi et al.,2022; Li,2020). Overall, social media provides a great platform for healthcare practitioners to interact, exchange knowledge, and cooperate on projects, hence increasing results from projects and healthcare service quality.

ROLE OF SOCIAL MEDIA IN ENHANCING TELEMEDICINE AND CONSULTATION

The scientific progress of using telecommunications for medical purposes began in the second half of the 18th century and persists to this day. As a result of decades of scientific knowledge growth, the concept and word "telemedicine" originated in the 1970s. Professor Kenneth Bird's research group at Massachusetts General Hospital was instrumental in developing the scientific basis for the telemedicine idea. Professor Bird's group undertook two scientific initiatives to establish a telemedicine network from 1968 to 1976, which included consistent research and the introduction of the word "telemedicine" into scholarly circulation. The group pioneered the measurement of telemedicine's success by evaluating the correctness of remote diagnostic choices made utilizing two-way television communication. Professor Bird's group's scientific research design during this period has become a telemedicine classic (Vladzymyrskyy,2022). Telemedicine is a type of healthcare delivery in which medical treatments are provided remotely using technology. It enables people to consult with healthcare specialists and obtain diagnosis, treatment, and monitoring without having to go to a physical location. Telemedicine makes use of numerous communication technologies to support virtual consultations and the sharing of medical information, such as video conferencing, smartphone applications, and internet portals. It has grown in importance in recent years, particularly with the rise of social media and other digital platforms. Telemedicine has various advantages, including enhanced access to healthcare, patient convenience, and improved healthcare delivery efficiency. It also allows medical practitioners to interact and communicate with one another, improving care coordination and knowledge exchange (Hjelm,2017). The telemedicine business began to rise in the 2000s and is expected to be worth $83.5 billion by 2022. The figure is expected to rise by $101.2 billion by 2023, and an astounding $455.3 billion by 2030 as shown in "Figure 2" (Vaniukov,2023).

Figure 2. Market statistics of telemedicine
Source: Adopted from Vanioukov,2023

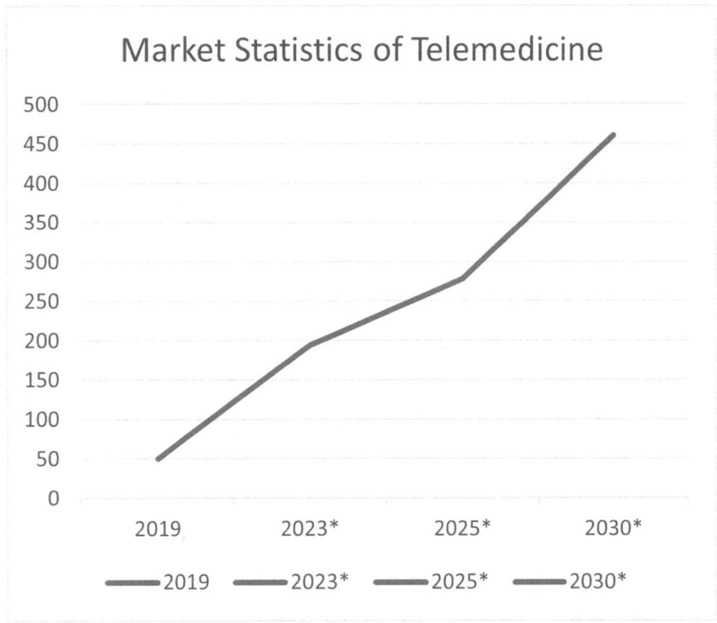

Although patients and health care providers are familiar with social media, which has been widely accessible and used in recent years for interaction and surveillance in healthcare. As a whole, medical treatment has been offered remotely via a variety of telemedicine programs, offering the best access to care for certain populations such as those that live in isolation, have limited access to expert care, or live in rural areas. Similarly, monitoring clients at home and in rural areas with limited access to healthcare may improve healthcare services for those individuals and their neighbourhoods. The majority of healthcare experts feel that social media is a fantastic way for healthcare professionals who want to improve their knowledge and abilities to exchange and spread scientific and technical information (Jayasinghe & Jayasinghe,2023). Social media platforms create a virtual community for medical professionals to network and share knowledge, boosting communication and cooperation in telemedicine. Medical practitioners can follow and analyze discussions on social media, which might be beneficial in telemedicine to keep track of patient progress and make educated choices. Medical practitioners may customize information for specific users via social media, providing that patients receive personalized treatment and guidance via telemedicine. Social media platforms have a vast reach and can swiftly spread information to a large audience, making them a useful tool for telemedicine communication. (Huo et al.,2019; Syed,2021). In line with Creation Pinpoint research, healthcare workers tweet over 152,000 times each day, totalling 208 million tweets since 2006.The study found that healthcare professionals are not just talking to patients, but also networking and exchanging research and resources. And the situation is the same with telemedicine. Social media is a wonderful networking tool for telemedicine and an effective way to communicate with clients; it's a way to learn about what works and what doesn't for providers. It's also possibly the quickest method to learn about anything and everything related to telemedicine happening throughout the world (Price,2014). Healthcare workers may use social media platforms to interact with colleagues, share expertise, and remain up to speed on scientific advances. Doctors, nurses, and other practitioners can participate in professional forums, promoting lifelong learning and helping to raise the level of patient care. Social media for doctors has aided the expansion of telemedicine, particularly during the COVID-19 epidemic. Telemedicine systems use social media networks to link patients and healthcare providers remotely. Patients may make appointments, conduct remote consultations, and get medical information using these platforms, minimizing the need for personal meetings. Social media has a tremendous impact on telemedicine and medical practitioner communication. It provides a public forum for the exchange of ideas, opinions, and material, allowing physicians, patients, and healthcare professionals to interact and debate health-related concerns. Professional networking platforms as well as social networking sites, media sharing platforms, and content production platforms, among others, enable effective communication and engagement between physicians and patients for consultation. During the COVID-19 epidemic, these platforms have grown more significant since they provide a secure and easy manner for healthcare delivery and patient-doctor engagement. Furthermore, social media may be used for teaching and learning, allowing trainees to gain from the skills and knowledge of experienced doctors. In general, social media improves communication and collaboration (Sultan et al.,2021). Social media platforms have become essential instruments in telemedicine and medical professional communication, enhancing elements of telemedicine delivery and professional cooperation. Furthermore, social media enables patient participation through forums, self-management of chronic illnesses, and support networks. On the clinical side, these gatherings allow for multidisciplinary collaboration and knowledge sharing. Also, hospitals and other healthcare organizations must establish their social media policies to join professional groups that offer social media support. Establish explicit procedures to ensure that your employees and contractors ethically use social media. The guidelines must provide clear boundaries to safeguard patients' privacy and security. Training seminars are an excellent way to ensure that everyone understands the rules. Some healthcare professionals may wish to communicate with patients via social media to offer encouragement or pleasant reminders. Healthcare administrators demonstrate to their personnel how to engage with their patients without causing privacy issues or other concerns by establishing regulations (Farsi,2021). Telemedicine, which includes remote counseling and healthcare services, makes use of social media as a tool to promote patient-physician contact to deliver clinical care, diagnosis, and treatment suggestions via digital channels. Medical practitioners combining social media with telemedicine and medical experts not only broadens the scope of health care delivery but also improves the professional atmosphere, encouraging cooperation and information exchange, and eventually improving patient care.rs utilize social media to participate in debates and to share information. Participatory on-the-ground learning and successful research dissemination Immediate and easy access to social media improve cooperation and decision-making, which eventually helps patients.

THE EVOLVING ROLE OF SOCIAL MEDIA IN MEDICAL FORUMS AND GROUPS: CONNECTING BEYOND BORDERS

Individuals can use social media platforms to share, generate, and trade information in a variety of formats, such as text, photographs, videos, voice, or document files. Delivering health information using social media platforms reduces constraints such as time and cost while allowing for information exchange across large distances. Social media platforms can assist in reducing the stigma associated with certain health problems such as epilepsy and obesity by facilitating healthcare education initiatives and encouraging patient self-esteem. Social networks in the form of social media platforms, such as Facebook

Groups and WhatsApp Groups, allow users to interact and communicate with others from all walks of life. Medical forums and organizations provide a space for medical practitioners to debate and share their perspectives, problems, and experiences, which can help to refine and enhance medical education and practice (Zulkefli et al.,2018). Social media platforms have grown from being primarily used for social interaction and news exchange to include lively virtual academic settings. Pathologists from all around the world may communicate, share expertise, and cooperate on these sites. Study reveals Pathology in Nigeria, as in most of Africa, suffers from major knowledge and practice gaps, as well as a lack of contemporary laboratory facilities. Social media is a potentially extremely useful route for addressing some of these shortcomings. Medical forums and groups among medical practitioners are greatly facilitated by social media platforms (Folaranmi et al.,2022). Social media use currently has a substantial influence on political, commercial, and scientific circles, in addition to promoting interactions between individuals. People of many ages, ethnicities, and locations utilise social media for a variety of medical objectives. It enable medical professionals to communicate, share information, and participate in conversations about medical education and practice. Medical forums and groups on social media enable a broader reach and involvement, allowing medical practitioners from all over the world to interact and share information and experiences. Social networking networks enable medical practitioners to seek advice, ask questions, and receive rapid replies from their peers in real time. Medical practitioners may use social media to remain up to speed on the newest research, recommendations, and breakthroughs in their area, increasing their professional growth. Medical practitioners may also use social media to advocate for significant healthcare problems, exchange resources, and cooperate on initiatives. The utilization of social media in medical forums and organizations encourages networking, cooperation, and the exchange of ideas, eventually helping to enhance medical education and practice (Dehmoobad et al.,2019). Professional networking is the practice of forming mutually advantageous relationships with other professionals. Professional networking between various operational units enhances knowledge transfer and the dissemination of ideas inside an organization, possibly leading to increased professional performance. Professional development may be done through collective learning within social groups or networks, according to evolving perspectives on learning such as community of practice and connectivism. Social media applications, through the formation of Web-based communities, may enhance networking and professional growth by allowing interactions between individuals independent of time, location, or region (Rolls et al.,2016). Through applications, websites, and networked devices, health platforms promote the creation, access, and exchange of health knowledge. These platforms attempt to connect self-care users with healthcare practitioners by sharing and reviewing data from sensors in smartphones or wearables. Social media may serve a similar function in facilitating cooperation and information exchange among healthcare professionals and medical students in the context of medical forums and groups. These platforms can provide a forum for conversations, resource sharing, and networking possibilities. Social media may build a feeling of community and ease the flow of information and ideas by linking people with similar interests and skills. Furthermore, social media may be used to disseminate medical research and instructional resources, boosting educational opportunities for medical professionals and students (Rothkrantz,2015). Individuals in comparable situations can contact with others in similar situations via online support groups and forums, fostering a feeling of community and mutual comprehension. Social media may also be used to link people with medical specialists or other resources that might help them. Doctors may utilize social media to form user-generated groups in which they can debate specific medical subjects, share experiences, and seek advice from other experts. User-created groups in health forums enable professionals to establish communities based on common interests or expertise, boosting rapport and involvement among members. Social media platforms enable more effective information exchange and community building throughout the medical profession by allowing professionals to develop their own groups (Rajashri & Malloy,2023). Social media is currently used in many healthcare organisations' marketing and communications initiatives. Over 99 percent of hospitals in the United States have a Facebook page, and an increasing number are also establishing a presence on sites such as Twitter and Instagram. Social networking is no longer considered a luxury. Social networking and advertising are key components of the overall digital marketing strategy for engaging not just with patients but also with medical practitioners on the platforms they choose (Kubheka,2017). Throughout the last decade, there has been an increase in the use of many social and business networking platforms on the web, including as Facebook, Doc2doc, iBibo, LinkedIn, Bharatstudent, and Twitter. In India, there are around 56 million users, and this number is expanding at a pace of 26% per six months. India ranks third in the world with 34 million users, after only the United States (165 million) and Brazil (57 million). Notably, the use of social networking sites by physicians and medical students has increased. According to studies, more than 90% of medical students utilise social networking sites like Facebook and Twitter. These systems have robust communication channels among medical physicians that may be used in several areas of public wellness (Grajales et al.,2014; Visser et al.,2012). Doctors and interns utilize medical forums and groups as platforms to share their tales and experiences, which act as data banks of experience, knowledge, and talent, benefiting both the writers and their colleagues, trainees, and students. Reflective writing in these venues helps practitioners to examine their own decision-making processes, interactions with colleagues, and patient responses, assisting them in analyzing hesitations, gaps in competence and knowledge, and dealing with difficult and traumatic experiences. Writing and debating experiences in a confidential environment also allows colleagues to contribute useful ideas, judgments, and points of view, increasing awareness and knowledge of ethical concerns. Through the writing and debate processes, these platforms may also be used to reduce professional stress (Lainson et al.,2019). Medical practitioners' forums provide a space for exchanging expertise and debating medical matters. Social media may assist in interacting with and engaging a larger audience. Medical professionals' social media platforms boost public health by providing excellent communication and education tools. Medical workers and pupils are increasingly connecting and learning using social media platforms like Facebook, Doc2doc, and LinkedIn. These networks have the ability to benefit public health through efficient interactions and teaching methods (Gulia,2017).

SOCIAL MEDIA IN LEVERAGING PATIENT EDUCATION AND AWARENESS

Social media networks such as Facebook, Twitter, Instagram, and LinkedIn have billions of active members. Healthcare organizations use these channels to reach a large audience. Patients may quickly obtain healthcare updates, suggestions, and resources across regional borders. Social media enables healthcare practitioners to deliver real-time information on health crises, epidemics, and emergency circumstances. During the COVID-19 epidemic, platforms like Twitter were critical for providing the public with real-time information and guidance. Social media acts as a hub for health education. Patients can see articles, films, and infographics about a variety of health subjects. Healthcare organizations utilize these channels to spread information about illnesses, preventive measures, and a nutritious diet. Social media has enabled patients to become more empowered and knowledgeable about their health. They can look up symptoms, remedies, and healthcare professionals' credentials. This knowledge allows people to make educated decisions regarding their health (Chirumamilla,2021). Social media may be used to disseminate critical public health details and educate the public, perhaps enhancing their responsiveness to developing public health challenges. Initially, public awareness campaigns reached their target audience through printed materials, in-person seminars, and television and radio ads. However, with social media being the primary source of information and entertainment for the general population, these platforms may be used to engage with and educate the public on critical public health issues. Public health organizations may use social media to reach new audiences and boost the public's reaction to growing public health challenges. This method can potentially contribute to the digitization of medicine by advancing telemedicine (Garcia et al.,2022). Social media may be used to spread essential public health information and educate the public, perhaps improving their response to emerging public health concerns. Social media has become a primary source of news and communication, with approximately 60% of the worldwide population utilizing it. Social media networks can offer patients selected instructional information about dermatologic disorders. However, it is critical to examine ethical issues and the possibility of disinformation on social media. As social media platforms update their algorithms and content filters, they may become a credible source of patient education in dermatology (Wojtara,2023). The study highlighted that social media is beneficial for patient education in neurosurgery since it improves knowledge by giving access to a diverse set of educational materials and information. Streamlines interaction between patients and neurosurgeons, allowing for a faster and more efficient interaction of information and clarification of questions. Patients and carers are empowered by having a platform to share their personal stories, connect with others going through similar struggles and access support networks. These advantages make social media an effective tool for patient education in neurosurgery, improving the entire patient experience and encouraging informed decision-making. To enable the most effective use of social media in outreach to patients, obstacles such as content accuracy, integrity, privacy, and time management must be addressed (Shlobin et al.,2022). By leveraging its accessibility and communication efficacy, social media may be utilized to execute infection prevention and control techniques in hospital settings through education and awareness campaigns. Social media has been used successfully for teaching and training, education initiatives, risk communication during epidemics, monitoring illnesses, and pharmacovigilance. It provides a rapid and effective manner of connecting with both the general public and health workers, enabling people to make educated decisions and modify their behavior patterns to implement infection control policies. Social media may be used to convey essential public health data as well as educate the public, perhaps increasing their response to emerging public health concerns and control of infections, which are accessible via social media platforms. Social media may play a vital role in generating awareness about infection control measures, helping disrupt the chain of transmission of illnesses, and averting subsequent outbreaks (Jayaprakasam et al.,2021). Social media platforms can promote health promotion and literacy by including people in the administration of their healthcare and treatment. Providing patients with access to pertinent health information and resources that will allow them to make educated health decisions. Providing a platform for healthcare organizations to exchange instructional content, such as films and instructive postings, can help people grasp complicated medical language and instructions. Allowing patients to actively engage in talks and ask questions can help them feel empowered and take control of their healthcare experience. Facilitating peer support and community participation, allowing patients to interact with people who share their health issues and exchange experiences, suggestions, and guidance (Marta et al.,2022). Social media platforms such as Facebook and WhatsApp can improve the reach and effectiveness of public health initiatives, such as patient education and awareness. Social media platforms have the potential to significantly expand the reach and efficiency of critical public health policies or initiatives via social networking mechanisms. Health practitioners, public health organizations, and researchers may use these platforms to gather people's voices, elicit textual descriptions, and create material on a variety of topics. Billions of people benefit from their timely and accessible public health information on illness prevention, diagnosis, treatment, and personal care. Throughout the COVID-19 pandemic, social media was critical in disseminating viral awareness and educating the public about preventative and control techniques like as social distancing, hand cleanliness, mask-wearing, and vaccination. Social media platforms like Twitter and Facebook helped the rapid dissemination of pandemic-related news, affecting a larger audience than the virus itself (Achrekar et al.,2023). During natural catastrophes or public health emergencies, healthcare organizations utilize social media to communicate crises. Urgent notifications, safety recommendations, and evacuation directions may be quickly distributed. Social media has become a crucial tool for healthcare promotion. It connects patients with information, enables people to take charge of their health, and develops a feeling of community. As social media evolves, its function in healthcare promotion will become even more important.

DIFFERENT SOCIAL MEDIA PLATFORMS FOR HEALTHCARE EXPERTS

Social media has influenced healthcare research by making it simpler to exchange data and recruit people. Wearables and personal health monitoring gadgets have become increasingly popular, allowing for remote clinical tracking and data collection. Artificial intelligence, particularly machine learning, has evolved to improve prediction algorithms and aid in decision-making. The confluence of social media, wearables, and artificial intelligence presents unprecedented opportunities for clinical investigation. These digital technologies enable patients to actively engage in their healthcare by monitoring their health and contributing to research (Korjian et al.,2022). Different social media platforms enable medical practitioners to cooperate and engage in a variety of ways. These platforms provide accessible and popular ways for dermatologists to share healthcare information, network, and reach out. They also allow patients, families, and professionals to work together to advance scientific understanding of uncommon illnesses. Social media may be used to obtain health information, and professional clinical knowledge, and participate in research initiatives (Szeto et al.,2023). In addition, social media channels enable the public publication and debate of one-of-a-kind ideas and materials. Doctors and healthcare professionals must communicate with their peers and colleagues to deal with complex health issues. Doctors and healthcare professionals can benefit from social networks specifically created for them. Believe it or not, social networking sites are a double-edged sword for many medical professionals, including doctors, nurses, and other healthcare workers. These channels are critical for communicating with current and prospective patients, obtaining expert guidance, and exploring partnership opportunities. To sum it up, healthcare-oriented social networking sites are particularly intended for healthcare workers to help them exchange advice, information, and other critical resources. Here are some social media channels for healthcare practitioners:

- Sermo - Sermo is the most popular online resource for healthcare workers worldwide. Sermo can build a community of qualified physicians from all over the world, including New Zealanders, Australians, Norwegians, French, Guatemalans, Dutch, Colombians, Irish, Mexicans, Danes, and Finns. This one-of-a-kind network brings together professionals from all around the country to discuss patients' healthcare issues. Sermo also facilitates thorough medical Q&A sessions guided by professionals, which is one of its primary advantages. Sermo now has over 500,000 active users.

- Doximity - In fact, the internet is regarded as one of the most effective communication platforms and marketing tactics available to any organisation. Similarly, to sites like LIhedcare, practitioners may remain in touch with friends, classmates, residents, and other persons they know. It is an online platform that links personnel at prominent hospitals to their colleagues while also allowing one-on-one interactions among users and direct connections with patients. Interestingly, healthcare workers on Doximity can also earn Category 1 CME credit units by reading online journal articles or using HIPAA-compliant private communications within the site.
- QuantiaMD - QuantiaMD offers a variety of brief lectures, as well as possibilities for professionals to address topics and other issues. QuantiaMD is available on any device, enabling for simple transmission of critical information even during morning coffee breaks and working hours. This website offers a variety of brief video presentations addressing various aspects of practice management and clinical concerns.
- Figure 1 - Figure 1 is a platform for healthcare practitioners to exchange illness pictures, including X-ray scans, and engage in conversations with their colleagues. This website allows professionals to network with other doctors while also increasing their understanding of uncommon diseases. Figure 1 is an essential resource for collaborative learning and expertise sharing, especially for healthcare staff attending to patients in remote places.
- Doctorshangout - Doctorshangout is an online social networking site where doctors, inhabitants, and medical students may meet people with similar interests. Doctorshangout members can join a variety of groups depending on their interests. It may help healthcare workers maintain current professional and personal links while also building new ones by linking them with other healthcare professionals worldwide.

CONCLUSION

Social networking sites are invaluable assets that enable healthcare practitioners from all over the world to interact and collaborate. These digital spaces enable unfettered information sharing among professionals as well as worldwide discourse on practice-related subjects. These platforms have a worldwide reach, allowing practitioners to gain cross-cultural knowledge and collaborate on research. At its finest, social media aids in the rapid dissemination of true and accurate information to various groups of people. When the information is scientifically true, clear, and useful, this can be beneficial. This allows for teamwork, information exchange, and advancement in their area. Doctors can learn about novel treatments through social media. It allows them to communicate with other physicians, patients, and anybody else involved in health care. As technology advances, more individuals can be reached through social media. It can assist everyone in healthcare to improve. In this day and age, information flows quickly across borders. A doctor's internet reputation benefits more than simply their employment. It has the potential to alter how we disseminate medical information and collaborate on health solutions. With new platforms and purposes appearing throughout time, these applications will evolve and extend, boosting accessibility and thus creating additional options to employ social media in conjunction with healthcare in the future.

REFERENCES

Abbasi, M. S., Lal, A., Das, G., Salman, F., Akram, A., Ahmed, A. R., . . . Ahmed, N. (2022, October). Impact of Social Media on Aesthetic Dentistry: General Practitioners' Perspectives. In Healthcare (Vol. 10, No. 10, p. 2055). MDPI.

Achrekar, G. C., & Batra, K. (2023). Applications of social media in qualitative research in diverse public health areas. In *Effective Use of Social Media in Public Health* (pp. 193–215). Academic Press. doi:10.1016/B978-0-323-95630-7.00016-0

Ahmed, Y. A., Ahmad, M. N., Ahmad, N., & Zakaria, N. H. (2019). Social media for knowledge-sharing: A systematic literature review. *Telematics and Informatics*, *37*, 72–112. doi:10.1016/j.tele.2018.01.015

Alali, H. (2018). Using Social Media to Improve Knowledge Sharing among Healthcare Practitioners. In *Recent Advances in Mathematical and Statistical Methods: IV AMMCS International Conference, Waterloo, Canada, August 20–25, 2017 IV* (pp. 411-418). Springer International Publishing. 10.1007/978-3-319-99719-3_37

Alasnag, M., Ahmed, W., & Mamas, M. (2021). Best Practices of Social Media for the Clinician. *Current Cardiology Reviews*, *17*(2), 118–121. doi:10.2174/1573403X16666200128101509 PMID:31994467

Bhasin, N. (2017). Why all doctors and medical institutions need to embrace social media: #socialmediadoctors. *Journal of Surgical Simulation*, *41–43*, 41–43. Advance online publication. doi:10.1102/2051-7726.2017.0008

Bosch, B., & Mansell, H. (2015). Interprofessional collaboration in health care: Lessons to be learned from competitive sports. *Canadian Pharmacists Journal/Revue des Pharmaciens du Canada, 148*(4), 176-179.

Campbell, L., Evans, Y., Pumper, M., & Moreno, M. A. (2016). Social media use by physicians: A qualitative study of the New Frontier of Medicine. *BMC Medical Informatics and Decision Making*, *16*(1), 91. Advance online publication. doi:10.1186/s12911-016-0327-y PMID:27418201

Chaudhuri, A., & Prendes, C. F. (2023). Social Media and EJVES 2013–2023: From Inception to Evolution. *European Journal of Vascular and Endovascular Surgery*, *65*(6), 769–771. doi:10.1016/j.ejvs.2023.04.012 PMID:37084879

Chiang, A. L. (2021). Navigating and Leveraging Social Media. *Gastrointestinal Endoscopy Clinics of North America*, *31*(4), 695–707. doi:10.1016/j.giec.2021.05.006 PMID:34538409

Chirumamilla, S., & Gulati, M. (2021). Patient education and engagement through social media. *Current Cardiology Reviews*, *17*(2), 137–143. PMID:31752656

Dehmoobad Sharifabadi, A., Clarkin, C., & Doja, A. (2019). Perceptions of competency-based medical education from medical student discussion forums. *Medical Education*, *53*(7), 666–676. doi:10.1111/medu.13803 PMID:30690769

El Kheir, D. Y., AlShammari, R. Z., Alamri, R. A., & AlShamsi, R. A. (2022). Social Media and medical applications in the healthcare context: Adoption by medical interns. *Saudi Journal of Health Systems Research, 2*(1), 32–41. doi:10.1159/000521635

Farsi, D. (2021). Social media and health care, part I: Literature review of social media use by health care providers. *Journal of Medical Internet Research, 23*(4), e23205. doi:10.2196/23205 PMID:33664014

Folaranmi, O. O., Ibiyeye, K. M., Odetunde, O. A., & Kerr, D. A. (2022). The influence of social media in promoting knowledge acquisition and pathology excellence in Nigeria. *Frontiers in Medicine, 9*, 906950. doi:10.3389/fmed.2022.906950 PMID:35721068

García, M. J. C., Ramírez, S. I. Q., Gómez, G. A. N., Serrano, E. V., García, D. L. C., Cantón, C. V., . . . de los Ángeles Segura-Azuara, N. (2022). Social Media Campaign as a Tool for Patient Education of Disease Prevention and Health Promotion: Digital Health Campaign on Osteoporosis Knowledge. In Advancing Health Education With Telemedicine (pp. 183-208). IGI Global.

Giroux, C. M., & Moreau, K. A. (2020). Leveraging social media for medical education: Learning from patients in online spaces. *Medical Teacher, 42*(9), 970–972. doi:10.1080/0142159X.2020.1779920 PMID:32552288

Grajales, F. J. III, Sheps, S., Ho, K., Novak-Lauscher, H., & Eysenbach, G. (2014). Social media: A review and tutorial of applications in medicine and health care. *Journal of Medical Internet Research, 16*(2), e2912. doi:10.2196/jmir.2912 PMID:24518354

Gulia, A. (2017). Social media in medical practice: A boon or bane. *Indian Journal of Medical Sciences, 69*(1), 1. doi:10.18203/issn.0019-5359.IndianJMedSci20170480

Hjelm, N. M. (2017). *Benefits and drawbacks of telemedicine* (2nd ed.). Introduction to Telemedicine.

Huo, J., Desai, R., Hong, Y. R., Turner, K., Mainous, A. G. III, & Bian, J. (2019). Use of social media in health communication: Findings from the health information national trends survey 2013, 2014, and 2017. *Cancer Control, 26*(1). doi:10.1177/1073274819841442 PMID:30995864

Jayaprakasam, M. (2021). Use of "Social Media"-an Option for Spreading Awareness in Infection Prevention. *Current Treatment Options in Infectious Diseases, 13*(1), 1–18. doi:10.1007/s40506-020-00244-3

Jayasinghe, R. M., & Jayasinghe, R. D. (2023). Role of social media in telemedicine. In *Effective Use of Social Media in Public Health* (pp. 317–338). Academic Press. doi:10.1016/B978-0-323-95630-7.00003-2

Korjian, S., & Gibson, C. M. (2022). Digital technologies and the democratization of clinical research: Social media, wearables, and artificial intelligence. *Contemporary Clinical Trials, 117*, 106767. doi:10.1016/j.cct.2022.106767 PMID:35462032

Kubheka, B. (2017). Ethical and legal perspectives on the medical practitioners use of social media. *South African Medical Journal, 107*(5), 386–389. doi:10.7196/SAMJ.2017.v107i5.12047 PMID:28492116

Lainson, K., Braun, V., & Clarke, V. (2019). Being both narrative practitioner and academic researcher: A reflection on what thematic analysis has to offer narratively informed research. *International Journal of Narrative Therapy & Community Work*, (4), 86–98.

Li, Z., & Xu, X. (2020). Analysis of network structure and doctor behaviors in e-health communities from a social-capital perspective. *International Journal of Environmental Research and Public Health*, *17*(4), 1136. doi:10.3390/ijerph17041136 PMID:32053913

Lopez, M., Chan, T. M., Thoma, B., Arora, V. M., & Trueger, N. S. (2019). The social media editor at medical journals: Responsibilities, goals, barriers, and facilitators. *Academic Medicine*, *94*(5), 701–707. doi:10.1097/ACM.0000000000002496 PMID:30334841

Magda, W. (2023). Use of Social Media for Patient Education in Dermatology: Narrative Review. *JMIR Dermatology*, *6*, e42609–e42609. doi:10.2196/42609 PMID:37632938

Marta, M. (2020). Social Media to Improve Health Promotion and Health Literacy for Patients Engagement. doi:10.1007/978-3-030-43993-4_10

Nyström, M. E., Karltun, J., Keller, C., & Andersson Gäre, B. (2018). Collaborative and partnership research for improvement of health and social services: Researcher's experiences from 20 projects. *Health Research Policy and Systems*, *16*(1), 1–17. doi:10.1186/s12961-018-0322-0 PMID:29843735

Patel, M. M., Moseley, T. W., Nia, E. S., Perez, F., Kapoor, M. M., & Whitman, G. J. (2021). Team science: A practical approach to starting collaborative projects. *Journal of Breast Imaging*, *3*(6), 721–726. doi:10.1093/jbi/wbab034 PMID:34805982

Popa, G. (2022, August 8). *Social Media in healthcare: Best practices for professionals*. Creatopy Blog. https://www.creatopy.com/blog/social-media-healthcare/

Price, Y. (2014, November 14). *Impact of social media in healthcare and telemedicine*. https://telemedicine.arizona.edu/blog/impact-social-media-healthcare-and-telemedicine

Quesenberry, K. A. (2020). *Social media strategy: Marketing, advertising, and public relations in the consumer revolution*. Rowman & Littlefield Publishers.

Rajshri, R., & Malloy, J. (2023). Evolving Role of Social Media in Health Promotion. In Health Promotion-Principles and Approaches. IntechOpen. doi:10.5772/intechopen.111967

Rothkrantz, L. (2015). How social media facilitate learning communities and peer groups around MOOCS. *International Journal of Human Capital and Information Technology Professionals*, *6*(1), 1–13. doi:10.4018/ijhcitp.2015010101

Shlobin, N. A., Patel, S., & Dahdaleh, N. S. (2022). Social media as a Tool for Patient Education in Neurosurgery: An overview. *World Neurosurgery*, *161*, 127–134. doi:10.1016/j.wneu.2022.02.054 PMID:35202876

Social media platforms for doctors and healthcare professionals. (2021, November 30). https://www.zealousweb.com/18-niche-social-media-platforms-for-doctors-nurses-and-healthcare-professionals/

Son, Y. J., Jeong, S., Kang, B. G., Kim, S. H., & Lee, S. K. (2015). Visualization of e-Health research topics and current trends using social network analysis. *Telemedicine Journal and e-Health*, *21*(5), 436–442. doi:10.1089/tmj.2014.0172 PMID:25885639

Stephens, H. (2014). Social media and engaging with health providers. *Rare Diseases in the Age of Health, 2*(0), 115–122. doi:10.1007/978-3-642-38643-5_12

Stukus, D. R., Patrick, M. D., Nuss, K. E., & Stukus, D. R. (2019). The role of medical professionals in social media. *Social Media for Medical Professionals: Strategies for Successfully Engaging in an Online World*, 65-82.

Sultan, M., Brown, E. M., & Thomas, R. H. (2021). Clinicians embracing social media: Potential and pitfalls. *Epilepsy & Behavior*, *115*, 106462. doi:10.1016/j.yebeh.2019.106462 PMID:31732329

Syed, S. A. (2021). Changing the paradigm of healthcare after Covid-19-A narrative review. *Pakistan Journal of Science*, *73*(2).

Szeto, M. D., Mamo, A., Afrin, A., Militello, M., & Barber, C. (2021). Social media in dermatology and an overview of popular social media platforms. *Current Dermatology Reports*, *10*(4), 1–8. doi:10.1007/s13671-021-00343-4 PMID:34692234

Vaniukov, S. (2023, August 8). *Telemedicine Trends & Telehealth market size statistics for 2023 - softermii blog*. Softermii. https://www.softermii.com/blog/telemedicine-trends-and-healthcare-market-statistics#form

Ventola, C. L. (2014). Social media and health care professionals: Benefits, risks, and best practices. *P&T*, *39*(7), 491. PMID:25083128

Visser, B. J., Huiskes, F., & Korevaar, D. A. (2012). A social media self-evaluation checklist for medical practitioners. *Indian Journal of Medical Ethics*, *9*(4), 245–248. doi:10.20529/IJME.2012.083 PMID:23099596

Vladzymyrskyy, A. V. (2022). History of the Scientific Rationale of the «Telemedicine» Concept: Professor KT Bird's Research Group Contribution. *History and Modern Perspectives*, *4*(2), 95–103. doi:10.33693/2658-4654-2022-4-2-95-103

Zalatoris, J. J., Scheerer, J. B., & Lebeda, F. J. (2017). Collaborative systems biology projects for the military medical community. *Military Medicine*, *182*(9-10), e1802–e1809. doi:10.7205/MILMED-D-16-00446 PMID:28885940

Zimba, O., & Gasparyan, A. Y. (2021). Social media platforms: a primer for researchers. *Reumatologia/Rheumatology, 59*(2), 68-72.

Zulkefli, N. A., Iahad, N. A., & Yusof, A. F. (2018). Benefits of Social Media Platform in Healthcare. *International Journal of Innovative Computing*, *8*(3). Advance online publication. doi:10.11113/ijic.v8n3.201

Compilation of References

Abantika, G. (2022, April 2). *How AI is changing India's healthcare — it is reading scans, predicting risks & a lot more.* The Print. https://theprint.in/health/how-ai-is-changing-indias-healthcare-its-reading-scans-predicting-risks-a-lot-more/896495/

Abbasi, M. S., Lal, A., Das, G., Salman, F., Akram, A., Ahmed, A. R., . . . Ahmed, N. (2022, October). Impact of Social Media on Aesthetic Dentistry: General Practitioners' Perspectives. In Healthcare (Vol. 10, No. 10, p. 2055). MDPI.

Abdel-Basset, M., Chang, V., & Nabeeh, N. A. (2021). An intelligent framework using disruptive technologies for COVID-19 analysis. *Technological Forecasting and Social Change*, *163*, 163–175. doi:10.1016/j.techfore.2020.120431 PMID:33162617

Abdelrahman, M. (2020). Personality traits, risk perception, and protective behaviors of Arab residents of Qatar during the COVID-19 pandemic. *International Journal of Mental Health and Addiction*, 1–12. PMID:32837433

Abid Haleem, M. J. (2022). Artificial intelligence (AI) applications for marketing: A literature-based study. *International Journal of Intelligent Networks*, 119-132.

Abid Haleem, M. J. (2022). *Medical 4.0 technologies for healthcare: Features, capabilities, and applications. Internet of Things and Cyber-Physical Systems.*

Abid, H., Mohd, J., Pratap, S. R., & Rajiv, S. (2022). Medical 4.0 technologies for healthcare: Features, capabilities, and applications. *Internet of Things and Cyber-Physical Systems, 2*, 12-30. doi:10.1016/j.iotcps.2022.04.001

Abouelmehdi, K., Beni-Hessane, A., & Khaloufi, H. (2018). Big healthcare data: Preserving security and privacy. *Journal of Big Data*, *5*(1), 1–18. doi:10.1186/s40537-017-0110-7

Aceto, G., & Persico, V. (2018). The role of Information and Communication Technologies in Healthcare : The role of Information and Communication Technologies in Healthcare. *Taxonomies, Perspectives, and Challenges.*, (February). Advance online publication. doi:10.1016/j.jnca.2018.02.008

Aceto, G., Persico, V., & Pescapé, A. (2020). Industry 4.0 and health: Internet of things, big data, and cloud computing for healthcare 4.0. *Journal of Industrial Information Integration*, *18*, 100129. doi:10.1016/j.jii.2020.100129

Acharya, A., & Vellakal, S. (2012). mpact of national health insurance for the poor and the informal sector in low- and middle-income countries. Evidence for Policy and Practice Information and Co-ordinating Centre (EPPI-Centre).

Achrekar, G. C., & Batra, K. (2023). Applications of social media in qualitative research in diverse public health areas. In *Effective Use of Social Media in Public Health* (pp. 193–215). Academic Press. doi:10.1016/B978-0-323-95630-7.00016-0

Adewole, K. S., Akintola, A. G., Jimoh, R. G., Mabayoje, M. A., Jimoh, M. K., Usman-Hamza, F. E., Balogun, A. O., Sangaiah, A. K., & Ameen, A. O. (2021). Intelligent IoT Systems in Personalized Health Care. Elsevier.

Adian, Y. A. P., & Budiarto, W. (2020). Literature Review: The Implementation of E-Health At Primary Healthcare Centers in Surabaya City. *Jurnal Administrasi Kesehatan Indonesia*, *8*(1), 40. Advance online publication. doi:10.20473/jaki.v8i1.2020.40-55

Afifah, K., Yulita, I. N., & Sarathan, I. (2021). Sentiment Analysis on Telemedicine App Reviews using XGBoost Classifier. *2021 International Conference on Artificial Intelligence and Big Data Analytics*, 22–27.

Agarkhed, J., Ashalatha, R., & Patil, S. R. (2019). Smart Healthcare Systems Using Cloud Computing Environments. In R. Bera, S. Sarkar, O. Singh, & H. Saikia (Eds.), *Advances in Communication, Devices and Networking. Lecture Notes in Electrical Engineering* (Vol. 537). Springer. doi:10.1007/978-981-13-3450-4_59

Aghdam, Z. N., Rahmani, A. M., & Hosseinzadeh, M. (2021). The role of the Internet of Things in healthcare: Future trends and challenges. *Computer Methods and Programs in Biomedicine*, *199*, 105903. doi:10.1016/j.cmpb.2020.105903 PMID:33348073

Agrawal, A. V., Shashibhushan, G., Pradeep, S., Padhi, S. N., Sugumar, D., & Boopathi, S. (2024). Synergizing Artificial Intelligence, 5G, and Cloud Computing for Efficient Energy Conversion Using Agricultural Waste. In B. K. Mishra (Ed.), Practice, Progress, and Proficiency in Sustainability. IGI Global. doi:10.4018/979-8-3693-1186-8.ch026

Ahmed, Y. A., Ahmad, M. N., Ahmad, N., & Zakaria, N. H. (2019). Social media for knowledge-sharing: A systematic literature review. *Telematics and Informatics*, *37*, 72–112. doi:10.1016/j.tele.2018.01.015

Ahsan, M. M., Ahad, M. T., Soma, F. A., Paul, S., Chowdhury, A., Luna, S. A., Yazdan, M. M. S., Rahman, A., Siddique, Z., & Huebner, P. (2021). Detecting SARS-CoV-2 From Chest X-Ray Using Artificial Intelligence. *IEEE Access : Practical Innovations, Open Solutions*, *9*, 35501–35513. doi:10.1109/ACCESS.2021.3061621 PMID:34976572

Akbari, A., Haghverd, F., & Behbahani, S. (2021). Robotic Home-Based Rehabilitation Systems Design: From a Literature Review to a Conceptual Framework for Community-Based Remote Therapy During COVID-19 Pandemic. *Frontiers in Robotics and AI*, *8*(June), 1–34. doi:10.3389/frobt.2021.612331 PMID:34239898

Akkaş, M. A., Sokullu, R., & Ertürk Çetin, H. (2020). Healthcare and patient monitoring using IoT. *Internet of Things : Engineering Cyber Physical Human Systems*, *11*, 100173. doi:10.1016/j.iot.2020.100173

Alali, H. (2018). Using Social Media to Improve Knowledge Sharing among Healthcare Practitioners. In *Recent Advances in Mathematical and Statistical Methods: IV AMMCS International Conference, Waterloo, Canada, August 20–25, 2017 IV* (pp. 411-418). Springer International Publishing. 10.1007/978-3-319-99719-3_37

Alasnag, M., Ahmed, W., & Mamas, M. (2021). Best Practices of Social Media for the Clinician. *Current Cardiology Reviews*, *17*(2), 118–121. doi:10.2174/1573403X16666200128101509 PMID:31994467

Albanians, L. (2023, September 14). *The importance of patient engagement: A comprehensive overview.* Retrieved from nasscom: https://community.nasscom.in/communities/application/importance-patient-engagement-comprehensive-overview

Alekya, R., Boddeti, N.D., Monica, K.S., Prabha, D.R., & Venkatesh, D.V. (2021). *IoT based Smart Healthcare Monitoring Systems: A Literature Review*. Academic Press.

Ali, O., Shrestha, A., Soar, J., & Wamba, S. F. (2018). Cloud computing-enabled healthcare opportunities, issues, and applications: A systematic review. *International Journal of Information Management*, *43*, 146–158. doi:10.1016/j.ijinfomgt.2018.07.009

Alshamrani, M. (2022). IoT and artificial intelligence implementations for remote healthcare monitoring systems: A survey. *Journal of King Saud University. Computer and Information Sciences*, *34*(8), 4687–4701. doi:10.1016/j.jksuci.2021.06.005

Altimier, L., & Phillips, R. (2016). The Neonatal Integrative Developmental Care Model: Advanced Clinical Applications of the Seven Core Measures for Neuroprotective Family-centered Developmental Care. *Newborn and Infant Nursing Reviews; NAINR, 16*(4), 230–244. doi:10.1053/j.nainr.2016.09.030

Amboage, E. S., Fernández, V. A., Boga, O. J., & Fernández, M. M. (2019). Redes sociales y promoción de destinos turísticos termales de la Eurorregión Galicia-Norte de Portugal. *Observatorio (OBS*), 13*(1), 137-152. doi:10.15847/obsOBS13120191108

Amlung, J., Huth, H., Cullen, T., & Sequist, T. (2020). Modernizing health information technology: Lessons from healthcare delivery systems. *JAMIA Open, 3*(3), 369–377. doi:10.1093/jamiaopen/ooaa027 PMID:33215072

Anaya-Aguilar, R., Gemar, G., & Anaya-Aguilar, C. (2021). Usability Analysis of Andalusian Spas' Websites. *Sustainability (Basel), 13*(4), 1–14. doi:10.3390/su13042307

Anderl, I. (2014, October 9). Industrie 4.0 – advanced engineering of smart products and smart production, technological innovations in product development. *19th International Seminar on High Technology*, 1-14.

Anderson, J. G., & Balas, E. A. (2006). Computerization of primary care in the United States. *International Journal of Healthcare Information Systems and Informatics, 1*(3), 1–23. doi:10.4018/jhisi.2006070101

Angell, B. J., Prinja, S., Gupt, A., Jha, V., & Jan, S. (2019). The Ayushman Bharat Pradhan Mantri Jan Arogya Yojana and the path to universal health coverage in India: overcoming the challenges of stewardship and governance in India: overcoming the challenges of stewardship and governance. *PLoS Medicine, 16*(3), e1002759. doi:10.1371/journal.pmed.1002759 PMID:30845199

Anitha, C., R, K. C., Vivekanand, C. V., Lalitha, S. D., Boopathi, S., & R, Revathi. (2023, February). Artificial Intelligence driven security model for Internet of Medical Things (IoMT). *IEEE Explore*. doi:10.1109/ICIPTM57143.2023.10117713

Antunes, J., & Rita, P. (2007). O marketing relacional e a fidelização de clientes - Estudo aplicado ao termalismo português. *Global Economics and Management Review, 12*(2), 109–132.

Arosa-Carrera, C., & Chica-Mesa, J. C. (2020). La innovación en el paradigma del marketing relacional. *Journal of Management and Economics for Iberoamerica, 36*(154), 114–122. doi:10.18046/j.estger.2020.154.3494

Ashish, R. (2010). A Model Based Approach to Implement Cloud Computing in E-Governance. *International Journal of Computer Application, 9*(7).

Ayesha Amjad, P. K. (2023). A Review on Innovation in Healthcare Sector (Telehealth) through Artificial Intelligence. *Sustainability*.

Ayodele, A. (2023, June 30). *Five Social Media Platforms That Can Help Healthcare Organizations Boost Their Online Presence.* Retrieved from Linkedin: https://www.linkedin.com/pulse/five-social-media-platforms-can-help-healthcare-boost-adedotun/

Azzawi, M. A., Hassan, R., & Bakar, K. A. A. (2016). A review on Internet of Things (IoT) in healthcare. *International Journal of Applied Engineering Research: IJAER, 11*, 10216–10221.

Babakerkhell & Pandey. (2019). Analysis of Different IOT Based Healthcare Monitoring Systems. *International Journal of Innovative Technology and Exploring Engineering, 8*(6S2).

Babar, M. I., Jehanzeb, M., Ghazali, M., Jawawi, D. N., Sher, F., & Ghayyur, S. A. K. (2016, October). Big data survey in healthcare and a proposal for intelligent data diagnosis framework. *2016 2nd IEEE International Conference on Computer and Communications (ICCC)*, 7-12. 10.1109/CompComm.2016.7924654

Babu, B. S., Kamalakannan, J., Meenatchi, N., M, S. K. S., S, K., & Boopathi, S. (2023). Economic impacts and reliability evaluation of battery by adopting Electric Vehicle. *IEEE Explore*, 1–6. doi:10.1109/ICPECTS56089.2022.10046786

Babu, S. K., Vasavi, S., & Nagarjuna, K. (2017, January). Framework for Predictive Analytics as a Service using ensemble model. *2017 IEEE 7th International Advance Computing Conference (IACC)*, 121-128. 10.1109/IACC.2017.0038

Bajaj, S. (2023). *Digital health for all: Importance of digital healthcare in India.* New Delhi: Times of India.

Bajdor, P., & Starostka-Patyk, M. (2021). The internet of things in healthcare management: Potential applications and challenges. *Smart Healthcare Monitoring Using IoT with 5G. Challenges, Directions, and Future Predictions*, *18*(3), 1–21. doi:10.1201/9781003171829-1

Baker, D. P., Salas, E., & Barach, P. (2006). *E Vidence -B Ased R Elation*. Academic Press.

Bakshi, H., Sharma, R., & Kumar, P. (2018). yushman Bharat Initiative (2018): What we stand to gain or lose! *Indian Journal of Community Medicine*, *43*, 63. PMID:29899601

Basiratzadeh, S., Lemaire, E. D., & Baddour, N. (2022). A Novel Augmented Reality Mobile-Based Application for Biomechanical Measurement. *BioMed*, *2*(2), 255–269. doi:10.3390/biomed2020021

Battineni, E. (2020). Factors affecting the quality and reliability of online health information. *Digital Health, 6.*

Bennett, C. L., & James, A. H. (2022). quality improvement. *Clinical Leadership in Nursing and Healthcare*, 337-353. doi:10.1002/9781119869375.ch16

Berlet, M., Vogel, T., Gharba, M., Eichinger, J., Schulz, E., Friess, H., Wilhelm, D., Ostler, D., & Kranzfelder, M. (2022). Emergency telemedicine mobile ultrasounds using a 5G-enabled application: Development and usability study. *JMIR Formative Research*, *6*(5), e36824. doi:10.2196/36824 PMID:35617009

Bernstein, C. (2022). *Digital health (digital healthcare).* Retrieved from TechTarget: https://www.techtarget.com/searchhealthit/definition/digital-health-digital-healthcare

Bhasin, N. (2017). Why all doctors and medical institutions need to embrace social media: #socialmediadoctors. *Journal of Surgical Simulation*, *41–43*, 41–43. Advance online publication. doi:10.1102/2051-7726.2017.0008

Bhattacharya, S. (2023). The impact of 5g technologies on healthcare. *Indian Journal of Surgery*, *85*(3), 531–535. doi:10.1007/s12262-022-03514-0

Birje, M. N. (2020). Internet of things based distributed healthcare systems: A reviewJ. Data. *Information & Management*, *2*(3), 149–165.

Birje, M. N., & Hanji, S. S. (2020). Internet of things based distributed healthcare systems: A review. *J. Data Inf. Manag.*, *2*(3), 149–165. doi:10.1007/s42488-020-00027-x

Black, A. D., Car, J., Pagliari, C., Anandan, C., Cresswell, K., Bokun, T., & Sheikh, A. (2011). The Impact of eHealth on the Quality and Safety of Health Care: A Systematic Overview. *PLoS Medicine*, *8*(1), e1000387. Advance online publication. doi:10.1371/journal.pmed.1000387 PMID:21267058

Blake, M. B. (2015). An internet of things for healthcare. *IEEE Internet Computing*, *19*(4), 4–6. doi:10.1109/MIC.2015.89

Boopathi, S., Arigela, S. H., Raman, R., Indhumathi, C., Kavitha, V., & Bhatt, B. C. (2023). Prominent Rule Control-based Internet of Things: Poultry Farm Management System. *IEEE Explore*, 1–6. doi:10.1109/ICPECTS56089.2022.10047039

Boopathi, S., Khare, R., Jaya Christiyan, K. G., Muni, T. V., & Khare, S. (2023). Additive manufacturing developments in the medical engineering field. In Development, Properties, and Industrial Applications of 3D Printed Polymer Composites (pp. 86–106). IGI Global. doi:10.4018/978-1-6684-6009-2.ch006

Boopathi, S. (2019). Experimental investigation and parameter analysis of LPG refrigeration system using Taguchi method. *SN Applied Sciences*, *1*(8), 892. Advance online publication. doi:10.1007/s42452-019-0925-2

Boopathi, S. (2022). An Extensive Review on Sustainable Developments of Dry and Near-Dry Electrical Discharge Machining Processes. *Journal of Manufacturing Science and Engineering*, *144*(5), 50801. doi:10.1115/1.4052527

Boopathi, S. (2023a). *Deep Learning Techniques Applied for Automatic Sentence Generation*. doi:10.4018/978-1-6684-3632-5.ch016

Boopathi, S. (2023b). *Internet of Things-Integrated Remote Patient Monitoring System*. doi:10.4018/978-1-6684-6894-4.ch008

Boopathi, S. (2023c). *Securing Healthcare Systems Integrated With IoT*. doi:10.4018/978-1-6684-6894-4.ch010

Boopathi, S., & Kanike, U. K. (2023). Applications of Artificial Intelligent and Machine Learning Techniques in Image Processing. In B. K. Pandey, D. Pandey, R. Anand, D. S. Mane, & V. K. Nassa (Eds.), Advances in Computational Intelligence and Robotics. IGI Global. doi:10.4018/978-1-6684-8618-4.ch010

Boopathi, S., Pandey, B. K., & Pandey, D. (2023). Advances in Artificial Intelligence for Image Processing: Techniques, Applications, and Optimization. In B. K. Pandey, D. Pandey, R. Anand, D. S. Mane, & V. K. Nassa (Eds.), Advances in Computational Intelligence and Robotics. IGI Global. doi:10.4018/978-1-6684-8618-4.ch006

Bosch, B., & Mansell, H. (2015). Interprofessional collaboration in health care: Lessons to be learned from competitive sports. *Canadian Pharmacists Journal/Revue des Pharmaciens du Canada, 148*(4), 176 179.

Bossen, C., & Piras, E. M. (2020). Introduction to the Special Issue on Information Infrastructures in Healthcare: Governance, Quality Improvement and Service Efficiency. *Computer Supported Cooperative Work*, *29*(4), 381–386. doi:10.1007/s10606-020-09381-1

Bouazzi, I., Zaidi, M., Usman, M., Shamim, M. Z., Gunjan, V. K., & Singh, N. (2022). Future Trends for Healthcare Monitoring System in Smart Cities Using LoRaWAN-Based WBAN. *Mobile Information Systems*, *2022*, 1–12. doi:10.1155/2022/1526021

Boyd, A., & Chaffee, B. (2019). Critical Evaluation of Pharmacy Automation and Robotic Systems: A Call to Action. *Hospital Pharmacy*, *54*(1), 4–11. doi:10.1177/0018578718786942 PMID:30718928

Braithwaite, J., Glasziou, P., & Westbrook, J. (2020). The three numbers you need to know about healthcare: The 60-30-10 challenge. *BMC Medicine*, *18*(1), 1–8. doi:10.1186/s12916-020-01563-4 PMID:32362273

Brenas, J. H., & Shaban-Nejad, A. (2020). Health intervention evaluation using semantic explainability and causal reasoning. *IEEE Access : Practical Innovations, Open Solutions*, *8*, 9942–9952. doi:10.1109/ACCESS.2020.2964802

Brenner, S. (2023). Government health insurance and spatial peer effects: New evidence from India. *Social Science & Medicine*, 196.

Bricci, L., Fragata, A., & Antunes, J. (2016). The Effects of Trust, Commitment and Satisfaction on Customer Loyalty in the Distribution Sector. Journal of Economics. *Business and Management*, *4*(2), 174–177. doi:10.7763/JOEBM.2016.V4.386

Burbano-Perez, Á. B., Velástegui-Carrasco, E. B., Villamarin-Padilla, J. M., & Novillo-Yaguarshungo, C. E. (2018). El marketing relacional y la fidelización del cliente. *Polo del conocimiento, 3*(8), 579-590. doi:10.23857/pc.v3i8.683

Burns, M., Bally, J., Burles, M., Holtslander, L., & Peacock, S. (2022). Constructivist grounded theory or interpretive phenomenology? Methodological choices within specific study contexts. *International Journal of Qualitative Methods, 21*, 16094069221077758. doi:10.1177/16094069221077758

Buyya, R., Yeo, C. S., Venugopal, S., Broberg, J., & Brandic, I. (2009). Cloud computing and emerging IT platforms: Vision, hype, and reality for delivering computing as the 5th utility. *Future Generation Computer Systems, 25*(6), 599–616. doi:10.1016/j.future.2008.12.001

C., S. (2023, June 23). *Wearable Devices and IoT in Healthcare: Revolutionizing Patient Monitoring and Transforming the Healthcare Industry.* Retrieved from Linkedin: https://www.linkedin.com/pulse/wearable-devices-iot-healthcare-revolutionizing-patient-chhabra/

Calabrò, R. S., Sorrentino, G., Cassio, A., Mazzoli, D., Andrenelli, E., Bizzarini, E., Campanini, I., Carmignano, S. M., Cerulli, S., Chisari, C., Colombo, V., Dalise, S., Fundarò, C., Gazzotti, V., Mazzoleni, D., Mazzucchelli, M., Melegari, C., Merlo, A., Stampacchia, G., ... Bonaiuti, D. (2021). robotic-assisted gait rehabilitation following stroke: A systematic review of current guidelines and practical clinical recommendations. *European Journal of Physical and Rehabilitation Medicine, 57*(3), 460–471. doi:10.23736/S1973-9087.21.06887-8 PMID:33947828

Campbell, L., Evans, Y., Pumper, M., & Moreno, M. A. (2016). Social media use by physicians: A qualitative study of the New Frontier of Medicine. *BMC Medical Informatics and Decision Making, 16*(1), 91. Advance online publication. doi:10.1186/s12911-016-0327-y PMID:27418201

Capraro, G. T. (2016). Artificial Intelligence (AI), Big Data, and Healthcare. *Proceedings of the International Conference on Artificial Intelligence (ICAI)*, 425.

Carvalho and Cazarini. (2020). *Industry 4.0 - What Is It?* Núbia Gabriela Pereira Carvalho and Edson Walmir Cazarini. IntechOpen., doi:10.5772/intechopen.90068

Castral, T. C., Bueno, M., Carvalho, J. C., Warnock, F., Sousa, J. C. G. D., Ribeiro, L. M., & Mendonça, A. K. M. S. (2023). Implementation of a knowledge translation and exchange intervention for pain management in neonates. *Acta Paulista de Enfermagem, 36*. Advance online publication. doi:10.37689/acta-ape/2023ARSPE024073

Chandra Saha, B., Sai Thrinath, B. V., Boopathi, S., Ramya, J., & Sudhakar, M. (n.d.). IOT BASED SMART ENERGY METER FOR. *Smart Grid.*

Chaudhuri, A., & Prendes, C. F. (2023). Social Media and EJVES 2013–2023: From Inception to Evolution. *European Journal of Vascular and Endovascular Surgery, 65*(6), 769–771. doi:10.1016/j.ejvs.2023.04.012 PMID:37084879

Chauhan, R., & Kumar, A. (2013). Cloud Computing for Improved Healthcare: Techniques, Potential, and Challenges. *4th IEEE International Conference on E-Health and Bioengineering*, 1-4. 10.1109/EHB.2013.6707234

Cheng, C. H., Kuo, Y. H., & Zhou, Z. (2018). Tracking nosocomial diseases at individual level with a real-time indoor positioning system. *Journal of Medical Systems, 42*(11), 1–21. doi:10.1007/s10916-018-1085-4 PMID:30284042

Chiang, A. L. (2021). Navigating and Leveraging Social Media. *Gastrointestinal Endoscopy Clinics of North America, 31*(4), 695–707. doi:10.1016/j.giec.2021.05.006 PMID:34538409

Chirumamilla, S., & Gulati, M. (2021). Patient education and engagement through social media. *Current Cardiology Reviews, 17*(2), 137–143. PMID:31752656

Chowdary, M. (2023). *The Future of Digital Health in India*. https://www.linkedin.com/pulse/future-digital-health-india-promising-trends-watch-meghana-chowdary-1c/

Christopher, M., Payne, A., & Ballantyne, D. (2013). *Relationship Marketing*. Elsevier. doi:10.4324/9780080516042

Christoph, J., Griebel, L., Leb, I., Engel, I., Kopcke, F., Toddenroth, D., Prokosch, H.-U., Laufer, J., Marquardt, K., & Sedlmayr, M. (2015). Secure secondary use of clinical data with cloud-based NLP services: Towards a highly scalable research infrastructure. *Methods of Information in Medicine*, *53*(6), 276–282. doi:10.3414/ME13-01-0133 PMID:25377309

Chuke, A., Hendricks, J., Wurz, J., & Shudes, C. (2021) Digital transformation, From a buzzword to an imperative for health systems. *Deloitte Insights*. https://www2.deloitte.com/us/en/insights/industry/health-care/digital-transformation-in-healthcare.html

Chute, D. C. (2022). *Chesapeake regional information system for our patients (CRISP)*. Retrieved from Johns Hopkins Institute for Clinical & Translational Research: https://ictr.johnshopkins.edu/service/informatics/crisp/

Classen, D. C., Holmgren, A. J., Newmark, L. P., Seger, D., Danforth, M., & Bates, D. W. (2020). National trends in the safety performance of electronic health record systems from 2009 to 2018. *JAMA Network Open*, *3*(5), e205547–e205547. doi:10.1001/jamanetworkopen.2020.5547 PMID:32469412

Crear-Perry, J., Correa-de-Araujo, R., Lewis Johnson, T., McLemore, M. R., Neilson, E., & Wallace, M. (2021). Social and structural determinants of health inequities in maternal health. *Journal of Women's Health*, *30*(2), 230–235. doi:10.1089/jwh.2020.8882 PMID:33181043

Cristobal-Fransi, E., Daries, N., del Rio-Rama, M., & Fuentes-Tierno, M. G. (2023). The challenge of digital marketing in health tourism: The case of Spanish health resorts. *Quality & Quantity*. Advance online publication. doi:10.1007/s11135-023-01744-2

Cunha, B., Ferreira, R., & Sousa, A. S. P. (2023). Home-Based Rehabilitation of the Shoulder Using Auxiliary Systems and Artificial Intelligence: An Overview. *Sensors (Basel)*, *23*(16), 1–22. doi:10.3390/s23167100 PMID:37631637

Currie, W., & Seddon, J. (2013). A cross-country study of cloud computing policy and regulation in healthcare. *The European Conference on Information Systems*, 1–16. 10.1016/j.hlpt.2013.09.003

da Rosa, V. M., Saurin, T. A., Tortorella, G. L., Fogliatto, F. S., Tonetto, L. M., & Samson, D. (2021). Digital technologies: An exploratory study of their role in the resilience of healthcare services. *Applied Ergonomics*, *97*, 103517. doi:10.1016/j.apergo.2021.103517 PMID:34261003

Darshan, K. R., & Anandakumar, K. R. (2015). A comprehensive review on usage of Internet of Things (IoT) in healthcare system. *2015 International Conference on Emerging Research in Electronics, Computer Science and Technology (ICERECT)*, 132–136. 10.1109/ERECT.2015.7499001

Darwish, A., Hassanien, A. E., Elhoseny, M., Sangaiah, A. K., & Muhammad, K. (2019). The impact of the hybrid platform of internet of things and cloud computing on healthcare systems: Opportunities, challenges, and open problems. *Journal of Ambient Intelligence and Humanized Computing*, *10*(10), 4151–4166. doi:10.1007/s12652-017-0659-1

Dash, S., Shakyawar, S. K., Sharma, M., & Kaushik, S. (2019). big data in healthcare: Management, analysis and future prospects. *Journal of Big Data*, *6*(1), 54. doi:10.1186/s40537-019-0217-0

Davenport, T., & Kalakota, R. (2019). The potential for artificial intelligence in healthcare. *Future Health J.*, *6*(2), 94-98. https://csd.columbia.edu/sites/default/files/content/docs/ICT%20India/Papers/ICT_India_Working_Paper_43.p doi:10.7861/futurehosp.6-2-94

De Silva, D., Burstein, F., Jelinek, H. F., & Stranieri, A. (2015). Addressing the complexities of big data analytics in healthcare: The diabetes screening case. *AJIS. Australasian Journal of Information Systems*, *19*, 99–115. doi:10.3127/ajis.v19i0.1183

Dehmoobad Sharifabadi, A., Clarkin, C., & Doja, A. (2019). Perceptions of competency-based medical education from medical student discussion forums. *Medical Education*, *53*(7), 666–676. doi:10.1111/medu.13803 PMID:30690769

Deliana, I. (2024, Jan. 12). *AI-Powered Genomic Analysis: Revolutioning the Detection of Genetic Mutations.* News Medical. https://www.news-medical.net/health/AI-Powered-Genomic-Analysis-Revolutioning-the-Detection-of-Genetic-Mutations.aspx

Desai, N. (2023). *Digital Health in India.* Nishith Desai Associates.

Deshpande, U. U., & Kulkarni, M. A. (2017). IoT based Real Time ECG Monitoring System using Cypress WICED. *International Journal of Advanced Research in Electrical*, *6*(2), 710–720.

Devi, D. H., Duraisamy, K., Armghan, A., Alsharari, M., Aliqab, K., Sorathiya, V., Das, S., & Rashid, N. (2023). 5g technology in healthcare and wearable devices: A review. *Sensors (Basel)*, *23*(5), 2519. doi:10.3390/s23052519 PMID:36904721

Dhanvijay, M. M., & Patil, S. C. (2019). Internet of Things: A survey of enabling technologies in healthcare and its applications. *Computer Networks*, *153*, 113–131. doi:10.1016/j.comnet.2019.03.006

Dhanya, D., Kumar, S. S., Thilagavathy, A., Prasad, D. V. S. S. V., & Boopathi, S. (2023). Data Analytics and Artificial Intelligence in the Circular Economy: Case Studies. In B. K. Mishra (Ed.), Advances in Civil and Industrial Engineering. IGI Global. doi:10.4018/979-8-3693-0044-2.ch003

Digital Transformation in Health Care: Accelerating Innovation and Efficiency. (2023). Retrieved from Evolved Metrics: https://evolvedmetrics.com/digital-transformation-in-health-care/

Dillete, A. K., Douglas, A. C., & Andrzejewski, C. (2020). Dimensions of holistic wellness as a result of international wellness tourism experiences. *Current Issues in Tourism*, *24*(6), 794–810. doi:10.1080/13683500.2020.1746247

Duan, A., Guo, L., Gao, H., Wu, X., & Dong, X. (2020). Deep Focus Parallel Convolutional Neural Network for Imbalanced Classification of Machinery Fault Diagnostics. *IEEE Transactions on Instrumentation and Measurement*, *69*(11), 8680–8689. doi:10.1109/TIM.2020.2998233

Durairaj, M., Jayakumar, S. M., Karpagavalli, V. S., Maheswari, B. U., & Boopathi, S. (2023). Utilization of Digital Tools in the Indian Higher Education System During Health Crises. In C. S. V. Negrão, I. G. P. Maia, & J. A. F. Brito (Eds.), Advances in Logistics, Operations, and Management Science (pp. 1–21). IGI Global. doi:10.4018/978-1-7998-9213-7.ch001

Dwivedi, A., Wickramasinghe, N., Bali, R. K., & Naguib, R. N. G. (2008). Designing intelligent healthcare organisations with KM and ICT. *International Journal of Knowledge Management Studies*, *2*(2), 198–213. doi:10.1504/IJKMS.2008.018321

Ebrahim, R. S. (2020). Articles The Role of Trust in Understanding the Impact of Social Media Marketing on Brand Equity and Brand Loyalty. *Journal of Relationship Marketing*, *19*(4), 287–308. doi:10.1080/15332667.2019.1705742

Edmond Li, J. C. (2021). Electronic Health Records, Interoperability and Patient Safety in Health Systems of High-income Countries: A Systematic Review Protocol. *BMJ Open*. PMID:34261679

Edworthy, S. M. (2001). Telemedicine in developing countries. *British Medical Journal*, *323*(7312), 524–525. doi:10.1136/bmj.323.7312.524 PMID:11546681

E-health resolution. (2005). World Health Organization. Retrieved from http://www.who.int/ healthacademy/ media/en/ eHealth_EB_Res-en.pdf

Ekin, K. (2023, Nov. 24). *The Six main subsets of AI: (Machine Learning, NLP, and more)*. https://www.akkio.com/post/the-five-main-subsets-of-ai-machine-learning--nlp-and-more

Ekso Bionics. (n.d.). *Robotic exoskeleton used during 4 weeks of inpatient gait training*. Ekso-GTWebsite: https://www.eksobionics.com/ekso

El Kheir, D. Y., AlShammari, R. Z., Alamri, R. A., & AlShamsi, R. A. (2022). Social Media and medical applications in the healthcare context: Adoption by medical interns. *Saudi Journal of Health Systems Research*, *2*(1), 32–41. doi:10.1159/000521635

Emeritus. (2023, July 21). *(Some of the) Benefits of AI in Healthcare and How It Improves Patient Care*. https://emeritus.org/blog/ai-andml-benefits-of-ai-in-healthcare/

Faridi, F., Sarwar, H., Ahtisham, M., Kumar, S., & Jamal, K. (2022). Cloud computing approaches in health care. *Materials Today: Proceedings*, *51*, 1217–1223. doi:10.1016/j.matpr.2021.07.210

Farsi, D. (2021). Social media and health care, part I: Literature review of social media use by health care providers. *Journal of Medical Internet Research*, *23*(4), e23205. doi:10.2196/23205 PMID:33664014

Fernandez, F., & Pallis, G. C. (2015). Opportunities and challenges of the Internet of Things for healthcare: Systems engineering perspective. *Proceedings of the 2014 4th International Conference on Wireless Mobile Communication and Healthcare - "Transforming Healthcare Through Innovations in Mobile and Wireless Technologies", MOBIHEALTH 2014*, 263–266. https://doi.org/10.1109/MOBIHEALTH.2014.7015961

FerrerE. C.RudovicO.HardjonoT.PentlandA. (2018). *RoboChain: A Secure Data Sharing Framework for Human-Robot Interaction*. http://arxiv.org/abs/1802.04480

Folaranmi, O. O., Ibiyeye, K. M., Odetunde, O. A., & Kerr, D. A. (2022). The influence of social media in promoting knowledge acquisition and pathology excellence in Nigeria. *Frontiers in Medicine*, *9*, 906950. doi:10.3389/fmed.2022.906950 PMID:35721068

Forestiero, A., & Papuzzo, G. (2018, December). Distributed algorithm for big data analytics in healthcare. In *2018 IEEE/WIC/ACM International Conference on Web Intelligence (WI)*. IEEE Computer Society. 10.1109/WI.2018.00015

Galetsi, P., & Katsaliaki, K. (2020). A review of the literature on big data analytics in healthcare. *The Journal of the Operational Research Society*, *71*(10), 1511–1529. doi:10.1080/01605682.2019.1630328

García, M. J. C., Ramírez, S. I. Q., Gómez, G. A. N., Serrano, E. V., García, D. L. C., Cantón, C. V., . . . de los Ángeles Segura-Azuara, N. (2022). Social Media Campaign as a Tool for Patient Education of Disease Prevention and Health Promotion: Digital Health Campaign on Osteoporosis Knowledge. In Advancing Health Education With Telemedicine (pp. 183-208). IGI Global.

Gassert, R., & Dietz, V. (2018). Rehabilitation robots for the treatment of sensorimotor deficits: A neurophysiological perspective. *Journal of Neuroengineering and Rehabilitation*, *15*(1), 46. doi:10.1186/s12984-018-0383-x PMID:29866106

Gatiti, P., Ndirangu, E., Mwangi, J., Mwanzu, A., & Ramadhani, T. (2021). Enhancing healthcare quality in hospitals through electronic health records: A systematic review. *Journal of Health Informatics in Developing Countries*, *15*(2), 1.

Gbadamosi, A. (2019). Marketing: The Paradigm Shift. In A. Gbadamosi (Ed.), *Contemporary Issues in Marketing* (pp. 1–480). SAGE.

GHA. (2023, January 17). Because both rich and poor countries deserve good health.... *Times of India*, p. 12.

Giroux, C. M., & Moreau, K. A. (2020). Leveraging social media for medical education: Learning from patients in online spaces. *Medical Teacher*, *42*(9), 970–972. doi:10.1080/0142159X.2020.1779920 PMID:32552288

Global Welness Institute. (2018). *The global wellness tourism economy report*. Obtido de https://globalwellnessinstitute.org/industry-research/global-wellness-tourism-economy/

Godinho, T. M., Viana-Ferreira, C., Silva, L. B., & Costa, C. (2016). A routing mechanism for cloud outsourcing of medical imaging repositories. *IEEE Journal of Biomedical and Health Informatics*, *20*(1), 367–375. doi:10.1109/JBHI.2014.2361633 PMID:25343773

Gottlieb, L. K., Stone, E. M., Stone, D., Dunbrack, L. A., & Calladine, J. (2005). Regulatory and Policy Barriers to Effective Clinical Data Exchange: Lessons Learned from Meds Info-ED. *Health Affairs*, *24*(5), 1197–1204. doi:10.1377/hlthaff.24.5.1197 PMID:16162563

Gowsalya, M., Krushitha, K., & Valliyammai, C. (2014, December). Predicting the risk of readmission of diabetic patients using MapReduce. In *2014 Sixth International Conference on Advanced Computing (ICoAC)*. IEEE. 10.1109/ICoAC.2014.7229729

Grajales, F. J. III, Sheps, S., Ho, K., Novak-Lauscher, H., & Eysenbach, G. (2014). Social media: A review and tutorial of applications in medicine and health care. *Journal of Medical Internet Research*, *16*(2), e2912. doi:10.2196/jmir.2912 PMID:24518354

Gravili, G., Benvenuto, M., Avram, A., & Viola, C. (2018). The influence of the Digital Divide on Big Data generation within supply chain management. *International Journal of Logistics Management*, *29*(2), 592–628. doi:10.1108/IJLM-06-2017-0175

Grogan, J. (2006). EHRs and information availability: Are you at risk? *Health Management Technology*, *27*(5), 8–16. PMID:16739432

Grönroos, C. (1997). Value-driven relational marketing: From products to resources and competencies. *Journal of Marketing Management*, *13*(5), 407–419. doi:10.1080/0267257X.1997.9964482

Gül, M., & Gül, K. (2016). Innovative Planning in Thermal Tourism Destinations: Balikesir-Güre Thermal Tourism Destination Case Study. In *Global Issues and Tourism* (pp. 149-162). Academic Press.

Gulia, A. (2017). Social media in medical practice: A boon or bane. *Indian Journal of Medical Sciences*, *69*(1), 1. doi:10.18203/issn.0019-5359.IndianJMedSci20170480

Guo, L., Chen, F., Chen, L., & Tang, X. (2010). The building of cloud computing environment for e-health. *2010 International Conference on E-Health Networking Digital Ecosystems and Technologies (EDT)*. 10.1109/EDT.2010.5496512

Hamdani, S. U., Huma, Z. E., Suleman, N., Warraitch, A., Muzzafar, N., Farzeen, M., Minhas, F. A., Rahman, A., & Wissow, L. S. (2021). Scaling-up school mental health services in low resource public schools of rural Pakistan: The Theory of Change (ToC) approach. *International Journal of Mental Health Systems*, *15*(1), 1–10. doi:10.1186/s13033-021-00435-5 PMID:33436049

Hameed, K., Bajwa, I. S., Sarwar, N., Anwar, W., Mushtaq, Z., & Rashid, T. (2021). Integration of 5G and block-chain technologies in smart telemedicine using IoT. *Journal of Healthcare Engineering*, *2021*, 1–18. doi:10.1155/2021/8814364 PMID:33824715

Han, H., Kiatkawsin, K., Jung, H., & Kim, W. (2018). The role of wellness spa tourism performance in building destination loyalty: The case of Thailand. *Journal of Travel & Tourism Marketing*, *35*(5), 595–610. doi:10.1080/10548408.2017.1376031

Hanley, T., Sefi, A., Grauberg, J., Prescott, J., & Etchebarne, A. (2021). A theory of change for web-based therapy and support services for children and young people: Collaborative qualitative exploration. *JMIR Pediatrics and Parenting*, *4*(1), e23193. doi:10.2196/23193 PMID:33749615

Hansen, S., & Baroody, A. J. (2023). Beyond the boundaries of care: Electronic health records and the changing practices of healthcare. *Information and Organization*, *33*(3), 100477. doi:10.1016/j.infoandorg.2023.100477

Harahap, N. C., Handayani, P. W., & Hidayanto, A. N. (2022). Barriers and facilitators of personal health record adoption in Indonesia: Health facilities' perspectives. *International Journal of Medical Informatics*, *162*, 104750. doi:10.1016/j.ijmedinf.2022.104750 PMID:35339888

Hassan, R. (2023). Digital Health Usage and Awareness among MedicalStudents: A Survey Study. *Open Access Macedonian Journal of Medical Sciences*.

Hathaliya, J. J., & Tanwar, S. (2020). An exhaustive survey on security and privacy issues in Healthcare 4.0. *Computer Communications*, *153*, 311–335. doi:10.1016/j.comcom.2020.02.018

Haux, R. (2006). Health information systems – past, present, future. *International Journal of Medical Informatics*, *75*(3-4), 268–281. doi:10.1016/j.ijmedinf.2005.08.002 PMID:16169771

Hayrinen, K., Saranto, K., & Nykanen, P. (2008). Definition, structure, content, use and impacts of electronic health records: A review of the research literature. *International Journal of Medical Informatics*, *77*(5), 291–304. doi:10.1016/j.ijmedinf.2007.09.001 PMID:17951106

HealthcareRadius. (2021). *Social determinants of health in India*. Retrieved from HealthcareRadius: https://www.healthcareradius.in/uncategorized/29442-social-determinants-of-health-in-india

Hema, N., Krishnamoorthy, N., Chavan, S. M., Kumar, N. M. G., Sabarimuthu, M., & Boopathi, S. (2023). A Study on an Internet of Things (IoT)-Enabled Smart Solar Grid System. In P. Swarnalatha & S. Prabu (Eds.), Advances in Computational Intelligence and Robotics. IGI Global. doi:10.4018/978-1-6684-8098-4.ch017

Heung, V. C., & Kucukusta, D. (2013). Wellness Tourism in China: Resources,Development and Marketing. *International Journal of Tourism Research*, *15*(4), 346–359. doi:10.1002/jtr.1880

Hjelm, N. M. (2017). *Benefits and drawbacks of telemedicine* (2nd ed.). Introduction to Telemedicine.

Hootsuite. (n.d.). *Social Media Analytics in Healthcare: A Complete Guide*. https://blog.hootsuite.com/social-media-analytics-healthcare/amp/

Hossain, M. S., & Muhammad, G. (2016). Cloud-assisted industrial internet of things (iiot)–enabled framework for health monitoring. *Computer Networks*, *101*, 192–202. doi:10.1016/j.comnet.2016.01.009

Howard, R. (2023, Feb. 7). *(Some of the) Opportunities and Challenges of AI in Healthcare*. Forbes Business Council. https://www.forbes.com/sites/forbesbusinesscouncil/2023/02/07/top-five-opportunities-and-challenges-of-ai-in-healthcare/amp/

Hribernik, M., Umek, A., Tomažic, S., & Kos, A. (2022). Review of Real-Time Biomechanical Feedback Systems in Sport and Rehabilitation. *Sensors (Basel)*, *22*(8), 3006. Advance online publication. doi:10.3390/s22083006 PMID:35458991

Hsieh, J. C., & Hsu, M. W. (2012). A cloud computing based 12-lead ECG telemedicine service. *BMC Medical Informatics and Decision Making*, *12*(77), 1–12. doi:10.1186/1472-6947-12-77 PMID:22838382

Huo, J., Desai, R., Hong, Y. R., Turner, K., Mainous, A. G. III, & Bian, J. (2019). Use of social media in health communication: Findings from the health information national trends survey 2013, 2014, and 2017. *Cancer Control*, *26*(1). doi:10.1177/1073274819841442 PMID:30995864

Hussain, W. (2020). Role of social media in COVID-19 pandemic. *The International Journal of Frontier Sciences*, *4*(2), 59–60. doi:10.37978/tijfs.v4i2.144

Ienca, M., & Vayena, E. (2020). On the responsible use of digital data to tackle the Covid-19 pandemic. *Nature Medicine*, *26*(4), 463–464. doi:10.1038/s41591-020-0832-5 PMID:32284619

Indian Express. (2023). *Achievements and challenges of Ayushman Bharat health scheme*. Indian Express.

Infosys, B. P. M. (2023). *The benefits of using predictive analytics in healthcare.* Retrieved from Infosys BPM: https://www.infosysbpm.com/blogs/bpm-analytics/the-benefits-of-using-predictive-analytics-in-healthcare.html#:~:text=Predictive%20analysis%20has%20proven%20effective,and%20prevent%20potentially%20negative%20outcomes

Ingle, R. B., Swathi, S., Mahendran, G., Senthil, T. S., Muralidharan, N., & Boopathi, S. (2023). Sustainability and Optimization of Green and Lean Manufacturing Processes Using Machine Learning Techniques. In N. Cobîrzan, R. Muntean, & R.-A. Felseghi (Eds.), Advances in Finance, Accounting, and Economics. IGI Global. doi:10.4018/978-1-6684-8238-4.ch012

IQVIA. (2023, January 11). IQVIA techies build AI avatar for remote healthcare. Times Techies supplement. *Times of India,* p. 15.

Istepanian, R. S. (2022). Mobile health (m-Health) in retrospect: The known unknowns. *International Journal of Environmental Research and Public Health*, *19*(7), 3747. doi:10.3390/ijerph19073747 PMID:35409431

ITU. (2008). *International Telecommunication Union Radio Communication Sector*. ITU-R.

Jacob, O., Theo, A., Deen, F., Ram, N., & Bryan, R. (2023, February 27). Digital Trace Data (DTD) Collection for Social Media Effects Research: APIs, Data Donation, and (Screen) Tracking. *Communication Methods and Measures*, 1–18. Advance online publication. doi:10.1080/19312458.2023.2181319

Jacobs, B., Ir, P., Bigdeli, M., Annear, P. L., & Van Damme, W. (2012). Addressing access barriers to health services: An analytical framework for selecting appropriate interven- tions in low-income Asian countries. *Health Policy and Planning*, *27*(4), 288–300. doi:10.1093/heapol/czr038 PMID:21565939

Jacofsky, D. J., & Allen, M. (2016). Robotics in Arthroplasty: A Comprehensive Review. *The Journal of Arthroplasty*, *31*(10), 2353–2363. doi:10.1016/j.arth.2016.05.026 PMID:27325369

Jacqueline, M., & Ferguson, J. J. (2021). Virtual care expansion in the Veterans Health Administration during the COVID-19 pandemic: Clinical services and patient characteristics associated with utilization. *Journal of the American Medical Informatics Association : JAMIA*, 453–462. PMID:33125032

Jaffar Abbas, J. A. (2019). The Impact of Social Media on Learning Behavior for Sustainable Education: Evidence of Students from Selected Universities in Pakistan. *Sustainability*.

Jain, S. (2020). Healthcare goes mobile: Evolution of teleconsultation and e-pharmacy in new Normal. *EY, 37*(5).

Jakovljevic, M., Lamnisos, D., Westerman, R., Chattu, V. K., & Cerda, A. (2022). Future health spending forecast in leading emerging BRICS markets in 2030: Health policy implications. *Health Research Policy and Systems*, *20*(1), 23. doi:10.1186/s12961-022-00822-5 PMID:35183217

Jalali, A., & Lee, M. (2020). Atrial Fibrillation Prediction with Residual Network Using Sensitivity and Orthogonality Constraints. *IEEE Journal of Biomedical and Health Informatics*, *24*(2), 407–413. doi:10.1109/JBHI.2019.2957809 PMID:31825883

Jamal, H., & Mahar, M. J. (2019, March 1). *The Future of Telemedicine (and What's in the Way).* Retrieved from Consult QD: https://consultqd.clevelandclinic.org/the-future-of-telemedicine-and-whats-in-the-way/

Javaid, M., & Haleem, A. (2019). Industry 4.0 applications in the medical field: A brief review. *Current Medicine Research and Practice*, *9*(3), 102–109. doi:10.1016/j.cmrp.2019.04.001

Javaid, M., Haleem, A., Singh, R. P., Rab, S., Suman, R., & Khan, I. H. (2022). Evolutionary trends in progressive cloud computing-based healthcare: Ideas, enablers, and barriers. *International Journal of Cognitive Computing in Engineering*, *3*, 124–135. doi:10.1016/j.ijcce.2022.06.001

Javaid, M., Haleem, A., Vaishya, R., Bahl, S., Suman, R., & Vaish, A. (2020). Industry 4.0 technologies and their applications in fighting the Covid-19 pandemic. *Diabetes & Metabolic Syndrome*, *14*(4), 419–422. doi:10.1016/j.dsx.2020.04.032 PMID:32344370

Jayaprakasam, M. (2021). Use of "Social Media"-an Option for Spreading Awareness in Infection Prevention. *Current Treatment Options in Infectious Diseases*, *13*(1), 1–18. doi:10.1007/s40506-020-00244-3

Jayaprinkya, J. (2023, June 30). Artificial Intelligence in Indian Healthcare: A promising future with challenges. *Hindu Business Line*. https://www.thehindubusinessline.com/news/science/artificial-intelligence-in-indian-healthcare-a-promising-future-with-challenges/article67015361.ccc/amp/

Jayasinghe, R. M., & Jayasinghe, R. D. (2023). Role of social media in telemedicine. In *Effective Use of Social Media in Public Health* (pp. 317–338). Academic Press. doi:10.1016/B978-0-323-95630-7.00003-2

Jean, C. H. (2008). *Implementing e-Health in developing countries, guidance, and principles*. Retrieved from www.itu.int/ITU-D/cyb/

Jeevanantham, Y. A., A, S., V, V., J, S. Isaac., Boopathi, S., & Kumar, D. P. (2023). Implementation of Internet-of Things (IoT) in Soil Irrigation System. *IEEE Explore*, 1–5. doi:10.1109/ICPECTS56089.2022.10047185

Jeong, S., Shen, J.-H., & Ahn, B. (2021). A Study on Smart Healthcare Monitoring Using IoT Based on Blockchain. *Wireless Communications and Mobile Computing*, *2021*, 9932091. doi:10.1155/2021/9932091

Jha Durgesh Nandan. (2022, December 29). AI is a force multiplier in medicine, but it is not about to replace doctors. *Times of India*, p. 10.

Jin, Q., Wu, B., Nishimura, S., & Ogihara, A. (2016, August). Ubi-Liven: a human-centric safe and secure framework of ubiquitous living environments for the elderly. In *2016 International Conference on Advanced Cloud and Big Data (CBD).* IEEE. 10.1109/CBD.2016.059

Johnson, P. M., Lin, D. J., Zbontar, J., Zitnick, C. L., Sriram, A., Muckley, M., Babb, J. S., Kline, M., Ciavarra, G., Alaia, E., Samim, M., Walter, W. R., Calderon, L., Pock, T., Sodickson, D. K., Recht, M. P., & Knoll, F. (2023, January 17). Deep learning reconstruction enables prospectively accelerated clinical knee MRI. *Radiology*, *307*(2), e220425. Advance online publication. doi:10.1148/radiol.220425 PMID:36648347

Joseph, N. (2023, Feb. 15). *Four Ways Artificial Intelligence Can Benefit Robotic Surgery*. Forbes Technology Council. https://www.forbes.com/sites/forbestechcouncil/2023/02/15/four-ways-artificial-intelligence-can-benefit-robotic-surgery/amp/

Kagermann, H., Anderl, R., Gausemeier, J., Schuh, G., & Wahlster, W. (2016). *Industrie 4.0 in a Global Context: Strategies for Cooperating with International Partners (Acatech Study).* https://www.acatech.de/wp-content/uploads/2018/03/acatech_STU_engl_KF_Industry40_Global_01.pdf

Kagermann, H. (2015). *Change through digitization - value creation in the age of Industry 4.0. Management of Permanent Change*. Springer. doi:10.1007/978-3-658-05014-6_2

Kamble, S. S., Gunasekaran, A., Goswami, M., & Manda, J. (2018). A systematic perspective on the applications of big data analytics in healthcare management. *International Journal of Healthcare Management, 12*(3), 226–240. doi:10.1080/20479700.2018.1531606

Kanore L, S. S. (2019). A study of awareness about Ayushyaman Bharat Yojana among low income urban families. An exploratory study. *Remarking an Analisation., 4*(1, part 1).

Karatas, M., Eriskin, L., Deveci, M., Pamucar, D., & Garg, H. (2022). Big Data for Healthcare Industry 4.0: Applications, challenges and future perspectives. *Expert Systems with Applications, 200*, 116912. doi:10.1016/j.eswa.2022.116912

KareExpert. (2023, January 13). How Nidhi Jain is helping hospitals become digital. Times Techies supplement. *Times of India*, p. 11.

Karthik, S. A., Hemalatha, R., Aruna, R., Deivakani, M., Reddy, R. V. K., & Boopathi, S. (2023). Study on Healthcare Security System-Integrated Internet of Things (IoT). doi:10.4018/978-1-6684-7684-0.ch013

Kassem, A., El Murr, S., Jamous, G., Saad, E., & Geagea, M. (2016). A smart lock system using Wi-Fi security. *2016 3rd International Conference on Advances in Computational Tools for Engineering Applications, ACTEA 2016*, 222–225. 10.1109/ACTEA.2016.7560143

Kaur, P. D., & Chana, I. (2014). Cloud based intelligent system for delivering health care as a service. *Computer Methods and Programs in Biomedicine, 113*(1), 346-359. doi:10.1016/j.cmpb.2013.09.013

Kaur, P., Kumar, R., & Kumar, M. (2019). A healthcare monitoring system using random forest and internet of things (IoT). *Multimedia Tools and Applications, 78*(14), 19905–199. doi:10.1007/s11042-019-7327-8

Kavitha, C. R., Varalatchoumy, M., Mithuna, H. R., Bharathi, K., Geethalakshmi, N. M., & Boopathi, S. (2023). Energy Monitoring and Control in the Smart Grid: Integrated Intelligent IoT and ANFIS. In M. Arshad (Ed.), Advances in Bioinformatics and Biomedical Engineering. IGI Global. doi:10.4018/978-1-6684-6577-6.ch014

Ke, H., Chen, D., Shi, B., Zhang, J., Liu, X., Zhang, X., & Li, X. (2020). Improving Brain E-Health Services via High-Performance EEG Classification with Grouping Bayesian Optimization. *IEEE Transactions on Services Computing, 13*(4), 696–708. doi:10.1109/TSC.2019.2962673

Keikhosrokiani, P. (Ed.). (2022). *Big data analytics for healthcare: datasets, techniques, life cycles, management, and applications*. Academic Press.

Khanra, S., Dhir, A., Islam, A. N., & Mäntymäki, M. (2020). Big data analytics in healthcare: A systematic literature review. *Enterprise Information Systems, 14*(7), 878–912. doi:10.1080/17517575.2020.1812005

KienyM.BekedamH. (n.d.). Strengthening health systems for universal health coverage and sustainable development. Bulletin of the World Health Organization, *537*(9).

Kim, E. D., Kuan, K. K., Vaghasiya, M. R., Penm, J., Gunja, N., El Amrani, R., & Poon, S. K. (2023). Passive resistance to health information technology implementation: The case of electronic medication management system. *Behaviour & Information Technology, 42*(13), 2308–2329. doi:10.1080/0144929X.2022.2117081

Kim, M., Yu, S., Lee, J., Park, Y., & Park, Y. (2020, May 21). Design of Secure Protocol for Cloud-Assisted Electronic Health Record System Using Blockchain. *Sensors (Basel)*, *20*(10), 2913. doi:10.3390/s20102913 PMID:32455635

Kishor, A., & Chakraborty, C. (2021). Artificial Intelligence and Internet of Things Based Healthcare 4.0 Monitoring System. *Wireless Personal Communications*, 1–17.

Kleinman & Dougherty. (2013). Assessing quality improvement in health care: Theory for practice. *Pediatrics*, *131*(1), S110–S119. PMID:23457146

Korjian, S., & Gibson, C. M. (2022). Digital technologies and the democratization of clinical research: Social media, wearables, and artificial intelligence. *Contemporary Clinical Trials*, *117*, 106767. doi:10.1016/j.cct.2022.106767 PMID:35462032

Koshariya, A. K., Kalaiyarasi, D., Jovith, A. A., Sivakami, T., Hasan, D. S., & Boopathi, S. (2023). AI-Enabled IoT and WSN-Integrated Smart. *Practice, Progress, and Proficiency in Sustainability*, 200–218. doi:10.4018/978-1-6684-8516-3.ch011

Kotler, P. (2000). *Marketing Management, Millenium Edition*. Prentice-Hall.

Krishnamoorthy, S., Dua, A., & Gupta, S. (2023, January). The Role of Emerging Technologies in the Future of IoT-driven Healthcare 4.0: A Survey, Current Challenges, and Future Directions. *Journal of Ambient Intelligence and Humanized Computing*, *14*(1), 361–407. doi:10.1007/s12652-021-03302-w

Krysik, A. (2023, September 25). *12 Types of Healthcare Software*. Retrieved from Stratflow: https://stratoflow.com/healthcare-software-types/

Kubheka, B. (2017). Ethical and legal perspectives on the medical practitioners use of social media. *South African Medical Journal*, *107*(5), 386–389. doi:10.7196/SAMJ.2017.v107i5.12047 PMID:28492116

Kumar, B. M., Kumar, K. K., Sasikala, P., Sampath, B., Gopi, B., & Sundaram, S. (2024). Sustainable Green Energy Generation From Waste Water: IoT and ML Integration. In B. K. Mishra (Ed.), Practice, Progress, and Proficiency in Sustainability. IGI Global. doi:10.4018/979-8-3693-1186-8.ch024

Kumar, P. R., Meenakshi, S., Shalini, S., Devi, S. R., & Boopathi, S. (2023). Soil Quality Prediction in Context Learning Approaches Using Deep Learning and Blockchain for Smart Agriculture. In R. Kumar, A. B. Abdul Hamid, & N. I. Binti Ya'akub (Eds.), Advances in Computational Intelligence and Robotics. IGI Global. doi:10.4018/978-1-6684-9151-5.ch001

Kumela, A. G., Gemta, A. B., Hordofa, A. K., Dagnaw, H., Sheferedin, U., & Tadesse, M. (2023). Quantum machine learning assisted lung cancer telemedicine. *AIP Advances*, *13*(7), 075301. doi:10.1063/5.0153566

Ladeiras, A., Mota, A., & Pardo, M. C. (2015). A Comparative Study of Thermal Legislation in the Galicia–North Portugal Euroregion. In Health and Wellness: Emergence of a New Market Segment (pp. 1-20). Springer. doi:10.1007/978-3-319-11490-3_1

Lagomarsino, G., & Garabrant, A. (n.d.). Moving towards universal health coverage: Health insurance reforms in nine developing countries in Africa and Asia. *Lancet*, 380. doi:10.1016/S0140-6736(12)61147-7 PMID:22959390

Lainson, K., Braun, V., & Clarke, V. (2019). Being both narrative practitioner and academic researcher: A reflection on what thematic analysis has to offer narratively informed research. *International Journal of Narrative Therapy & Community Work*, (4), 86–98.

Langer, A., Feingold-Polak, R., Mueller, O., Kellmeyer, P., & Levy-Tzedek, S. (2019). Trust in socially assistive robots: Considerations for use in rehabilitation. *Neuroscience and Biobehavioral Reviews*, *104*(July), 231–239. doi:10.1016/j.neubiorev.2019.07.014 PMID:31348963

Laszlo, C., Munari, D., Maggioni, S., Knechtle, D., Wolf, P., & De Bon, D. (2023). Feasibility of an Intelligent Algorithm Based on an Assist-as-Needed Controller for a Robot-Aided Gait Trainer (Lokomat) in Neurological Disorders: A Longitudinal Pilot Study. *Brain Sciences*, *13*(4), 612. Advance online publication. doi:10.3390/brainsci13040612 PMID:37190576

Laut, J., Porfiri, M., & Raghavan, P. (2016). The Present and Future of Robotic Technology in Rehabilitation. *Current Physical Medicine and Rehabilitation Reports*, *4*(4), 312–319. doi:10.1007/s40141-016-0139-0 PMID:28603663

Leandro, M., Nogueira, F., & Carvalho, A. (2015). Diversity and Interconnection: Spas, Health and Wellness Tourism. In Health and Wellness Tourism (pp. 153-164). doi:10.1007/978-3-319-11490-3_10

Lee, B. W., Min, S. D., Jeong, W., Choo, Y., & Lee, M. (2007). Construction of APEC e-Health Portal Site for e-Health Service Providers and Demanders in APEC area. *2007 9th International Conference on e-Health Networking, Application and Services*. 10.1109/HEALTH.2007.381657

Li, J. (2019, March 6). *Medical wearables offer new hope for diabetes patients*. Retrieved from TechTarget: https://www.techtarget.com/iotagenda/blog/IoT-Agenda/Medical-wearables-offer-new-hope-for-diabetes-patients

Lian, J. W. (2017). Establishing a cloud computing success model for hospitals in Taiwan. *Inquiry*, *54*(1/6), 1–6. doi:10.1177/0046958016685836 PMID:28112020

Liberato, D., Alén, E., Liberato, P., & Domínguez, T. (2018). Governance and cooperation in Euroregions: Border tourism between Spain and Portugal. *European Planning Studies*, *26*(7), 1347–1365. doi:10.1080/09654313.2018.1464129

Linder,, M. (2014). Program To Improve Arm Function Following Stroke : A Case Study. *Journal of Neurologic Physical Therapy; JNPT*, *37*(3), 125–132. doi:10.1097/NPT.0b013e31829fa808 PMID:23872687

Lin, T., Goyal, P., Girshick, R., He, K., & Dollár, P. (2020). Focal Loss for Dense Object Detection. *IEEE Transactions on Pattern Analysis and Machine Intelligence*, *42*(2), 318–327. doi:10.1109/TPAMI.2018.2858826 PMID:30040631

Lin, T.-W., & Hsu, C.-L. (2021). FAIDM for medical privacy protection in 5G telemedicine systems. *Applied Sciences (Basel, Switzerland)*, *11*(3), 1155. doi:10.3390/app11031155

Li, Z., & Xu, X. (2020). Analysis of network structure and doctor behaviors in e-health communities from a social-capital perspective. *International Journal of Environmental Research and Public Health*, *17*(4), 1136. doi:10.3390/ijerph17041136 PMID:32053913

Lohr, H., Sadeghi, A. R., & Winandy, M. (2010). Securing the e-health cloud. *Proceedings of the ACM International Conference on Health Informatics - IHI '10*, 220–229. 10.1145/1882992.1883024

Lopez, M., Chan, T. M., Thoma, B., Arora, V. M., & Trueger, N. S. (2019). The social media editor at medical journals: Responsibilities, goals, barriers, and facilitators. *Academic Medicine*, *94*(5), 701–707. doi:10.1097/ACM.0000000000002496 PMID:30334841

Lubner, M. G., Gettle, L. M., Kim, D. H., Ziemlewicz, T. J., Dahiya, N., & Pickhardt, P. (2021). Diagnostic and procedural intraoperative ultrasound: Technique, tips and tricks for optimizing results. *The British Journal of Radiology*, *94*(1121), 20201406. Advance online publication. doi:10.1259/bjr.20201406 PMID:33684305

Lupton, D. (2013). The digitally engaged patient: Self-monitoring and self-care in the digital health era. *Social Theory & Health*, *11*(3), 256–270. doi:10.1057/sth.2013.10

Lv, D., Wang, Z., Ji, S., Wang, X., & Hou, H. (2021). Plasma levels of homocysteine is associated with liver fibrosis in health check-up population. *International Journal of General Medicine*, *14*, 5175–5181. doi:10.2147/IJGM.S329863 PMID:34512000

Lv, Q., Chen, H., Zhong, W., Wang, Y., Song, J., Guo, S., Qi, L., & Chen, C. Y. (2020). A Multi-Task Group Bi-LSTM Networks Application on Electrocardiogram Classification. *IEEE Journal of Translational Engineering in Health and Medicine*, *8*, 1–11. doi:10.1109/JTEHM.2019.2952610 PMID:32082952

Macabasag, R. L. A., Mallari, E. U., Pascual, P. J. C., & Fernandez-Marcelo, P. G. H. (2023). Catching up with rapid technology implementation: Mobilities, electronic medical records, and primary care work in the Philippines. *Applied Mobilities*, *8*(2), 97–112. doi:10.1080/23800127.2022.2087014

MacEachern, S. J., & Forkert, N. D. (2021). Machine learning for precision medicine. *Genome*, *64*(4), 416–425. doi:10.1139/gen-2020-0131 PMID:33091314

Magaña-Espinoza, P., Aquino-Santos, R., Cárdenas-Benítez, N., Aguilar-Velasco, J., Buenrostro-Segura, C., Edwards-Block, A., & Medina-Cass, A. (2014). WiSPH: A wireless sensor network-based home care monitoring system. *Sensors (Basel)*, *14*(4), 7096–7119. doi:10.3390/s140407096 PMID:24759112

Magda, W. (2023). Use of Social Media for Patient Education in Dermatology: Narrative Review. *JMIR Dermatology*, *6*, e42609–e42609. doi:10.2196/42609 PMID:37632938

Maguluri, L. P., Ananth, J., Hariram, S., Geetha, C., Bhaskar, A., & Boopathi, S. (2023). Smart Vehicle-Emissions Monitoring System Using Internet of Things (IoT). In P. Srivastava, D. Ramteke, A. K. Bedyal, M. Gupta, & J. K. Sandhu (Eds.), Practice, Progress, and Proficiency in Sustainability. IGI Global. doi:10.4018/978-1-6684-8117-2.ch014

Maheshwari, T. (2023). *Business outlook and money.* Retrieved from Healthcare In India: Bridging The Gap Between Innovation And Access: https://business.outlookindia.com/news/healthcare-in-india-bridging-the-gap-between-innovation-and-access

Maheswari, B. U., Imambi, S. S., Hasan, D., Meenakshi, S., Pratheep, V. G., & Boopathi, S. (2023). Internet of Things and Machine Learning-Integrated Smart Robotics. In M. K. Habib (Ed.), Advances in Computational Intelligence and Robotics. IGI Global. doi:10.4018/978-1-6684-7791-5.ch010

Majedi, N., Naeem, M., & Anpalagan, A. (2016). Telecommunication integration in e-healthcare: Technologies, applications and challenges. *Transactions on Emerging Telecommunications Technologies*, *27*(6), 775–789. doi:10.1002/ett.3025

Majid, M. A. (2008). *Electronic-health in Saudi Arabia- just around the corner?* College of Public Health and Health Informatics, King Saud bin Abdul-Aziz University for Health Sciences.

Maria, S. (2009). *An Essential Guide to Possibilities and Risks of Cloud Computing*. Whitepaper. Retrieved from http://www.mariaspinola.com/whitepapers/An Essential Guide to Possibilities and Risks of Cloud Computing a Pragmatic Effective and Hype Free Approach for Strategic Enterprise Decision Making.pdf

Mariana, C. D., & Yusuf, D. (2021). Building Timeless. co Brand Awareness Through Influencer and Internet Marketing. *Management and Sustainable Development Journal*, *3*(1), 75–92. doi:10.46229/msdj.v3i1.247

Marta, M. (2020). Social Media to Improve Health Promotion and Health Literacy for Patients Engagement. doi:10.1007/978-3-030-43993-4_10

Marx, E. W., & Padmanabhan, P. (2020). *Healthcare digital transformation: How consumerism, technology and pandemic are accelerating the future*. CRC Press. doi:10.4324/9781003035695

Mathew, P. S., & Pillai, A. S. (2016). Innovations in Bio-Inspired Computing and Applications. Springer.

Mathews, S. C., McShea, M. J., Hanley, C. L., Ravitz, A., Labrique, A. B., & Cohen, A. B. (2019). Digital health: A path to validation. *NPJ Digital Medicine*, *2*(1), 38. doi:10.1038/s41746-019-0111-3 PMID:31304384

Ma, X., Wang, Z., Zhou, S., Wen, H., & Zhang, Y. (2018, June). Intelligent healthcare systems assisted by data analytics and mobile computing. In *In 2018 14th International Wireless Communications & Mobile Computing Conference (IWCMC)* (pp. 1317–1322). IEEE. doi:10.1109/IWCMC.2018.8450377

McEwen, A., & Cassimally, H. (2014). *Designing the Internet of things*. https://ebookcentral-proquest-com.pxz.iubh.de:8443/lib/badhonnef/detail.action?docID=1471865

McGill, E., Er, V., Penney, T., Egan, M., White, M., Meier, P., Whitehead, M., Lock, K., Anderson de Cuevas, R., Smith, R., Savona, N., Rutter, H., Marks, D., de Vocht, F., Cummins, S., Popay, J., & Petticrew, M. (2021). Evaluation of public health interventions from a complex systems perspective: A research methods review. *Social Science & Medicine*, *272*, 113697. doi:10.1016/j.socscimed.2021.113697 PMID:33508655

McParlin, Z., Cerritelli, F., Manzotti, A., Friston, K. J., & Esteves, J. E. (2023). Therapeutic touch and therapeutic alliance in pediatric care and neonatology: An active inference framework. *Frontiers in Pediatrics*, *11*(February), 1–15. doi:10.3389/fped.2023.961075 PMID:36923275

Mehrtak, M., SeyedAlinaghi, S. A., MohsseniPour, M., Noori, T., Karimi, A., Shamsabadi, A., Heydari, M., Barzegary, A., Mirzapour, P., Soleymanzadeh, M., Vahedi, F., Mehraeen, E., & Dadras, O. (2021). Security challenges and solutions using healthcare cloud computing. *Journal of Medicine and Life*, *14*(4), 448–461. doi:10.25122/jml-2021-0100 PMID:34621367

Meier, C. A., Fitzgerald, M. C., & Smith, J. M. (2013). E-Health: Extending, Enhancing, and Evolving Health Care. *Annual Review of Biomedical Engineering*, *15*(1), 359–382. doi:10.1146/annurev-bioeng-071812-152350 PMID:23683088

Meskó, B., Drobni, Z., Bényei, É., Gergely, B., & Győrffy, Z. (2017). Digital health is a cultural transformation of traditional healthcare. *mHealth*, *3*, 3. doi:10.21037/mhealth.2017.08.07 PMID:29184890

Metty Paul, L. M. (2023). Digitization of healthcare sector: A study on privacy and security concerns. *ICT Express*, 571-588.

Mheidly, N., & Fares, J. (2020). Leveraging media and health communication strategies to overcome the COVID-19 infodemic. *Journal of Public Health Policy*, *41*(4), 410–420. doi:10.1057/s41271-020-00247-w PMID:32826935

Ministry of Electronics and Information Technology. (2023). *e-shushrut*. Retrieved from Ministry of Electronics and Information Technology Government of India: https://apps.gov.in/content/e-shushrut-hospital-management-information-system

Mitchell, J. (1999). *From telehealth to e-health: the unstoppable rise of e-health: Commonwealth Department of Communications*. Information Technology, and the Arts.

Moghaddasi, H., Asadi, F., Hosseini, A., & Ebnehoseini, Z. (2011). E-Health: A Global Approach with Extensive Semantic Variation. *Journal of Medical Systems*, *36*(5), 3173–3176. doi:10.1007/s10916-011-9805-z PMID:22113437

Mohanty, A., Jothi, B., Jeyasudha, J., Ranjit, P. S., Isaac, J. S., & Boopathi, S. (2023). Additive Manufacturing Using Robotic Programming. In S. Kautish, N. K. Chaubey, S. B. Goyal, & P. Whig (Eds.), Advances in Computational Intelligence and Robotics. IGI Global. doi:10.4018/978-1-6684-8171-4.ch010

Mohd Javaid, A. H. (2022). Significance of machine learning in healthcare: Features, pillars and applications. *International Journal of Intelligent Networks*, 58-73.

Molteni, F., Gasperini, G., Cannaviello, G., & Guanziroli, E. (2018). Exoskeleton and End-Effector Robots for Upper and Lower Limbs Rehabilitation: Narrative Review. *PM & R*, *10*(9), S174–S188. doi:10.1016/j.pmrj.2018.06.005 PMID:30269804

Moreira, A. C., & Silva, P. M. (2015). The trust-commitment challenge in service quality-loyalty relationships. *International Journal of Health Care Quality Assurance*, *28*(3), 253–266. doi:10.1108/IJHCQA-02-2014-0017 PMID:25860922

Mosadeghrad, A. M. (2014). Factors influencing healthcare service quality. *nt J. Health Policy and Management*, 77–89.

Mostafa, S. M. G., Zaki, M., Islam, M. M., Alam, M. S., & Ullah, M. A. (2022). Design and Implementation of an IoT-Based Healthcare Monitoring System. *Proceedings of the 2022 International Conference on Innovations in Science, Engineering and Technology (ICISET)*, 362–366. 10.1109/ICISET54810.2022.9775850

Mouloudj, K., Bouarar, A. C., & Saadaoui, L. (2023). *Factors Influencing the Adoption of Digital Health Apps: An Extended Technology Acceptance Model (TAM)*. Integrating Digital Health Strategies for Effective Administration. doi:10.4018/978-1-6684-8337-4.ch007

Moutselos, K., Kyriazis, D., Diamantopoulou, V., & Maglogiannis, I. (2018, December). Trustworthy data processing for health analytics tasks. In *2018 IEEE International Conference on Big Data (Big Data)*. IEEE. 10.1109/BigData.2018.8622449

Muehlematter, U. J., Daniore, P., & Vokinger, K. N. (2021). Approval of artificial intelligence and machine learning-based medical devices in the USA and Europe (2015–20): A comparative analysis. *The Lancet. Digital Health*, *3*(3), e195–e203. doi:10.1016/S2589-7500(20)30292-2 PMID:33478929

Mukherjee, A., & McGinnis, J. (2007). E-healthcare: An analysis of key themes in research. *International Journal of Pharmaceutical and Healthcare Marketing*, *1*(4), 349–363. doi:10.1108/17506120710840170

Mullner, R. M., & Chung, K. (2006). Current issues in health care informatics. *Journal of Medical Systems*, *30*(1), 1–2. doi:10.1007/s10916-006-7390-3 PMID:16548407

Mumtaz, H., Riaz, M. H., Wajid, H., Saqib, M., Zeeshan, M. H., Khan, S. E., Chauhan, Y. R., Sohail, H., & Vohra, L. I. (2023, September 28). Current challenges and potential solutions to the use of digital health technologies in evidence generation: A narrative review. *Frontiers in Digital Health*, *5*, 1203945. doi:10.3389/fdgth.2023.1203945 PMID:37840685

Myint, C. Y., & Pavlova, M. (n.d.). A systematic review of the health-financing mechanisms in the Association of Southeast Asian Nations countries and the People's Republic of China: Lessons for the move towards universal health coverage. *PLoS One*, 14. doi:10.1371/journal.pone.0217278 PMID:31199815

Nair Mohit and Sethumadhavan Arathi. (2022, October 18). *AI in healthcare: India's trillion-dollar opportunity*. World Economic Forum. https://www.weforum.org/agenda/2022/10/ai-in-healthcare-india-trillion-dollar/

Nashwan, A. J., & Hani, S. B. (2023). Transforming cancer clinical trials: The integral role of artificial intelligence in electronic health records for efficient patient recruitment. *Contemporary Clinical Trials Communications*, *101223*. Advance online publication. doi:10.1016/j.conctc.2023.101223 PMID:38034843

National Informatics Centre. (2024). *eHospital*. Retrieved from NIC: https://www.nic.in/products/e-hospital/

National Strategy for e-Health. (2006). Retrieved from www.sweden.gov.se/health

Navaz, A. N., Serhani, M. A., Al-Qirim, N., & Gergely, M. (2018). Towards an efficient and Energy-Aware mobile big health data architecture. *Computer Methods and Programs in Biomedicine*, *166*, 137–154. doi:10.1016/j.cmpb.2018.10.008 PMID:30415713

Nayak, B., Padhi, S. K., & Pattnaik, P. K. (2017) Impact of Cloud Accountability on Clinical Architecture and Acceptance of Healthcare System. *6th International Conference on Frontiers of Intelligent Computing: Theory and applications, 701*, 149-157. 10.1007/978-981-10-7563-6_16

Nayak, B., Padhi, S. K., & Pattnaik, P. K. (2019). Cloud-based remote healthcare system environment. *Jour of Adv Research in Dynamical & Control Systems, 11*(5), 1772-1780. https://www.jardcs.org/abstract.php?id=1662

Nazir, Ali, Ullah, & Garcıa-Magariño. (2019). Internet of Things for Healthcare Using Effects of Mobile Computing: A Systematic Literature Review. *Hindawi Wireless Communications and Mobile Computing.*

Nelson, M. R. (2009). The cloud, the crowd, and public policy. *Issues in Science and Technology*, *25*(4), 71–76.

Neves, A. L., Freise, L., Laranjo, L., Carter, A. W., Darzi, A., & Mayer, E. (2020). Impact of providing patients access to electronic health records on quality and safety of care: A systematic review and meta-analysis. *BMJ Quality & Safety*, *29*(12), 1019–1032. doi:10.1136/bmjqs-2019-010581 PMID:32532814

News Medical. (2023, January 17). *Reconstructing MRI scans with AI promises to expand MRI access to more patients.* https://www.news-medical.net/news/20230117/Reconstructing-MRI-scans-with-AI-promises-to-expand-MRI-access-to-more-patients.aspx#:~:text=Reconstructing%20MRI%20scans%20with%20AI%2C%20which%20is%20four%20times%20faster,for%20appointments%2C%20the%20study%20says

Nie, D., Wang, L., Adeli, E., Lao, C., Lin, W., & Shen, D. (2019). 3-D Fully Convolutional Networks for Multimodal Isointense Infant Brain Image Segmentation. *IEEE Transactions on Cybernetics*, *49*(3), 1123–1136. doi:10.1109/TCYB.2018.2797905 PMID:29994385

Nilashi, M., Samad, S., Manaf, A. A., Ahmadi, H., Rashid, T. A., Munshi, A., ... Ahmed, O. H. (2019). Factors influencing medical tourism adoption in Malaysia: A DEMATEL-Fuzzy TOPSIS approach. *Computers & Industrial Engineering*, *106005*. Advance online publication. doi:10.1016/j.cie.2019.106005

Niramai. (2022). *Niramai announces 'Easy launch kits' for NGOs to enable Community Screening.* A blog article on their website. September 28, 2022. https://www.niramai.com/blog/

Nishanth, J. R., Deshmukh, M. A., Kushwah, R., Kushwaha, K. K., Balaji, S., & Sampath, B. (2023). Particle Swarm Optimization of Hybrid Renewable Energy Systems. In B. K. Mishra (Ed.), Advances in Civil and Industrial Engineering. IGI Global. doi:10.4018/979-8-3693-0044-2.ch016

Nishimura, Y. (2022). Primary Care, Burnout, and Patient Safety: Way to Eliminate Avoidable Harm. *International Journal of Environmental Research and Public Health*, *19*(16), 10–12. doi:10.3390/ijerph191610112 PMID:36011747

Nitesh. (2022, September 10). AI to transform the Indian Healthcare Sector. *Business World.*

Nyström, M. E., Karltun, J., Keller, C., & Andersson Gäre, B. (2018). Collaborative and partnership research for improvement of health and social services: Researcher's experiences from 20 projects. *Health Research Policy and Systems*, *16*(1), 1–17. doi:10.1186/s12961-018-0322-0 PMID:29843735

O'Malley, L. (2014). Relational marketing: Development, debates and directions. *Journal of Marketing Management*, *30*(11-12), 1220–1238. doi:10.1080/0267257X.2014.939592

Oleg Bestsennyy, G. G. (2021, July 9). *Telehealth: A quarter-trillion-dollar post-COVID-19 reality?* Retrieved from https://www.mckinsey.com/industries/healthcare/our-insights/telehealth-a-quarter-trillion-dollar-post-covid-19-reality

Osterhaus, L. (2010). Cloud Computing and Health Information. *U of I SLIS Journal.* Retrieved from http://ir.uiowa.edu/bsides/19

Ozgur, A. G., Wessel, M. J., Olsen, J. K., Cadic-Melchior, A. G., Zufferey, V., Johal, W., Dominijanni, G., Turlan, J. L., Mühl, A., Bruno, B., Vuadens, P., Dillenbourg, P., & Hummel, F. C. (2022). The effect of gamified robot-enhanced training on motor performance in chronic stroke survivors. *Heliyon*, *8*(11), e11764. Advance online publication. doi:10.1016/j.heliyon.2022.e11764 PMID:36468121

Padhy, R. P., Patra, M. R., & Satapathy, S. C. (2012). Design and Implementation of a Cloud based Rural Healthcare Information System Model. *UNIASCIT*, *2*(1), 149–157.

Padilla-Castañeda, M. A., Sotgiu, E., Barsotti, M., Frisoli, A., Orsini, P., Martiradonna, A., Laddaga, C., & Bergamasco, M. (2018). An Orthopaedic Robotic-Assisted Rehabilitation Method of the Forearm in Virtual Reality Physiotherapy. *Journal of Healthcare Engineering*, *2018*, 1–20. Advance online publication. doi:10.1155/2018/7438609 PMID:30154992

Palmatier, R., & Steinoff, L. (2019). *Relationship Marketing in the Digital Age*. Routledge. doi:10.4324/9781315143583

Parisi, D., & Jain, N. (2022). *Awareness of India's national health insurance scheme (PM-JAY): a cross-sectional study across six states*. Oxford.

Patel, M. M., Moseley, T. W., Nia, E. S., Perez, F., Kapoor, M. M., & Whitman, G. J. (2021). Team science: A practical approach to starting collaborative projects. *Journal of Breast Imaging*, *3*(6), 721–726. doi:10.1093/jbi/wbab034 PMID:34805982

Pawer, P. (2022). Implementation Of Cloud Computing in Healthcare. *International Research Journal of Modernization in Engineering Technology and Science, 4*(5). https://www.irjmets.com/uploadedfiles/paper//issue_5_may_2022/24414/final/fin_irjmets1653635314.pdf

Pennep. (2023). *Digital Healthcare in India: Challenges and Opportunities for Transformation*. Retrieved from https://www.linkedin.com/pulse/digital-healthcare-india-challenges-opportunities-transformation/

Perappadan, B. S. (2023). *Digital innovations in healthcare must be for public good: PM Modi*. Retrieved from The Hindu: https://www.thehindu.com/news/national/open-innovations-for-public-good-pm-tells-g-20-health-ministers/article67209733.ece

Pereira, D. (2020). *Estratégias e ações de marketing para o destino Galiza e Norte de Portugal: um contributo para a sua valorização turística*. Instituto Politécnico de Viana do Castelo.

Perez, R. R., Marques, A., & Mohammadi, F. (2016). The application of supervised learning through feed-forward neural networks for ECG signal classification. *Proceedings of the 2016 IEEE Canadian Conference on Electrical and Computer Engineering (CCECE),* 1–4. 10.1109/CCECE.2016.7726762

Pérez, R., Costa, Ú., Torrent, M., Solana, J., Opisso, E., Cáceres, C., Tormos, J. M., Medina, J., & Gómez, E. J. (2010). Upper limb portable motion analysis system based on inertial technology for neurorehabilitation purposes. *Sensors (Basel)*, *10*(12), 10733–10751. doi:10.3390/s101210733 PMID:22163496

Peter, M., & Tim, G. (2009). *The NIST definition of Cloud Computing, Version 15*. Information Technology Laboratory. Retrieved from http://www.hexistor.com/blog/bid/36511/The NIST Definition of Cloud Computing.

Petropoulos, G. (2020). Artificial Intelligence in the Fight against. https://www.bruegel.org/2020/03/artificial-intelligence-in-the-fight-against-covid-19/

Philip, K. (2000). *Marketing Management*. Academic Press.

Philip, Rodrigues, Wang, Fong, & Chen. (2021). Internet of Things for in-home health monitoring systems: current advances, challenges and future directions. *IEEE Journal on Selected Areas in Communications*, *39*(2), 300-310.

PIB. (2020). *A study of awareness about Ayushyaman Bharat Yojana among low income urban families. An exploratory study*. Retrieved from PRESS INFO BEUARUE: https://pib.gov.in/newsite/Printrelease.aspx?relid=159376#:~:text=The%20primary%20aim%20of%20the,of%20good%20health%20through%20cross

PIB. (2022). *Addressing access barriers to health services: an analytical framework for selecting appropriate interventions in low-income Asian countries. Health Policy and Planning*. Retrieved from Press Information Beaureu: https://pib.gov.in/PressReleaseIframePage.aspx?PRID=1809569

Piras, S., Tobiasz-Lis, P., Currie, M., Dmochowska-Dudek, K., Duckett, D., & Copus, A. (2022). Spatial justice on the horizon? A combined Theory of Change scenario tool to assess place-based interventions. *European Planning Studies*, *30*(5), 952–973. doi:10.1080/09654313.2021.1928057

Popa, G. (2022, August 8). *Social Media in healthcare: Best practices for professionals*. Creatopy Blog. https://www.creatopy.com/blog/social-media-healthcare/

Popov, V. V., Kudryavtseva, E. V., Katiyar, N. K., Shishkin, A., Stepanov, S. I., & Goel, S. (2022). Industry 4.0 and Digitalisation in Healthcare. *Materials (Basel)*, *15*(6), 2140. Advance online publication. doi:10.3390/ma15062140 PMID:35329592

Praditporn, Aranya, Jiang, & Yi. (2023, July 31). Challenges in Adopting Artificial Intelligence to Improve Healthcare Systems and Outcomes in Thailand. *Central. Healthc Inform Res.*, 280–282. . doi:10.4258/hir.2023.29.3.280

Pramila, P. V., Amudha, S., Saravanan, T. R., Sankar, S. R., Poongothai, E., & Boopathi, S. (2023). *Design and Development of Robots for Medical Assistance*. doi:10.4018/978-1-6684-8913-0.ch011

Prasad, A., Chaurasia, S., Singh, A., & Gour, D. (2011). Mapping Cloud Computing onto useful E-Governance. *International Journal of Computer Science and Information Security*, *8*(5).

Precedence Research. (n.d.). *Global artificial intelligence in the healthcare market is growing at ~37% CAGR from 2022 to 2030*. https://www.precedenceresearch.com

Price, Y. (2014, November 14). *Impact of social media in healthcare and telemedicine*. https://telemedicine.arizona.edu/blog/impact-social-media-healthcare-and-telemedicine

Prodhan, U. K., Rahman, M. Z., Jahan, I., Abid, A., & Bellah, M. (2017). Development of a portable telemedicine tool for remote diagnosis of telemedicine application. *Proceedings of the 2017 International Conference on Computing, Communication and Automation (ICCCA)*, 287–292. 10.1109/CCAA.2017.8229817

Proffitt, R., & Lange, B. (2015). Considerations in the efficacy and effectiveness of virtual reality interventions for stroke rehabilitation: Moving the field forward. *Physical Therapy*, *95*(3), 441–448. doi:10.2522/ptj.20130571 PMID:25343960

Pulido-Fernández, J. I., & Merinero-Rodríguez, R. (2018). Destinations' relational dynamic and tourism development. *Journal of Destination Marketing & Management*, *7*, 140–152. doi:10.1016/j.jdmm.2016.09.008

Qadri, Y. A., Nauman, A., Zikria, Y., Vasilakos, A. V., & Kim, S. W. (2020). The Future of Healthcare Internet of Things: A Survey of Emerging Technologies. *IEEE Communications Surveys and Tutorials*, *22*(2), 1121–1167. doi:10.1109/COMST.2020.2973314

Qi, J., Yang, P., Min, G., Amft, O., Dong, F., & Xu, L. (2017). Advanced internet, of things for personalized healthcare systems: A survey. *Pervasive and Mobile Computing*, *41*, 132–149. doi:10.1016/j.pmcj.2017.06.018

Quesenberry, K. A. (2020). *Social media strategy: Marketing, advertising, and public relations in the consumer revolution*. Rowman & Littlefield Publishers.

Radanliev, P., De Roure, D. C., Walton, R., Van Kleek, M., Montalvo, R. M., Santos, O., Maddox, L., & Cannady, S. (2020). COVID-19 What Have We Learned? The Rise of Social Machines and Connected Devices in Pandemic Management Following the Concepts of Predictive, Preventive and Personalised Medicine. SSRN *Electronic Journal*, 311–332. doi:10.2139/ssrn.3692585

Raghupathi, V., & Raghupathi, W. (2020, May 13). Healthcare Expenditure and Economic Performance: Insights from the United States Data. *Frontiers in Public Health*, *8*, 156. doi:10.3389/fpubh.2020.00156 PMID:32478027

Rahamathunnisa, U., Sudhakar, K., Murugan, T. K., Thivaharan, S., Rajkumar, M., & Boopathi, S. (2023). *Cloud Computing Principles for Optimizing Robot Task Offloading Processes*. doi:10.4018/978-1-6684-8171-4.ch007

Raj, J. S. (2020). A novel information processing in IoT based real time health care monitoring system. *Journal of Electronics (China)*, *2*, 188–196.

Rajshri, R., & Malloy, J. (2023). Evolving Role of Social Media in Health Promotion. In Health Promotion-Principles and Approaches. IntechOpen. doi:10.5772/intechopen.111967

Rajula, H. S. R., Verlato, G., Manchia, M., Antonucci, N., & Fanos, V. (2020). Comparison of conventional statistical methods with machine learning in medicine: Diagnosis, drug development, and treatment. *Medicina*, *56*(9), 455. doi:10.3390/medicina56090455 PMID:32911665

Rakheja. (2023). *Five Years of AB-PMJAY*. Retrieved from Drishti IAS: https://www.drishtiias.com/daily-updates/daily-news-editorials/five-years-of-ab-pmjay

Ramudu, K., Mohan, V. M., Jyothirmai, D., Prasad, D. V. S. S. S. V., Agrawal, R., & Boopathi, S. (2023). Machine Learning and Artificial Intelligence in Disease Prediction: Applications, Challenges, Limitations, Case Studies, and Future Directions. In G. S. Karthick & S. Karupusamy (Eds.), Advances in Healthcare Information Systems and Administration. IGI Global. doi:10.4018/978-1-6684-8913-0.ch013

Ranganathan, S. (2020). *Towards a Holistic Digital Health Ecosystem in India.* Retrieved from ORF ISSUE BRIEF: https://www.orfonline.org/wp-content/uploads/2020/04/ORF_IssueBrief_351_Digital_Health.pdf

Rao, N. (2022). Understanding and information failures: Lessons from a health microinsurance program in India. *Health Policy and Planning*, *38*(3).

Rashmi, M. (2022, May 31). Worldwide, less than 4% of the labs have adopted digital pathology: SigTuple CEO. *The Economic Times, Health World.*

Ravisankar, A., Sampath, B., & Asif, M. M. (2023). Economic Studies on Automobile Management: Working Capital and Investment Analysis. In C. S. V. Negrão, I. G. P. Maia, & J. A. F. Brito (Eds.), Advances in Logistics, Operations, and Management Science. IGI Global. doi:10.4018/978-1-7998-9213-7.ch009

Rebecca, B., Kumar, K. P. M., Padmini, S., Srivastava, B. K., Halder, S., & Boopathi, S. (2023). Convergence of Data Science-AI-Green Chemistry-Affordable Medicine: Transforming Drug Discovery. In B. B. Gupta & F. Colace (Eds.), Advances in Computational Intelligence and Robotics. IGI Global. doi:10.4018/978-1-6684-9999-3.ch014

Reddy N, B. Y. (2020). Awareness and readiness of health care workers in implementing Pradhan Mantri Jan Arogya Yojana in a tertiary care hospital at Rishikesh. *Nepal Journal of Epidemiology, 32*(4).

Reddy, M. A., Gaurav, A., Ushasukhanya, S., Rao, V. C. S., Bhattacharya, S., & Boopathi, S. (2023). Bio-Medical Wastes Handling Strategies During the COVID-19 Pandemic. In C. S. V. Negrão, I. G. P. Maia, & J. A. F. Brito (Eds.), Advances in Logistics, Operations, and Management Science. IGI Global. doi:10.4018/978-1-7998-9213-7.ch006

Reddy, M. A., Reddy, B. M., Mukund, C. S., Venneti, K., Preethi, D. M. D., & Boopathi, S. (2023a). Social health protection during the COVID-pandemic using IoT. In *The COVID-19 Pandemic and the Digitalization of Diplomacy* (pp. 204–235). IGI Global. doi:10.4018/978-1-7998-8394-4.ch009

Ren, J., Zhang, A. H., & Wang, X. J. (2020). Traditional Chinese medicine for COVID-19 treatment. *Pharmacol. Res., 155*, 104743. https://www.ncbi.nlm.nih.gov/pubmed/32145402 doi:10.1016/j.phrs.2020.104743

Report by secretariat. (2005). *Health – propose tools and services, Executive board, 117th Session 1, Provisional agenda item 4.13*. Retrieved from https://www.who.int/gb/e/e_eb117.html

Rhodes, R. E., McEwan, D., & Rebar, A. L. (2019). Theories of physical activity behaviour change: A history and synthesis of approaches. *Psychology of Sport and Exercise*, *42*, 100–109. doi:10.1016/j.psychsport.2018.11.010

Rice, W. S., Sowman, M. R., & Bavinck, M. (2020). Using Theory of Change to improve post-2020 conservation: A proposed framework and recommendations for use. *Conservation Science and Practice*, *2*(12), e301. doi:10.1111/csp2.301

Riener, R., Lünenburger, L., & Colombo, G. (2006). Human-centered robotics applied to gait training and assessment. *Journal of Rehabilitation Research and Development*, *43*(5), 679. doi:10.1682/JRRD.2005.02.0046 PMID:17123208

Riffat, M., Yasir, A., Naheen, I. T., Paul, S., & Ahad, M. T. (2021). Augmented Reality for Smarter Bangladesh. *Proceedings of the 2020 IEEE Green Technologies Conference (GreenTech),* 217–222. 10.1109/GreenTech46478.2020.9289699

Rodrigues, C., Ferreira, F., Costa, V., Alves, M. J., Vaz, M., Fernandes, P. O., & Nunes, A. (2022). User's profile of thermal establishments: A literature Review. *Proceedings of the 5th International Conference on Tourism Research,* 15, 344-350. 10.34190/ictr.15.1.129

Rolfe, D., & Hooper, N. (2020). Startup don't stop. *Company Director*, *36*(4), 65–68.

Romanova, G., Vetitnev, A., & Dimanche, F. (2015). Health and Wellness Tourism. In Tourism in Russia: A Management Handbook. Emerald.

Romero, L. E., Chatterjee, P., & Armentano, R. L. (2016). An IoT approach for integration of computational intelligence and wearable sensors for Parkinson's disease diagnosis and monitoring. *Health and Technology*, *6*(3), 167–172. doi:10.1007/s12553-016-0148-0

Rosario, A. T., & Casaca, J. A. (2023). Marketing relacional y satisfacción del cliente: Una revisión sistemática de la literatura. *Estudios Gerenciale*, *39*(169), 516–532. doi:10.18046/j.estger.2023.169.6218

Rothkrantz, L. (2015). How social media facilitate learning communities and peer groups around MOOCS. *International Journal of Human Capital and Information Technology Professionals*, *6*(1), 1–13. doi:10.4018/ijhcitp.2015010101

Ruan, Q., Yang, K., Wang, W., Jiang, L., & Song, J. (2020). Clinical predictors of mortality due to COVID-19 based on an analysis of data from 150 patients from Wuhan, China. *Intensive Care Medicine*, *2020*(46), 846–848. doi:10.1007/s00134-020-05991-x PMID:32125452

Rubin, H. (2010). Risk and reward: Health IT SAAS licensing models. *Licensing Journal*, *30*(1), 13–15.

Rueben, M., Aroyo, A. M., Lutz, C., Schmolz, J., Van Cleynenbreugel, P., Corti, A., Agrawal, S., & Smart, W. D. (2019). Themes and Research Directions in Privacy-Sensitive Robotics. *Proceedings of IEEE Workshop on Advanced Robotics and Its Social Impacts, ARSO,* 77–84. 10.1109/ARSO.2018.8625758

S., P. K., Sampath, B., R., S. K., Babu, B. H., & N., A. (2022). Hydroponics, Aeroponics, and Aquaponics Technologies in Modern Agricultural Cultivation. In *Trends, Paradigms, and Advances in Mechatronics Engineering* (pp. 223–241). IGI Global. doi:10.4018/978-1-6684-5887-7.ch012

Saba and Faheem. (2023). *Types of Artificial Intelligence and Future of Artificial Intelligence in Medical Sciences. Saba Noor Us and Faheem Mohd. June 2023.* IntechOpen. doi:10.5772/intechopen.112056

Sabharwal, S., Gupta, S., & Thirunavukkarasu, K. (2016, April). Insight of big data analytics in healthcare industry. In *2016 International Conference on Computing, Communication and Automation (ICCCA).* IEEE Xplore. 10.1109/CCAA.2016.7813696

Sabrina, G. (2022, July 26). *State of the art of Explainable AI in healthcare in 2022.* https://medium.com/@thinkdata/state-of-the-art-of-explainable-ai-in-healthcare-in-2022-c02225deba1

Sabyasachi Dash, S. K. (2019). Big data in healthcare: Management, analysis and future prospects. *Journal of Big Data*.

Safavi, K., & Michel, B. (2021). *Digital adoption: Reaction or revolution?* Accenture.

Saha, B., Gupta, S., Phung, D., & Venkatesh, S. (2017). A Framework for Mixed-Type Multioutcome Prediction with Applications in Healthcare. *IEEE Journal of Biomedical and Health Informatics*, *21*(4), 1182–1191. doi:10.1109/JBHI.2017.2681799 PMID:28328519

Sakr, S., & Elgammal, A. (2016). Towards a comprehensive data analytics framework for smart healthcare services. *Big Data Res.*, *4*, 44–58. doi:10.1016/j.bdr.2016.05.002

Salman, O. H., Taha, Z., Alsabah, M. Q., Hussein, Y. S., Mohammed, A. S., & Aal-Nouman, M. (2021). A review on utilizing machine learning technology in the fields of electronic emergency triage and patient priority systems in telemedicine: Coherent taxonomy, motivations, open research challenges and recommendations for intelligent future work. *Computer Methods and Programs in Biomedicine*, *209*, 106357. doi:10.1016/j.cmpb.2021.106357 PMID:34438223

Salomi, M., & Balamurugan, S. A. A. (2016). Need, application and characteristics of big data analytics in healthcare—A survey. *Indian Journal of Science and Technology*, *9*(16), 1–5. doi:10.17485/ijst/2016/v9i16/87960

Salunke, P., & Nerkar, R. (2017). IoT Driven Healthcare System for Remote Monitoring of Patients. *International Journal for Modern Trends in Science and Technology*, *03*(June), 100–103.

Samikannu, R., Koshariya, A. K., Poornima, E., Ramesh, S., Kumar, A., & Boopathi, S. (2023). *Sustainable Development in Modern Aquaponics Cultivation Systems Using IoT Technologies*. doi:10.4018/978-1-6684-4118-3.ch006

Sampath, B. C. S., & Myilsamy, S. (2022). Application of TOPSIS Optimization Technique in the Micro-Machining Process. In M. A. Mellal (Ed.), Advances in Mechatronics and Mechanical Engineering. IGI Global. doi:10.4018/978-1-6684-5887-7.ch009

Sánchez-Amboage, E., Martínez-Fernández, V.-A., Juanatey-Boga, O., & Rodríguez-Fernández, M.-M. (2017). Modelos de Gestión de los Balnearios de la Eurorregión Galicia-Norte de Portugal. *Revista Portuguesa de Estudos Regionais*, (44), 5–21. doi:10.59072/rper.vi44.455

Sankar, K. M., Booba, B., & Boopathi, S. (2023). Smart Agriculture Irrigation Monitoring System Using Internet of Things. In G. S. Karthick (Ed.), Advances in Environmental Engineering and Green Technologies. IGI Global. doi:10.4018/978-1-6684-7879-0.ch006

Sapci, A. H., & Sapci, H. A. (2020). Artificial intelligence education and tools for medical and health informatics students: Systematic review. *JMIR Medical Education*, *6*(1), e19285. doi:10.2196/19285 PMID:32602844

Saranya, E., & Maheswaran, T. (2019). IoT Based Disease Prediction and Diagnosis System for Healthcare. *International Journal of Engineering Development and Research, 7*(2), 232-237.

Saravanan, A., Venkatasubramanian, R., Khare, R., Surakasi, R., Boopathi, S., Ray, S., & Sudhakar, M. (2022). *Policy Trends of Renewable Energy and Non Renewable Energy*. Academic Press.

Sari, P. K., Handayani, P. W., & Hidayanto, A. N. (2020, July). Security value issues on eHealth implementation in Indonesia. In IOP Conference Series: Materials Science and Engineering (Vol. 879, No. 1, p. 012040). IOP Publishing. doi:10.1088/1757-899X/879/1/012040

Satav, S. D., Lamani, D. K. G., H., Kumar, N. M. G., Manikandan, S., & Sampath, B. (2024). Energy and Battery Management in the Era of Cloud Computing: Sustainable Wireless Systems and Networks. In B. K. Mishra (Ed.), Practice, Progress, and Proficiency in Sustainability (pp. 141–166). IGI Global. doi:10.4018/979-8-3693-1186-8.ch009

Satav, S. D., Hasan, D. S., Pitchai, R., Mohanaprakash, T. A., Sultanuddin, S. J., & Boopathi, S. (2024). Next Generation of Internet of Things (NGIoT) in Healthcare Systems. In B. K. Mishra (Ed.), Practice, Progress, and Proficiency in Sustainability. IGI Global. doi:10.4018/979-8-3693-1186-8.ch017

Sathish, T., Sunagar, P., Singh, V., Boopathi, S., Sathyamurthy, R., Al-Enizi, A. M., Pandit, B., Gupta, M., & Sehgal, S. S. (2023). *Characteristics estimation of natural fibre reinforced plastic composites using deep multi-layer perceptron (MLP) technique*. Elsevier. doi:10.1016/j.chemosphere.2023.139346

Sawicki, G. S., Beck, O. N., Kang, I., & Young, A. J. (2020). The exoskeleton expansion: Improving walking and running economy. *Journal of Neuroengineering and Rehabilitation*, *17*(1), 1–9. doi:10.1186/s12984-020-00663-9 PMID:32075669

Schillinger, D., Chittamuru, D., & Ramírez, A. S. (2020). From "infodemics" to health promotion: A novel framework for the role of social media in public health. *American Journal of Public Health*, *110*(9), 1393–1396. doi:10.2105/AJPH.2020.305746 PMID:32552021

Schünke, L. C., Mello, B., da Costa, C. A., Antunes, R. S., Rigo, S. J., de Oliveira Ramos, G., da Rosa Righi, R., Scherer, J. N., & Donida, B. (2022). A rapid review of machine learning approaches for telemedicine in the scope of COVID-19. *Artificial Intelligence in Medicine*, *129*, 102312. doi:10.1016/j.artmed.2022.102312 PMID:35659388

Schwab, K. (2016). *The Fourth Industrial Revolution*. Currency.

Schwartz, I., Sajin, A., Fisher, I., Neeb, M., Shochina, M., Katz-Leurer, M., & Meiner, Z. (2009). The Effectiveness of Locomotor Therapy Using Robotic-Assisted Gait Training in Subacute Stroke Patients: A Randomized Controlled Trial. *PM & R*, *1*(6), 516–523. doi:10.1016/j.pmrj.2009.03.009 PMID:19627940

Secinaro, S., Calandra, D., Secinaro, A., Muthurangu, V., & Biancone, P. (2021). The role of artificial intelligence in healthcare: A structured literature review. *BMC Medical Informatics and Decision Making*, *21*(1), 125. doi:10.1186/s12911-021-01488-9 PMID:33836752

Selvaraj, S., Karan, K. A., Srivastava, S., Bhan, N., & Mukhopadhyay, I. (2022). India Health System Review. New Delhi: World Health Organization, Regional Office for South-East Asia. 2022. *Health Systems in Transition*, *11*(1).

Sen, A. (2008). Why and how is health a human right? *Lancet Journal*, *372*(9655).

Sengeni, D., Padmapriya, G., Imambi, S. S., Suganthi, D., Suri, A., & Boopathi, S. (2023). Biomedical Waste Handling Method Using Artificial Intelligence Techniques. In P. Srivastava, D. Ramteke, A. K. Bedyal, M. Gupta, & J. K. Sandhu (Eds.), Practice, Progress, and Proficiency in Sustainability. IGI Global. doi:10.4018/978-1-6684-8117-2.ch022

Senthil, T. S., Ohmsakthivel, R., Puviyarasan, M., Babu, S. R., Surakasi, R., & Sampath, B. (2023). Industrial robot-integrated fused deposition modelling for the 3D printing process. In Development, Properties, and Industrial Applications of 3D Printed Polymer Composites (pp. 188–210). IGI Global. doi:10.4018/978-1-6684-6009-2.ch011

Shaji George, A. H. (2023). Telemedicine: A New Way to Provide Healthcare. *Partners Universal International Innovation Journal (PUIIJ)*, 98-129.

Shakil, K. A., Zareen, F. J., Alam, M., & Jabin, S. (2020). BAMHealthCloud: A biometric authentication and data management system for healthcare data in cloud. *Journal of King Saud University. Computer and Information Sciences*, *32*(1), 57–64. doi:10.1016/j.jksuci.2017.07.001

Shanmugasundaram & Sankarikaarguzhali. (n.d.). An investigation on IoT healthcare analytics. *International Journal of Information Engineering and Electronic*.

Sharma, M., Singla, M. K., Nijhawan, P., Ganguli, S., & Rajest, S. S. (2020). An Application of IoT to Develop Concept of Smart Remote Monitoring System. *EAI/Springer Innovations in Communication and Computing*, 233–239. doi:10.1007/978-3-030-44407-5_15

Sharma, D. M., Venkata Ramana, K., Jothilakshmi, R., Verma, R., Uma Maheswari, B., & Boopathi, S. (2024). Integrating Generative AI Into K-12 Curriculums and Pedagogies in India: Opportunities and Challenges. In P. Yu, J. Mulli, Z. A. S. Syed, & L. Umme (Eds.), Advances in Higher Education and Professional Development. IGI Global. doi:10.4018/979-8-3693-0487-7.ch006

Sheth, J. N., & Parvatiyar, A. (1995). The Evolution of Relationship Marketing. *International Business Review*, *4*(4), 397–413. doi:10.1016/0969-5931(95)00018-6

Sheth, J. N., Parvatiyar, A., & Sinha, M. (2012). The Conceptual Foundations of Relationship Marketing: Review and Synthesis. *The European Electronic Newsletter*, *13*(3), 4–26.

Shetty, D. (2023). Future Of Health Policy. In *India: Trends And Predictions*. Indian School of Public Policy.

Shlobin, N. A., Patel, S., & Dahdaleh, N. S. (2022). Social media as a Tool for Patient Education in Neurosurgery: An overview. *World Neurosurgery*, *161*, 127–134. doi:10.1016/j.wneu.2022.02.054 PMID:35202876

Siddarth, T. (2023, January 6). How simulation technology will transform medical education. Times Techies supplement. *Times of India*, p. 13.

Sikandar, H., Abbas, A. F., Khan, N., & Qureshi, M. I. (2022). Digital Technologies in Healthcare: A Systematic Review and Bibliometric Analysis. *International Journal of Online and Biomedical Engineering*, *18*(8), 34–38. doi:10.3991/ijoe.v18i08.31961

Singh, P. (2018). Internet of things based health monitoring system: Opportunities and challenges. *Int. J. Adv. Res. Comput. Sci.*, *9*(1), 224–228. doi:10.26483/ijarcs.v9i1.5308

Slamanig, D., & Stingl, C. (2008). Privacy Aspects of eHealth. *2008 Third International Conference on Availability, Reliability and Security*.10.1109/ARES.2008.115

Smith, O. D. D. (2019). *PM-JAY across India's states need and utilization PM-JAY policy brief 2*. National Health Authority.

Social media platforms for doctors and healthcare professionals. (2021, November 30). https://www.zealousweb.com/18-niche-social-media-platforms-for-doctors-nurses-and-healthcare-professionals/

Solà, J., Castoldi, S., Chételat, O., Correvon, M., Dasen, S., Droz, S., Jacob, N., Kormann, R., Neumann, V., Perrenoud, A., Pilloud, P., Verjus, C., & Viardot, G. (2006). SpO2 sensor embedded in a finger ring: Design and implementation. *Annual International Conference of the IEEE Engineering in Medicine and Biology - Proceedings*, 4295–4298. 10.1109/IEMBS.2006.260820

Son, Y. J., Jeong, S., Kang, B. G., Kim, S. H., & Lee, S. K. (2015). Visualization of e-Health research topics and current trends using social network analysis. *Telemedicine Journal and e-Health*, *21*(5), 436–442. doi:10.1089/tmj.2014.0172 PMID:25885639

Sousa, B. B., & Barros, C. (2021). Encouraging Relational Marketing in the Wellness and Thermalism Segments. *Економічний вісник Національного технічного університету України «Київський політехнічний інститут»*, (28), 98-102. doi:10.20535/2307-5651.18.2021.240453

Sousa, B. M., & Alves, G. M. (2019). he role of relationship marketing in behavioural intentions of medical tourism services and guest experiences. *Journal of Hospitality and Tourism Insights*, *2*(3), 224–240. doi:10.1108/JHTI-05-2018-0032

Sriram, R. D., & Subrahmanian, E. (2020). Transforming health care through digital revolutions. *Journal of the Indian Institute of Science, 100*(4), 753–772. doi:10.1007/s41745-020-00195-0 PMID:33132546

Sriwastva, S. (2023). Implementation of PM-JAY in India: a qualitative study exploring the role of competency, organizational and leadership drivers shaping early roll-out of publicly funded health insurance in three Indian states. *Health Research Policy and Systems, 21*(65).

Srushti, A. (2022, June 14). Creating quality and affordable healthcare for every Indian. *Times of India*, p. 14.

Stakeholders In Indian Healthcare Sector 2023: An Overview . (2023). Retrieved from Watch doq: https://watchdoq.com/blog/post/stakeholders-in-indian-healthcare-sector-2023:-an-overview

Steinhoff, L., Arli, D., Weaven, S., & Kozlenkova, I. V. (2019). Online Relationship Marketing. *Journal of the Academy of Marketing Science*, *47*(3), 369–393. doi:10.1007/s11747-018-0621-6

Steinhoff, L., & Palmatier, R. W. (2021). Commentary: Opportunities and challenges of technology in relationship marketing. *Australasian Marketing Journal*, *29*(2), 111–117. doi:10.1016/j.ausmj.2020.07.003

Stellefson, M., Paige, S. R., Chaney, B. H., & Chaney, J. D. (2020). Evolving role of social media in health promotion: Updated responsibilities for health education specialists. *International Journal of Environmental Research and Public Health, 17*(4), 1153. doi:10.3390/ijerph17041153 PMID:32059561

Stephens, H. (2014). Social media and engaging with health providers. *Rare Diseases in the Age of Health*, *2*(0), 115–122. doi:10.1007/978-3-642-38643-5_12

Stoumpos, A. I., Kitsios, F., & Talias, M. A. (2023, February 15). Digital Transformation in Healthcare: Technology Acceptance and Its Applications. *International Journal of Environmental Research and Public Health*, *20*(4), 3407. = doi:10.3390/ijerph20043407 PMID:36834105

STPI. (2022). *Artificial Intelligence in the healthcare sector*. STPI KnowledgeUp Series.

Stukus, D. R., Patrick, M. D., Nuss, K. E., & Stukus, D. R. (2019). The role of medical professionals in social media. *Social Media for Medical Professionals: Strategies for Successfully Engaging in an Online World*, 65-82.

Subha, S., Inbamalar, T. M., R, K. C., Suresh, L. R., Boopathi, S., & Alaskar, K. (2023, February). A Remote Health Care Monitoring system using internet of medical things (IoMT). *IEEE Explore*. doi:10.1109/ICIPTM57143.2023.10118103

Sultan, M., Brown, E. M., & Thomas, R. H. (2021). Clinicians embracing social media: Potential and pitfalls. *Epilepsy & Behavior*, *115*, 106462. doi:10.1016/j.yebeh.2019.106462 PMID:31732329

Sundaramoorthy, K., Singh, A., Sumathy, G., Maheshwari, A., Arunarani, A. R., & Boopathi, S. (2023). A Study on AI and Blockchain-Powered Smart Parking Models for Urban Mobility. In B. B. Gupta & F. Colace (Eds.), Advances in Computational Intelligence and Robotics. IGI Global. doi:10.4018/978-1-6684-9999-3.ch010

Sustainable Development Goals, Good Health and Wellbeing. (n.d.). https://www.un.org/sustainabledevelopment/health

Syafa'Ah, L., Minarno, A. E., Sumadi, F. D. S., & Rahayu, D. A. P. (2019). ESP 8266 for Control and Monitoring in Smart Home Application. *Proceedings - 2019 International Conference on Computer Science, Information Technology, and Electrical Engineering, ICOMITEE 2019*, 123–128. 10.1109/ICOMITEE.2019.8921287

Syamala, M. (2023). Machine Learning-Integrated IoT-Based Smart Home Energy Management System. doi:10.4018/978-1-6684-8098-4.ch013

Syed, S. A. (2021). Changing the paradigm of healthcare after Covid-19-A narrative review. *Pakistan Journal of Science*, *73*(2).

Szeto, M. D., Mamo, A., Afrin, A., Militello, M., & Barber, C. (2021). Social media in dermatology and an overview of popular social media platforms. *Current Dermatology Reports*, *10*(4), 1–8. doi:10.1007/s13671-021-00343-4 PMID:34692234

Taati, B., Wang, R., Huq, R., Snoek, J., & Mihailidis, A. (2012). Vision-based posture assessment to detect and categorize compensation during robotic rehabilitation therapy. *Proceedings of the IEEE RAS and EMBS International Conference on Biomedical Robotics and Biomechatronics*, 1607–1613. 10.1109/BioRob.2012.6290668

Tabassum, S., Zaman, M. I. U., Ullah, M. S., Rahaman, A., Nahar, S., & Islam, A. M. (2019). The cardiac disease predictor: IoT and ML driven healthcare system. *Proceedings of the 2019 4th International Conference on Electrical Information and Communication Technology (EICT)*, 1–6. 10.1109/EICT48899.2019.9068821

Tao, H., Bhuiyan, M. Z. A., Abdalla, A. N., Hassan, M. M., Zain, J. M., & Hayajneh, T. (2019). Secured Data Collection with Hardware-Based Ciphers for IoT-Based Healthcare. *IEEE Internet of Things Journal*, *6*(1), 410–420. doi:10.1109/JIOT.2018.2854714

Tekeste, T., Saleh, H., Mohammad, B., & Ismail, M. (2019). Ultra-Low Power QRS Detection and ECG Compression Architecture for IoT Healthcare Devices. *IEEE Transactions on Circuits and Systems. I, Regular Papers*, *66*(2), 669–679. doi:10.1109/TCSI.2018.2867746

Thibaud, M., Chi, H., Zhou, W., & Piramuthu, S. (2018). Internet of Things (IoT) in high-risk Environment, Health and Safety (EHS) industries: A comprehensive review. *Decision Support Systems*, *108*, 79–95. doi:10.1016/j.dss.2018.02.005

Thimbleby H. (2013). Technology and the future of healthcare. *J Public Health Res.*, *2*(3), e28. Doi: doi:10.4081/jphr.2013

Tsao, S.-F., Chen, H., Tisseverasinghe, T., Yang, Y., Li, L., & Butt, Z. A. (2021). What social media told us in the time of COVID-19: A scoping review. *The Lancet. Digital Health*, *3*(3), e175–e194. doi:10.1016/S2589-7500(20)30315 0 PMID:33518503

Tubaishat, A. (2019). The effect of electronic health records on patient safety: A qualitative exploratory study. *Informatics for Health & Social Care*, *44*(1), 79–91. doi:10.1080/17538157.2017.1398753 PMID:29239662

Ugandar, R. E., Rahamathunnisa, U., Sajithra, S., Christiana, M. B. V., Palai, B. K., & Boopathi, S. (2023). Hospital Waste Management Using Internet of Things and Deep Learning: Enhanced Efficiency and Sustainability. In M. Arshad (Ed.), Advances in Bioinformatics and Biomedical Engineering. IGI Global. doi:10.4018/978-1-6684-6577-6.ch015

Ugwu, C. I., Ekere, J. N., & Onoh, C. (2021). Research paradigms and methodological choices in the research process. *Journal of Applied Information Science and Technology*, *14*(2), 116–124.

UNF. (n.d.). *Artificial Intelligence Definitions.* Office of Faculty Excellence, University of North Florida. https://www.unf.edu/ofe/ai/definitions.html

Vaidya, A. (2023). *What Are Digital Therapeutics and Their Use Cases.* https://mhealthintelligence.com/features/what-are-digital-therapeutics-and-their-use-cases

Valle, G., Saliji, A., Fogle, E., Cimolato, A., Petrini, F. M., & Raspopovic, S. (2021). Mechanisms of neuro-robotic prosthesis operation in leg amputees. *Science Advances*, *7*(17), eabd8354. Advance online publication. doi:10.1126/sciadv.abd8354 PMID:33883127

Vanitha, S. K. R., & Boopathi, S. (2023). Artificial Intelligence Techniques in Water Purification and Utilization. In *Human Agro-Energy Optimization for Business and Industry* (pp. 202–218). IGI Global. doi:10.4018/978-1-6684-4118-3.ch010

Vaniukov, S. (2023, August 8). *Telemedicine Trends & Telehealth market size statistics for 2023 - softermii blog.* Softermii. https://www.softermii.com/blog/telemedicine-trends-and-healthcare-market-statistics#form

Varkey, B. (2021). Principles of Clinical Ethics and Their Application to Practice. *Medical Principles and Practice*, *30*(1), 17–28. doi:10.1159/000509119 PMID:32498071

Varoquaux, G., & Cheplygina, V. (2022). Machine learning for medical imaging: Methodological failures and recommendations for the future. *NPJ Digital Medicine*, *5*(1), 48. doi:10.1038/s41746-022-00592-y PMID:35413988

Varshney, U. (2007). Pervasive Healthcare and Wireless Health Monitoring. *Mobile Networks and Applications*, *12*(2-3), 113–127. doi:10.1007/s11036-007-0017-1

Venkateswaran, N., Kumar, S. S., Diwakar, G., Gnanasangeetha, D., & Boopathi, S. (2023). Synthetic Biology for Waste Water to Energy Conversion: IoT and AI Approaches. In M. Arshad (Ed.), Advances in Bioinformatics and Biomedical Engineering. IGI Global. doi:10.4018/978-1-6684-6577-6.ch017

Venkateswaran, N., Vidhya, K., Ayyannan, M., Chavan, S. M., Sekar, K., & Boopathi, S. (2023). *A Study on Smart Energy Management Framework Using Cloud Computing*. doi:10.4018/978-1-6684-8634-4.ch009

Venkateswaran, N., Vidhya, R., Naik, D. A., Michael Raj, T. F., Munjal, N., & Boopathi, S. (2023). *Study on Sentence and Question Formation Using Deep Learning Techniques*. doi:10.4018/978-1-6684-6782-4.ch015

Ventola, C. L. (2014). Social media and health care professionals: Benefits, risks, and best practices. *P&T*, *39*(7), 491. PMID:25083128

Vignais, N., Miezal, M., Bleser, G., Mura, K., Gorecky, D., & Marin, F. (2013). Innovative system for real-time ergonomic feedback in industrial manufacturing. *Applied Ergonomics*, *44*(4), 566–574. doi:10.1016/j.apergo.2012.11.008 PMID:23261177

Visser, B. J., Huiskes, F., & Korevaar, D. A. (2012). A social media self-evaluation checklist for medical practitioners. *Indian Journal of Medical Ethics*, *9*(4), 245–248. doi:10.20529/IJME.2012.083 PMID:23099596

Vladzymyrskyy, A. V. (2022). History of the Scientific Rationale of the «Telemedicine» Concept: Professor KT Bird's Research Group Contribution. *History and Modern Perspectives*, *4*(2), 95–103. doi:10.33693/2658-4654-2022-4-2-95-103

Washington, P., Leblanc, E., Dunlap, K., Penev, Y., Kline, A., Paskov, K., Sun, M. W., Chrisman, B., Stockham, N., Varma, M., Voss, C., Haber, N., & Wall, D. P. (2020). Precision telemedicine through crowdsourced machine learning: Testing variability of crowd workers for video-based autism feature recognition. *Journal of Personalized Medicine*, *10*(3), 86. doi:10.3390/jpm10030086 PMID:32823538

What is HIE ? (2020, July 24). Retrieved from Breadcrumb: https://www.healthit.gov/topic/health-it-and-health-information-exchange-basics/what-hie

Wilson, E. V., & Lankton, N. K. (2004). Modelling Patients' Acceptance of Provider-delivered E-health. *Journal of the American Medical Informatics Association : JAMIA*, *11*(4), 241–248. doi:10.1197/jamia.M1475 PMID:15064290

Wong, B. K. M., & Hazley, S. A. S. A. (2020). The future of health tourism in the industrial revolution 4.0 era. *Journal of Tourism Futures*, *7*(2), 267–272. doi:10.1108/JTF-01-2020-0006

World Health Organization. (2005). *58th World Health Assembly Report*. WHO.

World Health Organization. (2020). *Constitution of the World Health Organization*. Obtido de https:// www.who.int/about/who-we-are/constitution

World Health Organization. (2021). *Global strategy on digital health 2020-2025*. World Health Organization.

World Health Organization. (n.d.). Leave no one behind: strengthening health systems for UHC and the SDGs in Africa. Brazzaville: WHO Regional Office for Africa.

World Population Review. (2024). Retrieved from world population review: https://worldpopulationreview.com/world-cities/delhi-population

Wright, A., Stone, K., Martinelli, L., Fryer, S., Smith, G., Lambrick, D., Stoner, L., Jobson, S., & Faulkner, J. (2021). Effect of combined home-based, overground robotic-assisted gait training and usual physiotherapy on clinical functional outcomes in people with chronic stroke: A randomized controlled trial. *Clinical Rehabilitation*, *35*(6), 882–893. doi:10.1177/0269215520984133 PMID:33356519

Wright, D. W. M., & Zascerinska, S. (2023). Becoming immortal: Future wellness and medical tourism markets. *Journal of Tourism Futures*, *9*(2), 168–195. doi:10.1108/JTF-05-2021-0119

Wu, J., Li, H., Liu, L., & Zheng, H. (2017). Adoption of big data and analytics in mobile healthcare market: An economic perspective. *Electronic Commerce Research and Applications*, *22*, 24–41. doi:10.1016/j.elerap.2017.02.002

Wu, S., Li, G., Deng, L., Liu, L., Wu, D., Xie, Y., & Shi, L. (2019). L1-Norm Batch Normalization for Efficient Training of Deep Neural Networks. *IEEE Transactions on Neural Networks and Learning Systems*, *30*(7), 2043–2051. doi:10.1109/TNNLS.2018.2876179 PMID:30418924

Wynne, R., Davidson, P. M., Duffield, C., Jackson, D., & Ferguson, C. (2021). Workforce management and patient outcomes in the intensive care unit during the COVID-19 pandemic and beyond: A discursive paper. *Journal of Clinical Nursing*, jocn.15916. Advance online publication. doi:10.1111/jocn.15916 PMID:34184349

Xu, G. (2020). IoT-Assisted ECG Monitoring Framework with Secure Data Transmission for Health Care Applications. *IEEE Access : Practical Innovations, Open Solutions*, *8*, 74586–74594. doi:10.1109/ACCESS.2020.2988059

Yadav, S., Bhole, G. P., & Sharma, A. (2022). Telemedicine using Machine Learning: A Boon. *Emerging Computational Approaches in Telehealth and Telemedicine: A Look at The Post COVID-19 Landscape*, 70.

Yagi, M., Yamanouchi, K., Fujita, N., Funao, H., & Ebata, S. (2023). Revolutionizing Spinal Care: Current Applications and Future Directions of Artificial Intelligence and Machine Learning. *Journal of Clinical Medicine*, *12*(13), 4188. Advance online publication. doi:10.3390/jcm12134188 PMID:37445222

Yang, Y., Wang, H., Jiang, R., Guo, X., Cheng, J., & Chen, Y. (2022). A Review of IoT-enabled Mobile Healthcare: Technologies, Challenges, and Future Trends. *IEEE Internet of Things Journal*, *9*(12), 9478–9502. doi:10.1109/JIOT.2022.3144400

Yang, Z., Zhou, Q., Lei, L., Zheng, K., & Xiang, W. (2016). An IoT-cloud Based Wearable ECG Monitoring System for Smart Healthcare. *Journal of Medical Systems*, *40*(12), 1–11. doi:10.1007/s10916-016-0644-9 PMID:27796840

Yasmyne Ronquillo, A. M. (2023, May 1). *Digital Health.* Retrieved from National Library of Medicine: https://www.ncbi.nlm.nih.gov/books/NBK470260/

Yegin, T. (2021). Brand Loyalty in Creating Relationship Marketing Practices: A Study on GMS Operators. *Electronic Journal of Social Sciences*, *20*(77), 201–216. doi:10.17755/esosder.661291

Yeole, A. S., & Kalbande, D. R. (2016). Use of Internet of Things (IoT) in healthcare: A survey. *Proceedings of the ACM Symposium on Women in Research*, 71–76. 10.1145/2909067.2909079

Young, D. P., Keller, C. M., Bliss, D. W., & Forsythe, K. W. (2003). Ultra-wideband (UWB) transmitter location using time difference of arrival (TDOA) techniques. *The Thrity-Seventh Asilomar Conference on Signals, Systems & Computers,* 2, 1225–1229. 10.1109/ACSSC.2003.1292184

Yu, X., Yu, Z., & Ramalingam, S. (2018). Learning Strict Identity Mappings in Deep Residual Networks. *Proceedings of the 2018 IEEE/CVF Conference on Computer Vision and Pattern Recognition*, 4432–4440. 10.1109/CVPR.2018.00466

Zalatoris, J. J., Scheerer, J. B., & Lebeda, F. J. (2017). Collaborative systems biology projects for the military medical community. *Military Medicine*, *182*(9-10), e1802–e1809. doi:10.7205/MILMED-D-16-00446 PMID:28885940

Zekrifa, D. M. S., Kulkarni, M., Bhagyalakshmi, A., Devireddy, N., Gupta, S., & Boopathi, S. (2023). Integrating Machine Learning and AI for Improved Hydrological Modeling and Water Resource Management. In V. Shikuku (Ed.), Advances in Environmental Engineering and Green Technologies. IGI Global. doi:10.4018/978-1-6684-6791-6.ch003

Zhang, J. Z., Watson, G. F., Dant, R. P., & Palmatier, R. W. (2016). Dynamic Relationship Marketing. *Journal of Marketing*, *80*(5), 53–75. doi:10.1509/jm.15.0066

Zhang, J., Yang, L., Cao, W., & Wang, Q. (2020). Formal Analysis of 5G EAP-TLS Authentication Protocol Using Proverif. *IEEE Access : Practical Innovations, Open Solutions*, *8*, 23674–23688. doi:10.1109/ACCESS.2020.2969474

Zhang, L. J., & Zhou, Q. (2009). CCOA: *Cloud Computing Open Architecture. IEEE International Conference on Web Services.* 10.1109/ICWS.2009.144

Zhou, K., Liu, T., & Liang, L. (2016). From cyber-physical systems to industry 4.0: Make future manufacturing become possible. *International Journal of Manufacturing Research*, *11*(2), 167–188. doi:10.1504/IJMR.2016.078251

Zhuravel, H. (2023, August 15). *Telemedicine and Remote Patient Monitoring: Use Cases & Best Practices.* Retrieved from Binariks: https://binariks.com/blog/telemedicine-remote-patient-monitoring/

Zimba, O., & Gasparyan, A. Y. (2021). Social media platforms: a primer for researchers. *Reumatologia/Rheumatology*, *59*(2), 68-72.

Zobair, K. M., Sanzogni, L., Houghton, L., & Islam, M. Z. (2021). Forecasting care seekers satisfaction with telemedicine using machine learning and structural equation modeling. *PLoS One*, *16*(9), e0257300. doi:10.1371/journal.pone.0257300 PMID:34559840

Zuccon, G., Lenzo, B., Bottin, M., & Rosati, G. (2022). Rehabilitation robotics after stroke: A bibliometric literature review. *Expert Review of Medical Devices*, *19*(5), 405–421. doi:10.1080/17434440.2022.2096438 PMID:35786139

Zulkefli, N. A., Iahad, N. A., & Yusof, A. F. (2018). Benefits of Social Media Platform in Healthcare. *International Journal of Innovative Computing*, *8*(3). Advance online publication. doi:10.11113/ijic.v8n3.201

Zurynski, Y., Smith, C. L., Vedovi, A., Ellis, L. A., Knaggs, G., Meulenbroeks, I., & Braithwaite, J. (2020). *Mapping the learning health system: a scoping review of current evidence*. Australian Institute of Health Innovation and the NHMRC Partnership Centre for Health System Sustainability.

About the Contributors

Sukanta Kumar Baral is an acclaimed global academician, closely associated with several National and Foreign universities for multiple academic and research activities. Prof. Baral has been applauded as a pragmatic visionary, who works to comprehend the social and economic factors that sustain poverty cycles and sustainable marketing practices globally in order to assist in the development and assessment of different successful social programmes. He has developed a novel approach to deliver by elucidating the connections and contributory ties between policy, poverty, behaviour, entrepreneurship and socio-economic status through the combination of creative field experiments and rigorous empirical analysis through international collaborations. Prof. Baral has working exposure with governments, multinational non-governmental organisations, corporations & academic institutions through different programmes. He is also a NAAC Assessor (Peer-team Member), Ministry of HRD, Govt. of India and significantly, has contributed a National Level Policy Paper on Higher Education Scenario of Chhattisgarh State to the Ministry of HRD, Government of India. Prof. Baral has contributed more than 150 Research Papers in different referred National and International Journals (including Scopus, ABDC & UGC Care Listed) to his credit. He has authored 14 books and edited 18 books (out of which 7 are at Scopus). He has worked with the renowned global publishers like Emerald, IGI Global, Taylor & Francis, Sage, Springer, etc. Prof. Baral has 28 years of rich experience in academia by holding several important positions at various levels and is currently working as Senior Professor, Department of Commerce, Faculty of Commerce & Management at Indira Gandhi National Tribal University (A Central University of Government of India), Amarkantak, Madhya Pradesh, India. He has authored 18 reference books, edited 16 books (out of 7 are at Scopus) and contributed 12 e-Resources. He has conferred with 35 National and International Awards and has earned 6 Indian Copyrights & 5 Patents to his credit. He is the Chief Editor of the 'Splint International Journal of Professionals', a Quarterly Peer Reviewed Multidisciplinary Journal, ISSN 2349 – 6045 (P), 2583 – 3561 (O). He is also a NAAC Assessor, Ministry of HRD, Govt. of India and working as Professor, Department of Commerce, Faculty of Commerce & Management at Indira Gandhi National Tribal University, Madhya Pradesh, India.

Richa Goel is Associate Professor-Economics and International Business at SCMS Noida, Symbiosis International University, Pune. She is a Gold Medalist in her Master of Economics and Ph.D. in Management where she had worked for almost 6 years on area of Diversity Management. She has a journey of almost 23+ years in academic. She is working in joint collaborations with few International Researchers on various projects and one of her project on Business Model for Inclusive banking sector has been appreciated by the Ministry of Finance, New-Zealand and has been proposed further to Reserve Bank of New-Zealand. She has to her credit numerous Research Papers in UGC Care Listed, Scopus, ABDC publications in reputed National and International journals accompanied with hundreds of Research participation in International/National Conferences including FDP, MDP and Symposiums along serving as a member of review committee for conferences and journals. She is handling many Scopus International Peer Reviewed Journals as Lead Editor for regular and special issue journals She is acting as the special issue Editor of Journal of Sustainable Finance and Investment, JSFI is abstracted and indexed in the Chartered Association of Business Schools Academic Journal Guide (2018 edition) and Scopus, Print ISSN: 2043-0795 Online ISSN: 2043-0809. According to SCImago Journal Rank (SJR), this journal is ranked 0.52 under Q1 category. She was also acting as the Editor for Amity Global Business Review Journal. Issn No 0975-511x Listed by ULRICH And EBSCO Of USA, International Peer Reviewed for past 10 years. She has many Books to her credit by Springer, IGI Global, Nova, De-Gruyters, Emerald, Bloombury's, Ocean etc. and also acting as the Book Series Editor for Taylor's & Francis Group.

* * *

Radhakrishna Batule holds the position of Senior Faculty at the Department of Management within Vishwakarma University, a State Private University located in Pune, India, operating under the jurisdiction of the Government of Maharashtra. He brings to this role 18 years of expertise in Marketing and Branding. Dr. Batule's extensive experience encompasses teaching, research, and consultancy, contributing significantly to the academic and practical dimensions of the university. His contributions make him an essential figure within the university's educational and research landscape, particularly in the domain of Marketing and Branding.

S. Bhavana is Asst. Professor, Department of Computer Science and Engineering- Internet of Things, Sreenidhi Institute of Science and Technology, Hyderabad, Telangana, India.

Bhubaneswari Bisoyi is Assistant Professor, School of Law, KIIT University, India.

Das Biswajit is Professor, School of Management, KIIT University, India.

Sampath Boopathi is an accomplished individual with a strong academic background and extensive research experience. He completed his undergraduate studies in Mechanical Engineering and pursued his postgraduate studies in the field of Computer-Aided Design. Dr. Boopathi obtained his Ph.D. from Anna University, focusing his research on Manufacturing and optimization. Throughout his career, Dr. Boopathi has made significant contributions to the field of engineering. He has authored and published over 180 research articles in internationally peer-reviewed journals, highlighting his expertise and dedication to advancing knowledge in his area of specialization. His research output demonstrates his commitment to conducting rigorous and impactful research. In addition to his research publications, Dr. Boopathi has also been granted one patent and has three published patents to his name. This indicates his innovative thinking and ability to develop practical solutions to real-world engineering challenges. With 17 years of academic and research experience, Dr. Boopathi has enriched the engineering community through his teaching and mentorship roles. He has served in various engineering colleges in Tamilnadu, India, where he has imparted knowledge, guided students, and contributed to the overall academic development of the institutions. Dr. Sampath Boopathi's diverse background, ranging from mechanical engineering to computer-aided design, along with his specialization in manufacturing and optimization, positions him as a valuable asset in the field of engineering. His research contributions, patents, and extensive teaching experience exemplify his expertise and dedication to advancing engineering knowledge and fostering innovation.

Vijit Chaturvedi is a professor in OB, HR&Psychology with Industry experience in Manufacturing and Academia experience of 21 years. She is Doctorate in Management, MBA(HR) M.Phil. in Management, Diploma Labor Laws, Certified teacher for Strategic management from IIM Indore with She is an accredited trainer from Indian Society of Training and Development, Ministry of Human Resource Development, and Industrial Psychologist. She is currently working as Professor in the area of HR and Psychology and Head of Department-Pratyahara "Department of Spirituality, Research &Consciousness" which conducts Certificate Programs in Spirituality, consciousness matched in a scientific way. She is also Research Coordinator - Funded Projects of the Institution. Her Research area includes -Strategic, administrative, and behavioural aspects of Human resource/People management. She has to her credit more than 91 publications in different areas (Including Indexed and Peer Reviewed Journal). She has published 8 Books in Talent management, ethical leadership, Organization behaviour and Emotional intelligence. Seven Scholars are pursuing their Doctoral program and 8 have been awarded Ph.D. Training and Consultancy experience includes both PSU's and Private organization in Behavioural, Technical and psychological aspects as MDP, EDP and consultancy assignment in training effectiveness measurement few organizations where trainings were conducted includes -NPTI, SEWA Exports, Sunland Alloys DAVIM, World Bank, Apollo Indraprastha Hospitall,NHRC, KRIBHCO, Election Commission of India, CFAI, Sleep well Foundation, IOCL.

Rocky J. Dwyer, PhD, FRSA, FCPA, CPA, FCMA, CMA, is a Core Faculty at Walden University – College of Managment & Human Potential. He is an award winning writer, editor, reviewer, and educator, who has consulted and undertaken research for private, not-for profit, and public sector organizations to examine and validate Corporate Social Responsibility, Poverty Reduction initiatives, strategic organizational capacity, performance management and ethics. His research has been presented and published for conferences and symposiums in Canada, the United States, South America, Germany, the Russian Federation; and, the Peoples Republic of China.

Tarun Madan Kanade stands out as a distinguished young author who has enriched the academic and literary worlds with his profound insights and prolific writings. His vast contributions span multiple books, insightful chapters, and groundbreaking research papers. A fervent traveller at heart, Dr. Kanade possesses a zest for discovery and exploration. His journeys, which have taken him to over 11 countries, are more than mere travels; they are quests for knowledge, which he meticulously documents for the benefit of educators and practitioners alike.

Rita Komalasari is a lecturer at YARSI University. Her current work is focused on Bridging the Gap: Theory of Change Guided Digital Health Implementation in Indonesian Primary Care.

L. Melita is Associate Professor Department of Computer Applications School of Science and Computer Studies (Lakeside), CMR University, Bengaluru. Karnatka Pin: 562149 Orcid Id: 0000-0001-9874-9180.

Lahari Mothukuri is a student, B.Tech, CSE-IOT, Sreenidhi Institute of Science and Technology, Hyderabad.

Biswajit Nayak is Assistant Professor, Sri Sri University, Cuttack, India.

B. C. M. Patnaik is Professor at KIIT University for Economics and Finance. Specialise in Rural development, Developmental Economics, Behavioral Economics and Micro-Finance.

Ana Teresa Pedreiro is a PhD Student in Public Health at Escola Nacional de Saúde Pública - Universidade Nova de Lisboa. PhD Thesis in Adjustment to Retirement (Gender). Science and Technology Management Fellow.

Sreekanth Rallapalli is Professor Department of Master of Computer Application Nitte Meenakshi Institute of Technology Yelahanka, Bengaluru, Karnataka Bengaluru Karnataka 560064. https://orcid.org/0000-0002-1626-0320.147d8f67-0e3f-4bec-852e-1910c25009d2

Sudha Ramesh is Professor Department of Master of Computer Applications Hindustan Institute of Technology and Science Kancheepuram Chennai Tamil Nadu 603103.

R. Renugadevi completed her PhD in 2022 from Anna University, Chennai. She has published many papers in International journals and Conferences. She is currently working as Associate professor in R.M.K Engineering College. She has more than 16 years of teaching experience in engineering colleges. Her interest includes Machine learning, Internet of Things, Wireless Sensor Networks and Cloud computing.

S. Reshma is Associate Professor Department of AI&ML, Dayananda Sagar College of Engineering Bangalore, Karnataka, 560111. Orchid Id: 0000-0002-7849-0543.

Maderametla Roja Rani is Assistant Professor Department of Microbiology & FST GITAM Deemed to be University Rushikonda, Visakhapatnam, Andhrapradesh. Orchid Id: 0000-0002-2473-8953.

Asma Saqib is Associate professor Department of Biochemistry, Maharani Cluster University, Bangalore.

Ipseeta Satpathy is a senior professor at KIIT University. Specializes in Psychology, Behavioral Science, and Organisational Behaviour.

P. Siva Satya Sreedhar is Associate Professor Department of Information Technology Seshadri Rao Gudlavalleru Engineering College, Gudlavalleru (Village & Mandal), Krishna (dist), Andhra Pradesh, India. Orchid ID: 0000-0002-1799-6022.

Bruno Barbosa Sousa is Adjunct Professor of Marketing at Polytechnic Institute of Cávado and Ave (IPCA), Portugal and PhD in Marketing and Strategy in Universidade do Minho, Portugal. Head of Masters Program - Tourism Management and Marketing Tourism (IPCA); CiTUR – Center for Tourism Research, Development and Innovation and UNIAG research member. He has published in the Journal of Enterprising Communities, Tourism Management Perspectives, Current Issues in Tourism, Journal of Organizational Change Management, World Review of Entrepreneurship, Management and Sust. Development, among others. https://orcid.org/0000-0002-8588-2422.aac5d92a-6e64-4f88-8f01-362429bd4dc7

V. Sujay is an Assistant Professor Department of Computer Science and Engineering Krishna University College of Engineering and Technology, Rudraram, Machilipatnam-, Krishna (dist), Andhra Pradesh, India. Orchid ID: 0009-0000-1944-9658.

Venkat T. is Professor, Department of Computer Science and Engineering- Internet of Things, Sreenidhi Institute of Science and Technology, Hyderabad, Telangana, India.

Ajay Upadhyaya is an Associate Professor, Department of Computer Engineering, SAL Engineering & Technical Institute, SAL Education, Ahmedabad Gujarat. Orchid Id: 0000-0002-7583-6430.

J. Vimala Devi is an Associate Professor Department of Computer Science Engineering Dayananda Sagar college of Engineering Kumaraswamy Layout, Bengaluru Bangalore Urban Karnataka.

Index

U

V

W

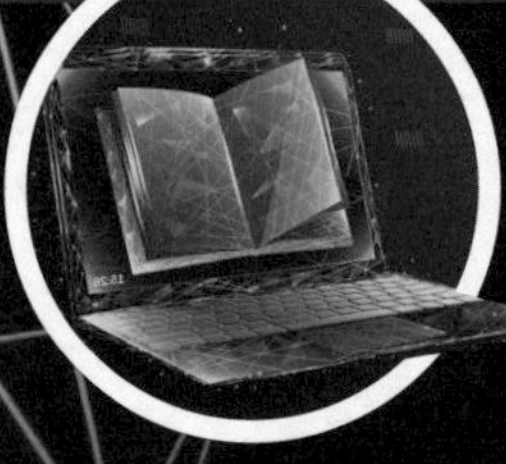

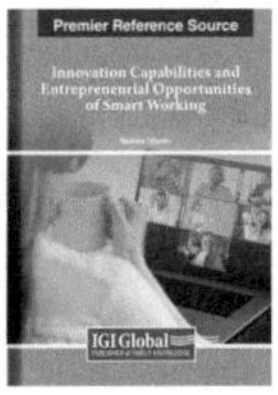

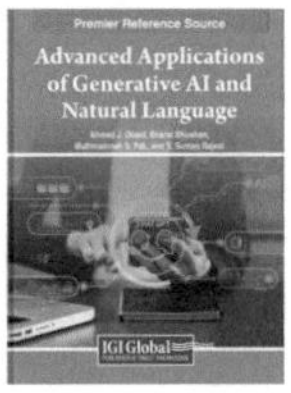

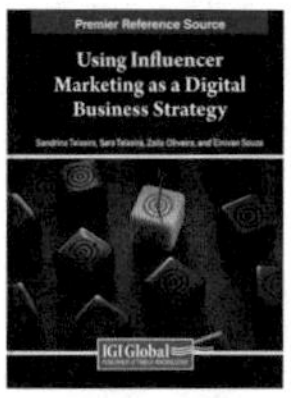

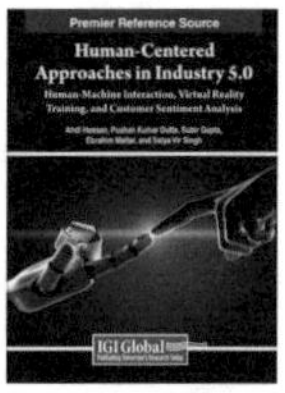

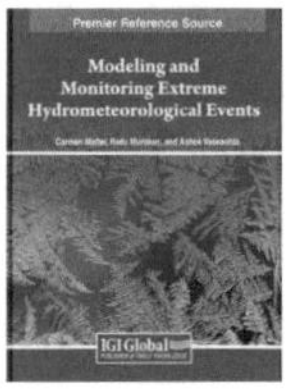

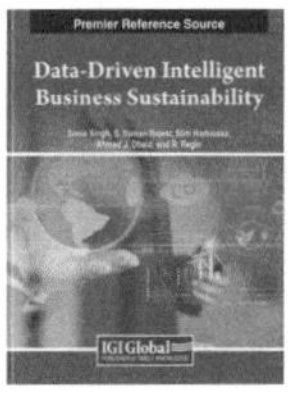

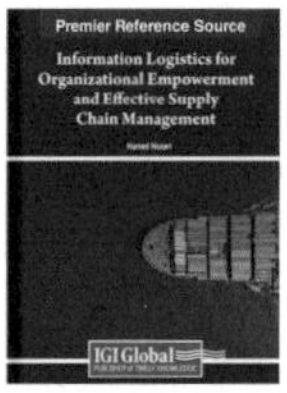

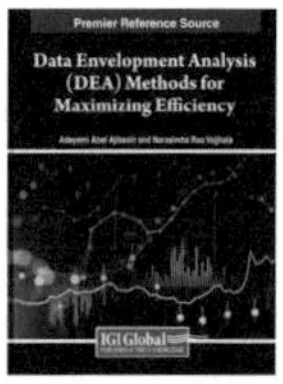